Accounting for health

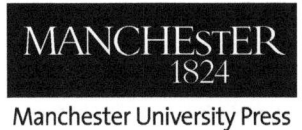

Manchester University Press

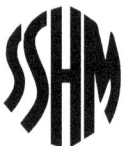

SOCIAL HISTORIES OF MEDICINE

Series editors: *David Cantor, Elaine Leong* and *Keir Waddington*

Social Histories of Medicine is concerned with all aspects of health, illness and medicine, from prehistory to the present, in every part of the world. The series covers the circumstances that promote health or illness, the ways in which people experience and explain such conditions, and what, practically, they do about them. Practitioners of all approaches to health and healing come within its scope, as do their ideas, beliefs, and practices, and the social, economic and cultural contexts in which they operate. Methodologically, the series welcomes relevant studies in social, economic, cultural, and intellectual history, as well as approaches derived from other disciplines in the arts, sciences, social sciences and humanities. The series is a collaboration between Manchester University Press and the Society for the Social History of Medicine.

Previously published

Migrant architects of the NHS *Julian M. Simpson*

Mediterranean quarantines, 1750–1914 Edited by *John Chircop and Francisco Javier Martínez*

Sickness, medical welfare and the English poor, 1750–1834 *Steven King*

Medical societies and scientific culture in nineteenth-century *Belgium Joris Vandendriessche*

Vaccinating Britain *Gareth Millward*

Madness on trial *James E. Moran*

Early Modern Ireland and the world of medicine Edited by *John Cunningham*

Feeling the strain *Jill Kirby*

Rhinoplasty and the nose in early modern British medicine and culture *Emily Cock*

Communicating the history of medicine Edited by *Solveig Jülich and Sven Widmalm*

Progress and pathology Edited by *Melissa Dickson, Emilie Taylor-Brown and Sally Shuttleworth*

Balancing the self Edited by *Mark Jackson and Martin D. Moore*

Global health and the new world order Edited by *Jean-Paul Gaudillière, Claire Beaudevin, Christoph Gradmann, Anne M. Lovell and Laurent Pordié*

Accounting for health

Calculation, paperwork,
and medicine, 1500–2000

Edited by Axel C. Hüntelmann and Oliver Falk

Manchester University Press

Copyright © Manchester University Press 2021

While copyright in the volume as a whole is vested in Manchester University Press, copyright in individual chapters belongs to their respective authors, and no chapter may be reproduced wholly or in part without the express permission in writing of both author and publisher.

Published by Manchester University Press
Altrincham Street, Manchester M1 7JA

www.manchesteruniversitypress.co.uk

British Library Cataloguing-in-Publication Data
A catalogue record for this book is available from the British Library

ISBN   978 1 5261 3516 2 hardback

First published 2021

The publisher has no responsibility for the persistence or accuracy of URLs for any external or third-party internet websites referred to in this book, and does not guarantee that any content on such websites is, or will remain, accurate or appropriate.

Typeset
by New Best-set Typesetters Ltd

Contents

List of figures	page vii
List of contributors	xiii
Introduction Axel C. Hüntelmann and Oliver Falk	1
Part I: Keeping the books	**33**
1 Accounting, religion, and the economics of medical care in sixteenth-century Germany: Hiob Finzel's *Rationarium praxeos medicae*, 1565–89 Michael Stolberg	35
2 'Making a living': Accounting and the medical market in and around Geneva, 1760–1820 Philip Rieder	56
3 Accounted bodies and counted cases: Elliott Joslin's diabetes research, 1898–1950 Oliver Falk	82
Part II: Household	**107**
4 Economies of the hospital, 1790–1910 Axel C. Hüntelmann	109
5 Contrasting accounting practices in the urban hospitals of England and France, 1890s to 1930s Barry M. Doyle	143

6 Reforming on paper: Accounting practices in the Leuven
   Academic Hospitals, 1920–60   166
   Joris Vandendriessche

7 Asylum accounts in health and in money   189
   Theodore M. Porter

Part III: Production   207
8 Charitable accounting: The Royal Jennerian Society
   and vaccine production   209
   Andrea Rusnock

9 The industry of clinical trials and the rise of medico-
   economic accounting: The case of antidepressants,
   1970–90   230
   Jean-Paul Gaudillière and Volker Hess

10 Accounting for Esther Smucker: The Mennonite
   church, the US National Institutes of Health, and
   the trade in healthy bodies, 1950–70   254
   Laura Stark

Part IV: Polity   281
11 States of healing in early modern Germany: Military
   health care and the management of manpower   283
   Sebastian Pranghofer

12 Miners' chest: How performative accounting forged
   the ills of industry   305
   J. Andrew Mendelsohn

13 Administrating sickness: The workings of an all-female
   sickness fund, 1898–1931   337
   Helene Castenbrandt

14 The health of nations: International health accounting in
   historical perspective, 1925–2011   359
   Christopher Sirrs

Index   386

List of figures

0.1	Poor Box at St. Bartholomew Hospital, London (photograph by Axel C. Hüntelmann)	page 2
1.1	Double page from Hiob Finzel's *Rationarium* (RSBZ QQQQ1a, 128–9)	39
1.2	Finzel's annual income 1573–88 in *gulden*	40
1.3	Double page from Hiob Finzel's *Rationarium* (RSBZ QQQQ1, 158–9)	45
2.1	Three practitioners in and around Geneva	59
2.2	Page of Joseph Despine's ledger (Archives départementales de Savoie, Fonds Despine, 11 J 106)	61
2.3	First page of Catherin Pichollet's ledger (Archives d'Etat de Genève, Manuscrit historique 201)	65
2.4	Page of Louis Odier's ledger/Livre de comptes de Louis Odier (Bibliothèque de Genève, Ms. Fr. 5647/9)	67
2.5	Page of Odier's clinical pocket books (Musée d'histoire des sciences, Z 92/2 Diarium clinicum)	72
3.1	Cases under observation 1 May 1914 to 1 May 1915 (Joslin, *Present-day Treatment and Prognosis in Diabetes*, p. 486)	87
3.2	Reporting scheme for results of urine sugar tests (Joslin, *A Diabetic Manual for the Mutual Use of Doctor and Patient*, 4th edn, p. 54)	96

3.3 Drawing by Mr Rainsford showing the colours of his urine sample in correlation with his daily diet (JDCHA, Box 20, Folder 6) Copyright © Joslin Diabetes Center. All rights reserved. Reprinted with permission. 97
3.4 Equivalency table for determining the quantities of carbohydrates, fats, and proteins and their caloric value in common foods. (Joslin, *A Diabetic Manual for the Mutual Use of Doctor and Patient* (6th edn), p. 51) 98
3.5 Post-treatment history of patient no. 16158 (front and back side). These file cards brought together registration categories, examination results, and the cause of death onto a single card (JDCHA, Box 5, Folder 2) Copyright © Joslin Diabetes Center. All rights reserved. Reprinted with permission. 100
4.1 Royal Charité Hospital in Berlin, hospital and *Ökonomie* buildings, surrounded by fields and garden, around 1730 (Eller, *Nützliche und auserlesene medicinische und chirurgische Anmerckungen*, Berlin 1730) 110
4.2 'Consumptions-Etat' – Designation of meals for '*Officianten*' and '*Deputanten*', June 1800 (HUA CD Nr. 1357, fol. 121) 117
4.3 Normal diet schemes (*Hauptdiätverordnung*), compiled and accumulated for all patients (Esse, *Krankenhäuser*, Beilage II, p. 271) 121
4.4 Form III breaking down the quantities of single ingredients (here i.e. coffee, sugar [...], herring, various baked fruits, cabbage) for the calculation of the daily diets (Esse, *Krankenhäuser*, Beilage III, pp. 278–9) 122
4.5 Calculation of catering days for 1902 (HUA CD No. 1200) 126
4.6 Recalculation of diet schemes (*Speisezettel*) 1st table, January 1897 (HUA CD No. 1259) 128
5.1 Expenditure, General Voluntary Hospitals Leeds and Sheffield, 1913–28 153
5.2 Expenditure, Lille Hospital Commission, 1910–28 153
6.1 Forms such as this 'Subscription Ticket' were used during the fundraising campaign for the Institute of Cancer in Leuven during the 1920s (UAL, ACA, 1046) 173

List of figures ix

6.2	A standardised form, filled out for the service of Pediatrics, 1952 (UAL, AVDS, 272)	180
8.1	*A Comparative View of the Natural Small-Pox, Inoculated Small-Pox, and Inoculated Cow-Pox*, by John Addington, by Order of the Medical Council of the Royal Jennerian Society for the Extermination of the Small-Pox (London: Nichols and Son, [1803], Library of the Royal College of Surgeons)	217
8.2	Register of Inoculations, *Address of the Royal Jennerian Society, for the Extermination of the Small-Pox. With the Plan, Regulations, and Instructions for Vaccine Inoculation. To Which is Added, a List of the Subscribers* (London: W. Phillips, 1803, p. 52, Wellcome Library)	219
8.3	Excerpt from RJS vaccination register, September 1804 (Minutes of the Medical Committee of the RJS, Wellcome MS 4304, 6 September 1804)	222
9.1	The CRF of the Levoprotiline study: Depressive mood, anxiety, agitation, inhibition, apathy, insomnia, and physical complaints (Courtesy of IGM Berlin, Arzneimittelforschung)	234
9.2	Target symptoms shape the efficacy of the CG antidepressant Ludiomil® (Maprotiline). Five items on the Hamilton-Scale affected significantly by the three drugs in different ways (compare Kielholz, *Depressive Zustände*, p. 256)	236
10.1	Esther Smucker and Mary Warye were admitted to the NIH Clinical Center in September 1965. Delbert Nye was director of NIH's Normal Volunteer Patient Program, which Esther and Mary joined to serve as 'normal control' research subject for the Mennonite church. They agreed to be the unit leaders for the Mennonite Voluntary Service group placed at the Clinical Center, which involved serving as the church's local accountants. This staged arrival scene, dated nine months after their actual admission, was likely photographed for publicity, though it was never ultimately used in promotional materials. The original	

photo caption reads: 'Esther Smucker shakes hands with Mr. Delbert Nye, director of the normal control patient program. Mary Warye watches in the background' (MCC, National Institutes of Health, 1955–66, box 4, file 74, MCC Photos, Voluntary Service, Photograph, IX-13.25) 255

10.2 The NIH Clinical Center opened in 1953 on the agency's main campus in Bethesda, Maryland, and started a new programme, the Normal Volunteer Patient Program, to get essential research material for scientists: healthy human subjects for medical experiments. Esther and Mary, like other 'Normals', lived in hospital rooms for weeks, months, or years alongside sick patients (US NIH National Library of Medicine, IHM database, Image ID: A014533, Unique ID: 10144118) 258

10.3 To get healthy human subjects for scientists' research in the Clinical Center, the NIH established a legal instrument for buying research supplies from vendors: the 'procurement contract'. The second line item under 'renewal contracts' in the NIH's 1956 inventory of contracts is contract 103-55, 'Volunteer Service' from Mennonite Central Committee (National Archives and Research Administration, College Park, Maryland, Contracts continuing 1955 and 1956, box 15, record group 511) 261

10.4 The Mennonite church and the Church of the Brethren signed the first contracts with the NIH for healthy human subjects, which were recruited through the churches' 'voluntary service' programs. The NIH paid the church organisations the cost of a stipend for voluntary service workers and a 10 per cent 'processing fee'. The churches also reimbursed voluntary service workers at NIH for their additional expenses, such as 'education and recreation' activities, and 'operation and administration' costs including phone and postage for church business. From among the group of voluntary service workers living at the Clinical Center, the

List of figures   xi

       churches assigned a 'unit leader', who worked as a vernacular accountant for the church to manage its local finances (MCC, Folder NIH MSU, Series MCC IX-6-3, Mennonite 'Report of unit income and expenses', c. 1966)   270
11.1 Aggregate manpower tables of the Hanoverian regiments in the Netherlands from May 1745 to April 1746 (NLA Hann, Hann 41 III, Nr. 16, fol. 178–9)   291
11.2 Monthly return from the Prussian field hospitals in Saxony during the Seven Years' War for the period from 6 November to 2 December 1760 (GStA PK, I HA Rep. 96, Nr. 85 U 2)   295
12.1 'Penny box' of a smelters' society (Hüttenknappschaft Freiberg) (Stadt- und Bergbaumuseum, Freiberg, Inv.-Nr. 51/92, photo by Wolfgang Thieme)   306
12.2 House of the Mining Brotherhood, Schwaz, Tyrol, showing hospital and sickbeds, c. 1510–50 ('Schwazer Bergbuch' [1556], illustrated in Bartels, Bingener, and Slotta [eds], *Schwazer Bergbuch*, Bochum 2006)   309
12.3 Quarterly invoice for medications given to miners, 1750 (Bergarchiv Freiberg, 40006, Bergamt Altenberg, No. 290)   325
12.4 Quarterly register of medications given to miners, with auditing annotation at bracket in the upper left margin, 1806–11 (Bergarchiv Freiberg, 40013 Bergamt Marienberg, No. 224)   327
13.1 Members and sickness funds in Gothenburg, 1901–40 (Kommerskollegium, *Arbetsstatistik. B, Registrerade sjukkassors verksamhet* [Stockholm: 1905–1912]; Socialstyrelsen, *Registrerade sjukkassor* [Stockholm: 1915–1936]. Pensionsstyrelsen, *Erkända sjukkassor år 1940, Sveriges officiella statistik: Försäkringsväsen* [Stockholm, 1943])   343
13.2 Income, expenditure, and financial assets in SSBK 1899–1930 (GLA, SSBK, vol. 42, annual statistic reports)   345
14.1 Health budgets in the *International Health Yearbooks*. Left: Germany, 1927 (extract); right: Italy, 1928   364–365

14.2 Comparative tables of health expenditure in *The Cost of Medical Care*, pp. 202–3 (International Labour Organization 1959)   369

14.3 Examples of comparative health expenditure data from the WHO Global Health Expenditure Database: Current health expenditure as a percentage of gross domestic product, selected OECD countries, 2000–15 (Source: http://apps.who.int/nha/database/ViewData/Indicators/en [accessed 21 May 2018])   376

List of contributors

Helene Castenbrandt is a researcher in the Department of Economic History at Lund University in Sweden where she is working on the history of long-term sickness absence. Castenbrandt's dissertation (2012) dealt with dysentery in Sweden between 1750 and 1900 as a demographic and medical history of a disease. Her main research interests involve medical history, demographic changes, and population history. Recently she published an article in *Economic History Review* (2018) on 'Trends in morbidity: national statistics on sickness claims among the working population in Sweden, 1892–1954'.

Barry M. Doyle is Professor of Health History at the University of Huddersfield. His teaching and research interests cover the political, social, and economic history of urban Britain in the late nineteenth and twentieth centuries. He has a particular interest in the development of health care systems before welfare states and the history of hospitals in Britain and Europe; the history of first aid and voluntary health care; and the development of maternity services in a global context. In 2014 he published *The Politics of Hospital Provision in Early Twentieth Century Britain* (Routledge).

Oliver Falk is Research Associate at the Institute of Biomedical Ethics and History of Medicine (IBME), University of Zurich. His main research areas are the history of diabetes therapy, doctor–patient relationships throughout the twentieth century, the epistemology of therapeutic self-techniques and medical writing, as well as sociology of knowledge in medicine. He recently published an article on the patient as an epistemic factor: 'Der Patient als epistemische Größe', *Medizinhistorisches Journal* 53 (2018).

Jean-Paul Gaudilliere is Senior Researcher at the Center for Research in Medicine, Science, Mental Health, and Society (CERMES 3) of the French Institute of Health and Medical Research. In 2015, he received an Advanced Grant from the European Research Council on the historical transformation 'From international public health to global heath: knowledge, diseases, and the government of health since 1945'. He has also worked and published on the relationships between science, medicine, and the pharmaceutical industry and the regulation of drugs in the twentieth century, as well as on medicine and risk management in cancer-related environmental health since the 1960s. He is involved in the volume *Global Health and the New World Order* that will be published in 2020 in the same book series as the current volume (Social Histories of Medicine).

Volker Hess is Chair of the Institute for the History of Medicine at the Charité Medical School in Berlin and Affiliated Professor in the History Department of the Humboldt University. In 2011, he received the Advanced Investigator Grant from the European Research Council for a collaborative project with J. Andrew Mendelsohn in reconstructing the 'paper technologies' of medical practices, based on their article in the journal *History of Science* (2010). In 2019, he was awarded an ERC Synergy Grant to study Europe's postwar history through the lens of medicine. With regard to the topic of the current volume, he edited with Alexa Geisthövel a volume on medical expertise (*Medizinisches Gutachten. Geschichte einer neuzeitlichen Praxis*, Göttingen 2017).

Axel C. Hüntelmann is Postdoctoral Research Fellow at the Institute for the History of Medicine at the Charité Medical School in Berlin. He has worked and published on the German Imperial Health Office (PhD 2007) and other European public health institutions between 1850 and 1950; scientific infrastructures; the history of laboratory animals; the production, marketing, and regulation of pharmaceuticals in Germany and France; and has written a biography on the immunologist Paul

Ehrlich (2011). He trained in accounting as well as history and is currently finishing a book on accounting and bookkeeping in medicine (1730–1930).

J. Andrew Mendelsohn is Reader in History of Science and Medicine at Queen Mary University of London. He co-led with Volker Hess the ERC-funded research project 'How physicians know, 1550–1950'. His research focuses on ways of writing and knowing and their effects in science and medicine; observation, experimenting, classifying, and predicting; and industrializing life and its sciences from the eighteenth to the twentieth century. Recent publications include the co-edited volume *Civic Medicine: Physician, Polity and Pen in Early Modern Europe* (2020).

Theodore M. Porter is Distinguished Professor of History at University of California, Los Angeles. His research integrates history of data, statistics, and quantification within the history of the human sciences. His most recent book is *Genetics in the Madhouse: The Unknown History of Human Heredity* (Princeton University Press, 2018).

Sebastian Pranghofer is Lecturer in Early Modern History at the Helmut-Schmidt-University in Hamburg. His main areas of research are early modern military administration and logistics; war, medicine, and disease; as well as the history of early modern anatomy. On military medicine, he recently published 'Zur Anatomie beurlaubt. Qualifizierung und Karrieren von Feldscheren in Berlin und Hannover im 18. Jahrhundert', in Johanna Bleker, Petra Lennig, and Thomas Schnalke (eds), *Tiefe Einblicke: Das anatomische Theater im Zeitalter der Aufklärung* (Berlin 2018).

Philip Rieder is Senior Lecturer (maître d'enseignement et de recherché) at the Institut Ethique Histoire Humanités (IEH2), University of Geneva. He has published widely on a variety of topics pertaining to the social and cultural history of medicine in the early modern period, namely the history of the patient, of medical practices, and of healers. Recently he edited with François Zanetti a volume on *Materia Medica: savoirs et usages des médicaments aux époques médiévales et modernes* (Geneva 2018), with his chapter on the history of the apothecary.

Andrea Rusnock is Professor in the Department of History at the University of Rhode Island and was the editor of *Osiris* between 2009 and 2017. She has worked and published widely on science and medicine in the Enlightenment; the history of quantification; public health and the environment; and on the history of vaccination. In 2002, she published *Vital Accounts: Quantifying Health and Population in Eighteenth-Century England and France* (Cambridge University Press).

Christopher Sirrs is Postdoctoral Fellow in the Department of History, University of Warwick. At the time of writing, he was a Research Fellow at the Centre for History in Public Health, London School of Hygiene and Tropical Medicine. An historian of medicine and public health, his research encompasses the history of global health, health systems, and occupational health and safety. In 2020, he started a research project funded by the Wellcome Trust, exploring the history of safety in the British National Health Service. His most recent publication is a journal article in the *International History Review*, exploring the International Labour Organization's approach towards health system financing in the second half of the twentieth century.

Laura J. M. Stark is Associate Professor at Vanderbilt University, Associate Editor of the journal *History & Theory*, and creator of the Vernacular Archive of Normal Volunteers housed at the Countway Center for the History of Medicine. Her research focuses on science and technology studies; social theory; and the history of science and medicine from feminist and postcolonial perspectives. In 2012, she published *Behind Closed Doors: IRBs and the Making of Ethical Research* with the University of Chicago Press and in 2019 she won the Freidson Prize from the American Sociological Association for her article in *Social History of Medicine*: 'Contracting health: procurement contracts, total institutions, and the problem of virtuous suffering in post-war human experiment'.

Michael Stolberg is Chair of History of Medicine in Würzburg, Germany. He has published widely on the history of early modern medicine. His most recent book is *Gelehrte Medizin und ärztlicher Alltag in der Renaissance* (Berlin: DeGruyter Oldenburg, 2020) and will be published in English (2021) as: *Learned Physicians and the World of Medical Practice in the Renaissance*.

Joris Vandendriessche is Postdoctoral Fellow of the Flanders Research Foundation (FWO) in the Cultural History since 1750 Research Group of the University of Leuven (Belgium). His research focusses on the history of scientific knowledge, medicine, and universities in the nineteenth and twentieth centuries. He is the author of *Medical Societies and Scientific Culture in Nineteenth-Century Belgium* (Manchester University Press, 2018) and *Zorg en wetenschap. Een geschiedenis van de Leuvense academische ziekenhuizen in de twintigste eeuw* (Leuven University Press, 2019). His current project engages with publishing practices and piracy in nineteenth-century science.

Introduction

Axel C. Hüntelmann and Oliver Falk

On 30 May 1751, after seven more people were admitted to a newly founded infirmary in Newcastle, the hospital's so-called poor boxes were opened, and '£9 18s. 10d. found therein'. In one of the boxes, there was a shilling, enclosed in a piece of paper with a short poem on it:

> To serve the needy, sick and lame,
> This splendid shilling freely came,
> From one who knows the want of wealth,
> And what is more – the want of health.
>
> Beneath this roof may thousands find,
> The greatest blessing of mankind;
> And hence may millions learn to know,
> That to do good's our end below;
> That Vice and Folly must decay
> Ere we can reach eternal day![1]

Poor boxes were common in many parts of Europe. They were located in front of hospitals, churches, and other places, notably as a part of poor relief systems. For instance, a similar box was located at the entrance of the Charité Hospital in Berlin in the eighteenth and nineteenth century. And as a relic of the past, even today a hospital visitor or patient who is entering or leaving St. Bartholomew Hospital in London from West Smithfield through the King Henry VIII gate can find a poor box opposite the former 'Counting House'. On the surface of the heavy box is a slot to insert a donation to the hospital and those who cannot afford proper treatment (Figure 0.1).

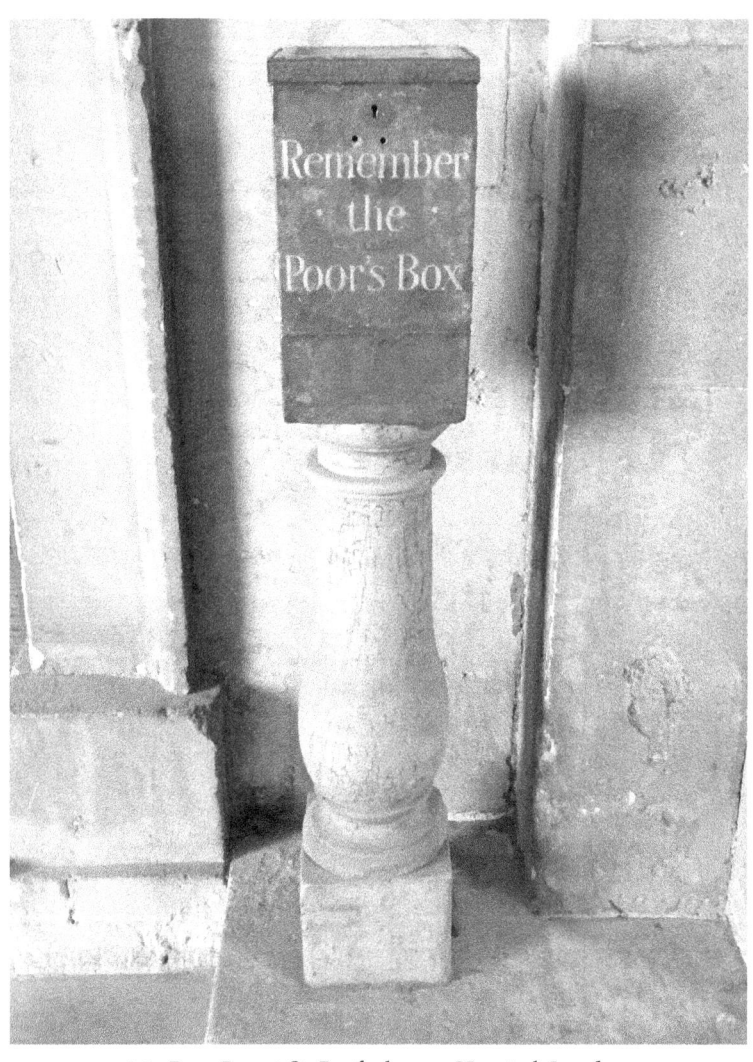

0.1 Poor Box at St. Bartholomew Hospital, London.

In the past, the sealed poor box was opened at regular intervals by the key holders and in the presence of several witnesses. The box was emptied, the money counted, the amount registered, and the donation then put to use. Detailed and itemised information about how the money was spent was kept in account books and each year the hospital's treasurer reported all income and expenditures in a published 'Annual Account'.

Although the revenue generated by poor boxes constituted only a small fraction of overall hospital income, these boxes illustrate the essence of accounting or, more specifically, accounting for health. Fundamentally, poor boxes represent accounting as a process of (countable) things going *in* and *out*, linking social and cultural preconditions and intentions (e.g. a system of poor relief), people (donors, processors, receivers), and the objects and materials involved. In this sense, poor boxes drew things together that, in their aggregate, reflect our understanding of accounting for health.

In this introduction, we will first frame what we mean by accounting for health by returning to the example of the poor box (1) and then summarise the current state of historical research (2). Then, after we have elaborated the volume's methodological approach (3), we will outline the book's structure (4) and sketch the different, deeply entwined dimensions of accounting for health (5).

Framing accounting for health

How does our understanding of accounting for health differ from other fields of accounting? What is so specific about accounting for health?

Accounting is about 'how much' and is usually assumed to be about money. It is viewed as a financial technology related to the administration of money, cost and costing, and the calculation of efficiency.[2] But the term 'accounting for health' involves both money and medicine and raises moral issues, given that making a living from medical treatment has ethical ramifications. Profiting from the 'pain and suffering of other people' (Chapter 1) was as problematic in 1500 as it is in today's debates about the economisation of medicine and the admissibility of for-profit hospitals.

The poor box illustrates that inserting a shilling into a slot is not just about money. Donations were made for a certain purpose and were laden with moral or social intentions. Because donors expected their money to be used for a specific purpose, treasurers had to provide information about the donor's gift – for instance, in published 'Annual Accounts' – and to account for its efficient and legitimate use. This accounting for health was not merely a matter of financial probity, but also about best medical practice, not least because it helped elicit further donations and encourage other prospective donors. For this reason, monetary income and medical outcome were correlated. Accounting for health involved information being collected, listed, and compiled in tables (for instance, about the number of patients treated and cured, about cure rates, and about changes in revenue sources or health outcomes over time) in order to demonstrate good medical practice.[3]

But what did good medical practice mean and who defined it? What was health and what was disease, and at what point did 'not so healthy' turn into 'sick'? What criteria determined healthiness, and how and by whom were those criteria developed? In society as well as interpersonal communication, such criteria have regulatory functions that enable (or necessitate) action and that therefore have to be plausible and comprehensible. Inasmuch as health, disease, and medicine have a socio-political and moral dimension, disease and illness couldn't simply be described in vague and subjective terms – such as an absence of disease or a comprehensive physical, mental, and social well-being – but instead had to be objectified and legitimised according to general, enumerable criteria. In this transformation process, calculative practices like reckoning, counting, computing, or evaluating played an important role.

For centuries, accounting and calculative practices have comprised an essential part of medicine. As early as the sixteenth century, health and disease had been described in terms of a balance or imbalance of bodily fluids. In the eighteenth century, patients' diets were calculated in grams, grains, or ounces of bread, meat, or fat, and pints of milk. Descriptions of human metabolism and internal secretions in the mid-nineteenth century likewise underscored the importance of calculative practices in medicine. And ever since, the once fluid transitions between 'still healthy' and 'already ill' have been clearly demarcated using threshold values. The normal and the pathological, and therefore the state of health and of medicine in general, have come to be determined by numbers. For instance, the number of blood cells or the proportion of blood sugar or uric acid in the blood has come to determine the state of health and disease in cases of anaemia, gout, or diabetes. At the end of the nineteenth century, new disciplines like nutritional science and calorimetry helped to establish methods for computing balanced diets as part of therapeutic approaches to stabilise and improve a person's health using precisely defined daily quantities of fats, proteins, and carbohydrates. Whether in research, therapy, or prevention, it became crucial to measure, count, or correlate everything that enters or exits the body.

Against this medical backdrop, accounting for health is a set of calculative practices and administrative techniques in which not only money but also goods and other countable objects are transformed into specific codes and formats that appear in (account- or case-) books, (double-entry) ledgers, lists, and tables. In this transposition, the status of the objects recorded is changed insofar as their availability is now no longer bound to their physical materiality; the countable objects have turned into manageable units, figures, and numbers that enable subsequent practices of reckoning, calculating, valuing, controlling, justifying, communicating, or researching. In this sense, accounting can be considered an administrative, scientific, and social technique. But this transposition generates not only a variety of figures and numbers, but also paper tools like ledgers and account books – the production of numbers itself was closely linked to accounting techniques and depended on, and was influenced by, the chosen form of recordkeeping.

State of research

Accounting for health brings together related perspectives and lines of research that have so far remained surprisingly unconnected. There are reams of literature on knowledge production in medicine or the life sciences, like the countless studies on laboratory science and historical epistemology from the Max Planck Institute for the History of Science or the Pickstone series on Science, Technology, and Medicine in modern history. In addition, scholars working in the field of health economics and other related areas have written extensively on the economisation of health and medicine,[4] on the commercialisation of medicine, on the commodification of the body and of health, as well as on the history of the drug and health markets.[5]

But we aim to describe a more detailed accounting for health that incorporates calculative practices, paper technologies, medicine, and medical knowledge. In the following summary of current research, we first review the literature on the sociology and history of calculative practices. We then outline several research perspectives within the history of accounting. And, finally, we turn specifically to the history of hospital accounting.

(1) Following in the footsteps of Werner Sombart's and Max Weber's classical work on organisations, sociologists have recently been eager to provide a better, broader, and more realistic understanding of the significance of numbers and figures. According to these approaches, the social character of figures needs to be explored in terms of the conditions, possibilities, boundaries, as well as the conflicts evoked within organisations and society. Moreover, their social context and the social integration and interlacing of their use – from measurement to management, from reckoning to governing, or from calculating to constructing – needs to be analysed.[6] At the same time, this approach attempts to compensate for a long interruption in theoretical debates and for a lack of systematic interest in calculative practices, as well as to answer the questions of whether and to what extent the massive mobilisation of numbers, measurements, and calculations might impair, support, or undermine social order.[7]

In this respect, Uwe Vormbusch's study *Die Herrschaft der Zahlen* is especially revealing because it illustrates how the cultural legitimacy of calculative practices varied widely over the course of their historical development. Thus, in the eighteenth century there were bitter debates about whether statistics on births and deaths should be produced, just as today we face the question of whether knowledge of prenatal and genetic diagnostics should be used to make life and death decisions.[8] This illustrates, for example, the extent to which calculative practices can be connected with genuinely medical–historical questions that inform studies about the rise of political arithmetic and vital statistics, about risk calculation, about medical quantification, about calculative practices in clinical medicine, and about public health and epidemiology.[9] The expanding influence of statistics from the eighteenth century onwards thus undermined the notion of mortality as a universal constant or as divine predestination, to the point that life and death could be seen not only to vary across regions, but also to depend on someone's sex and behaviour. Statistics thus became part of everyday social awareness. Their narrative expression can be found in the innumerable eighteenth-century prints that conveyed the emerging bourgeoisie's understanding of the connection between one's own behaviour and prospects for a long and healthy life[10] and that eventually influenced the construction of the modern body in nineteenth-century hygienic and physiological discourse.[11]

The arrival of a Foucauldian 'quantitative dispositive' was accompanied by a shift in the meaning of numbers, from a rather symbolic, mystical designation of size to a tool of 'world surveying' by state authorities in the early modern era, with considerable effects on social, economic, and scientific practices. That numbers produced by statisticians and accountants came to be regarded as 'objective', trustworthy, and reliable enough to serve as a basis for decision-making, was a process that developed over centuries.[12] For a number of years, early modern studies focused on the importance of statistics for the evolving absolutist territorial state, in particular with an emphasis on the emergence of quantifying and calculative practices related to natural resource acquisition, spatial perceptions, population surveys, military preparedness, tax surveys, etc. However, Lars Behrisch has pointed out that early modern studies have used the concept of statistics rather uncritically by tending to classify any form of numerical administrative technique as statistics. As a consequence, the question of *why* and *when* numbers, tables, and calculations began to influence perceptual patterns, arguments, and actions remains partly obscured. During the course of this shift in the meaning of counting and arithmetic practices, various forms of administrative manipulation came to be used as information collection practices, creating new forms for the non-statistical representations of numbers, such as tax lists, military recruitment lists, community registers, or catalogue entries. 'Statistics does not create more or better knowledge; it first and foremost creates an entirely new kind of knowledge.'[13] But the question is, what does this new knowledge mean for an important part of a society like medicine?

(2)   Aside from sociological work on calculative practices, there are also numerous studies on the history of accounting, most recently

by cultural historians like Jacob Soll and Jane Gleeson-White.[14] An overview of this research is provided by the compendium on the history of bookkeeping published by John R. Edwards and Stephen P. Walker.[15] In addition to the development of accounting practices (in particular double-entry bookkeeping), the focus lies on the historical development of accounting systems and the professionalisation and institutionalisation of those systems in corporate organisations and academic institutions,[16] as well as on the gender-specific aspects of accounting.[17] Furthermore, several publications from the London School of Economics around the group of Anthony G. Hopwood, Peter Miller, and Michael Power have, partly from a Foucauldian perspective, examined discourses on accounting, auditing, and governmentality.[18] However, the number of publications directly related to the subject of medicine and the generation of medical knowledge is far smaller. Alistair M. Preston's 'The birth of clinical accounting' is worthy of special mention. Preston examines the extent to which the history of bookkeeping should not be seen merely as a continuous 'improvement' and development of calculative techniques resulting from shifting socio-environmental conditions, but instead, conversely, as a governmental technique in itself by which certain social conditions are regulated and influenced.[19] Preston examines accounting in US hospitals and highlights two particular transformation processes: at the beginning of the twentieth century, the primary concern was to manage and control hospital costs, whereas the 1960s and 1970s were characterised by attempts to increase revenues and implement cost–benefit analyses. Preston shows 'how changes in accounting thought and practice over the past 100 years are intertwined with changes in medical knowledge and practice, the establishment of hospitals as the primary sites for medical treatment, the emergence of private insurance, changing forms of government regulation and shifting socio-political attitudes towards the cost and provision of health care.'[20] In this respect, Preston's investigation relies mainly on discourses in health policy and (hospital) bookkeeping and can be included among numerous other studies on governmentality. However, the mathematical practices themselves – counting, measuring, calculating, and tabulating – receive little notice. Nevertheless, Preston's study is an important landmark for this volume, but it is also a solitary one in the research landscape, since Foucauldian studies on the history of double-entry bookkeeping and auditing ended abruptly in the mid-1990s. In this context, Uwe Vormbusch has written of the long interruption 'in the theoretical discussion of calculative practices in economy and society'.[21] And ever since, according to Peter Miller, 'no more than rudimentary approaches of a sociology of calculative practices' can be identified.[22]

(3) Over the last twenty years, rich and substantial studies on the history of accounting in hospitals have been published. Focusing mainly on the monetary aspects of hospital funding and hospital finance, these studies take a completely different perspective and have little in common with the aforementioned sociological works. A good overview of the existing literature has been written by Florian Gebreiter and William J. Jackson.[23] The range of hospital finance and accounting practices is explored in the edited volumes by Martin Gorsky and Sally Sheard (2006, for Great Britain) and Alfons Labisch and Reinhard Spree (2001, for Germany).[24] These studies analyse the sources of income and (to a lesser extent) the structure of hospital expenditures mainly in the nineteenth and twentieth century. Both studies are social histories that strive to explain the emergence of welfare states and that deal with numerous questions about how social and institutional change influenced hospital finance. Those question include, for example: the rise of voluntary, charitable hospitals in Britain in the early eighteenth century (Croxson, see below Berry), the development and problems of their funding system, and that system's influence on hospital care during the nineteenth and twentieth century; the growing influence of state and local authorities, for instance due to the New Poor Law; the creation of national health insurance in Germany (1883)[25] and Britain (1911) as well as earlier or similar forms of funding, such as friendly societies and their payment schemes; and finally the establishment and development of the NHS (1948) and its influence on British health care.[26] Furthermore, there are specific studies on hospital contributory schemes in Britain, the importance of philanthropy in British health care, and patients' payments in interwar Britain.[27] There are also some publications about the use of Henry Burdett's *Uniform System of Accounts* in hospitals and other health institutions and its influence on the structure and administration of hospital finances.[28] But as Florian Gebreiter and William J. Jackson have noted, these studies have been almost exclusively 'UK-centric'[29], whereas American,[30] French,[31] or German[32] contributions are few and far between.

Furthermore, several studies are situated at the interface between economic history, the history of accounting, and cultural history, and have been published in journals like *Accounting, Business & Financial History*,[33] *Accounting, Organisations and Society*,[34] *Accounting, Auditing & Accountability Journal*,[35] or *Accounting History*.[36] They deal with various aspects of hospital accounting and appear to comprise a subfield of accounting history. Amanda Berry, for instance, investigates the financial management and funding of voluntary hospitals in Bristol, Northampton, Devon, and Exeter in the second half of the eighteenth and the early nineteenth centuries. In these hospitals, which were funded by donations, accounting was intended not just to administer and manage financial resources. In a competitive marketplace of charities, accounting as manifested in public 'accounts' and reports was also needed to prove and justify financial transactions and to demonstrate that donations were being properly and efficiently used for the common good. Furthermore, in order to elicit donations from potential benefactors and to exert pressure on members of 'polite society' who had not yet contributed, donors were acknowledged by publishing their names in the accounts. Berry's study shows that even mid-sized hospitals employed sophisticated accounting practices in the mid-eighteenth century. Moreover, Berry's work illustrates how accounting went beyond the mere managing of finances and could also serve to set exemplary standards within a gift economy,[37] as a social and cultural function designed to solicit further donations.[38] Andy Holden et al. analyse the moral economies of hospital accounting in the context of welfare and poor relief, using the example of the Newcastle infirmary in the second half of the nineteenth century.[39] The many aims of hospital accounting have also been emphasised by Paolo Quattrone, who has studied the accounting system of the Jesuits in the sixteenth and seventeenth centuries, and Enrico Bracci et al., who investigate the accounting system of Saint Anna Hospital in Ferrara at the end of the sixteenth century.[40] Again, accounting was more than simply the administration of financial transactions or of the hospital's (or the religious order's) economy; it also attested to and manifested institutional charity. Bookkeeping and accounting were involved in and part of a divine economy (*göttliche Ökonomie*).[41] Keeping accounts made the bookkeeper accountable both to himself and to God. James Aho argues that in the late medieval and early modern eras, when official

Church dogma regarded profit-making as morally suspect, bookkeeping allowed people to justify their actions vis-à-vis the state (or the investor), the community, and God, and to certify 'that for everything [...] earned something of equal value had been returned, and that for everything meted out something else was deserved'.[42] Further studies on hospital accounting in early modern Bologna, Verona, and Düsseldorf also refer to the multi-dimensional aspects of bookkeeping and its 'calculating with eternity' [Rechnen mit der Ewigkeit], as the title of Brigitte Pohl-Resl's book on a medieval Viennese hospital implies.[43] Yet these studies also demonstrate just how sophisticated accounting had already become by the sixteenth century, both generally[44] and in hospitals.

The studies on hospital accounting deal with hospital finances in all their different and multi-dimensional functions, at the interface between charity, philanthropy, medical profession, local government, welfare, and national health. But these multi-disciplinary perspectives are often disconnected, leaving an important gap at the interface between different fields of research: specifically, they fail to explore the reciprocal relationship and mutual interactions between accounting and its calculative practices and administrative techniques on the one hand, and medicine and medical knowledge on the other.

Methodological approach

This volume aims to combine these different perspectives. Spanning a period of nearly five centuries (1500–2000), the contributions address questions of how calculative practices changed over time and for what reasons, and what effects these changes have had on medicine and medical knowledge. More precisely, we are asking: who is doing the accounting in hospitals and other health institutions? What logic are they following? Why and for whom are health institutions engaged in accounting? And what are the effects of accounting on medicine, health, and medical knowledge? These questions can be summed up as follows: what roles have accounting and similar economic practices played in everyday medical modes of knowing? How do such practices generate information about medical costs, and in what ways are such data transformed into economic knowledge? Under what conditions have these relationships and processes become visible and contested or consciously shaped by actors toward specific ends? What changes can be observed over time, and what differences exist between countries or political and economic systems?

The chapters examine the different meanings of accounting with the aim of answering the key question of how accounting and calculative practices affected medical knowledge and practice, i.e. how they affected diagnosis and disease classification, the conceptual and economic organisation of medical research, the nature of prognosis and treatment, patients' self-observation and self-medication, and not least the power of hospital or national health budgets to shape everyday medical issues.

The link between accounting and medicine, between calculative practices and the generation of medical knowledge, will be discussed from a praxeological perspective that focuses on practices and processes. Hitherto unconnected research strands will thereby be brought together, including both general historical and social science studies on health economics, health markets, and their regulation, as well as more specific explorations in the history of hospital accounting. The methodological conceptualisation of this volume combines four approaches:

(1) Since accounting is examined as a calculative *practice*, praxeological considerations have to be taken on board. In the sense of 'looking at paperwork',[45] calculative practices as well as the practice of bookkeeping and the associated *paper technologies* between the sixteenth and the end of the twentieth century will be examined in detail. In recent years, numerous publications from different disciplines like the history of science or cultural and media studies have appeared on the epistemic effects of *paperwork* or *paper technologies* on writing practices and their materiality in science and medicine.[46] In his article 'Paperwork: the state of the discipline', Ben Kafka argues that mostly Anglo-American historiography in the 1960s and 1970s produced a series of important and interesting studies. 'By looking *through* paperwork', these social-scientific studies succeeded in reconstructing the lives of ordinary men and women. But at the same time, the studies were not 'looking *at* paperwork', i.e. at the conditions of production and reproduction of the sources. In addition to processes and practices, we turn our attention to the production of numbers and to the very objects and materiality of accounting systems, focusing not so much on numbers themselves

as the mere result or output of accounting practices, but rather on *how* the numbers, the balance sheets, the tables, and statistics emerge, for *what* reasons the counting is done, and *what* effects writing, reckoning, and calculating practices produce?

But our perspective is not limited to the purpose and function of accounting: we are also interested in the context of the individual figures, tables, lists, etc. in which they were actually created. As the example of the poor box shows, the question of how and why something has been collected cannot be separated from subsequent administrative processes. If we want to understand these processes, including all of their financial, moral, and epistemological implications, it is also necessary to ask how and why certain objects were collected and counted. In this sense, the contributions to this volume engage questions of how and for what purpose money, goods, and data were gathered, how these objects were subsequently processed and used, and what implicit and explicit effects they had. And so we intend to illustrate the importance of accounting in the making of (medical) knowledge and to decouple it from merely economic and monetary issues, without, however, neglecting its significance for those issues.

(2) As noted, accounting commonly is about figures that compare and analyse revenue and expenses. In handbooks, accounting is likewise defined as the measurement and processing of financial information about economic entities.[47] Reduced in this way, accounting tends to be treated merely as a 'body of technically refined calculations used by organisations to efficiently accomplish goals such as profit maximisation'.[48] We maintain that an understanding of accounting simply as the administration of money and the recording and reporting of financial or business transactions is too narrow. Instead, we understand accounting as a *combination* of different kinds of calculative and administrative practices[49] that have been established over time. These practices are a central element of the medical rationality that drives medicine and they are deeply entwined with the development of medical knowledge. In light of current debates about the 'economisation' of medicine, this link between accounting (in the broadest sense) and medicine and health is often overlooked. This may be due to the fact that calculative practices are deeply embedded within society as a whole, in everyday life-routines and institutionalised infrastructures.

As a result, they can easily evade critical and historical reflection. In this extended sense, accounting has long been an integral feature of medicine: confronted with calculative practices as implicitly objective, ineluctable factors in the interpretation of reality,[50] we often forget that the desire to quantify and measure has a long and complex history.[51]

We favour a broader understanding of accounting for two reasons. First, we feel that accounting for health comprises practices such as reckoning, computing, the calculation of risk, the (e)valuation of scientific results and clinical trials, the recording of patient data, the balancing of alternative therapies, the management of information and data processing as the basis for decision-making or, more traditionally, for the reasonable and efficient management of resources. With a broader definition of accounting (for health) we are able to focus on a variety of practices at the interface of finance, administration, or data management that are very common in medicine, yet beyond the logic of monetisation. An understanding of accounting as a financial technology requires the valuation of activities and objects and their transformation into monetary units. Only after this transformation has occurred can those activities and objects be accounted for. This warps or even excludes from medical practice certain kinds of social and health care activities and raises the vexing question of how to put a price on the priceless?[52] Furthermore, this leads to misguided discussions about the commodification of health and medicine, which are not the focal point of this book.

Second, according to literature on accounting (history), our current understanding of accounting as a financial technology is the result of a long and ongoing process that started in the late eighteenth century with the institutionalisation and professionalisation of accounting, business management, and economics and which eventually developed into today's master narrative. Within this process, the definition of accounting in the 'accountant's sense' has been separated from the 'general meanings of the word',[53] and the wider and more traditional socio-cultural practices and meanings of accounting have been purged and forgotten.[54] Arguably, this was a process of purification similar to that described in Bruno Latour's 'grand partage'. In his influential book *We Have Never Been Modern*, Latour critiques how science, economics, culture, and society became discrete domains ('neatly separated drawers') and how problems are discussed in isolation within these different domains.[55] When discussing accounting for *health* and the entangled calculative practices embedded within medicine, we must also include the social and cultural meanings and practices of accounting in a broader sense.[56] Especially in medicine, we find numerous examples of counting, measuring, and generating numbers that are recorded and kept in books, but that have only indirectly to do with finances. As contributions to this volume demonstrate, the outcome of clinical trials can be quantified, processed, and calculated, just as the physiological functions of the human body can be measured and brought into balance. Without neglecting financial bookkeeping and its importance for medicine, we hope to expand the definition of accounting beyond strictly fiscal issues and to thereby incorporate social norms such as accountability[57] and other more general notions of justification or legitimisation as denoted in the *Oxford English Dictionary*.[58]

(3) The epistemic effects of these calculative practices on medicine and medical knowledge also need to be investigated. In other words, in addition to studies on the history of bookkeeping and accounting, the historical epistemology of calculative practices – their connections, relations, and exchanges with the production of medical knowledge – deserves greater attention. For this reason, the contributions to this volume examine an expanded understanding of accounting. They are not about accounting systems as such, but about calculative practices (counting, measuring, calculating, cumulating) in a broader sense.[59]

(4) To penetrate the complex history of accounting, we take a structuralist, 'longué durée' perspective in order to show that medical accounting, like every epistemic culture,[60] is bound to special forms of the production and communication of knowledge. In other words, calculative practices have a long history, but are historically contingent in their specific manifestations. Thus, accounting practices served different purposes and have had different meanings over time. Hans Blumenberg has pointed to the constitutive character of calculative practices with regard to social perception. He argues that these practices replaced the category of substance with that of quantity as early as the fourteenth century, thus establishing the ideal of a calculative treatment of all

possible problems, not least in medicine.[61] In this sense, it is worth considering Michel Foucault's *The Order of Things*. His analysis of knowledge systems or *epistemes* of the renaissance, classical, and modern eras reveals the epistemic breaks in the respective epochal thresholds. According to Foucault, the Renaissance episteme of 'resemblance' becomes an episteme of 'representation' at the beginning of the classical epoch with the emerging idea that the world had a natural order that is completely displayable by means of an artificial system of signs: the tableau.

Cornelia Vismann, in her book on *Files: Media, Technology and Law*, also describes the orderly function of tables in the early modern age. As an early form of data processing, files created objects of knowledge that were not already present in this form in the visible world.[62] Vismann's work shows that specific forms of accounting not only generate new knowledge, but that accounting itself and its purpose are always dependent on the respective knowledge systems of an epoch. This may sound trivial, but it has consequences for the definition of what accounting actually is because it asks not only what accounting is in its practical dimensions, but also for what purposes it was used in different times or epistemic contexts.

Finally, we feel that a broader definition of accounting is necessary given that the chapters of this volume cover a period of nearly 500 years. Viewed through the lens of history, it becomes obvious that accounting is and has been much more than simply a financial technology. In its broader sense of 'good household practice' or 'good economy', accounting has involved the balancing and valuation not just of money, but also of goods, humours, moralities, and so forth, alongside societal demands to be accountable not only to investors but also to oneself and to God, as Michael Stolberg illustrates in his Chapter 1.[63] These are only a few examples of the range and original meaning of medically relevant accounting and economic practices. Accounting has its own temporality, facing both backward and forward in time, holding accountable for past actions and forecasting the trajectory of future ones; accounting puts to paper a variety of values and expectations and it does so in ways that have immediate and long-term effects on disease and survival thanks to the knowledge it generates. Accounting and other related practices thus shape what medicine is and, for actors in specific times and places, what it ought to be, for instance in terms of drug production, diagnosis, treatment, life insurance, hospitals, and more.

Structure of *Accounting for health*

In answering the aforementioned questions, the chapters of this book span a period of nearly 500 years, starting with the accounting ledger (*rationarium praxeos medicae*) of a German physician in the mid-sixteenth century (Chapter 1) and ending with the development of an international system of health accounting in the twentieth and the early twenty-first century (Chapter 14).

In their aggregate, the chapters cover a large geographic area. With a focus on the Western world, they include case studies drawn from the United States (Chapter 3, Chapter 7), Great Britain (Chapter 5, Chapter 8), France (Chapter 5), Germany (Chapters 1, 4, 11, and 12), Belgium (Chapter 6), Sweden (Chapter 13), Switzerland (Chapter 2), and supranational public health institutions like the World Health Organisation (Chapter 14).

Paper technologies as well as the administrative, writing, and calculative practices related to accounting figure prominently in the volume. First and foremost – and not surprisingly – a number of chapters describe bookkeeping and financial accounting in private practice (Chapter 1, Chapter 2) and in the hospital (Chapter 4, Chapter 5), or the evaluation of national health budgets (Chapter 14). Moreover, the authors examine calculative practices like the tabulation of vital and health statistics (Chapters 7, 8, and 11), the calculation of daily ratios of food for diabetic patients (Chapter 3) and in the hospital (Chapter 4), the collection and processing of data for clinical testing (Chapters 8, 9, and 10), and the balancing of hospitals' institutional economies as well as patients' bodily ones.

In the individual chapters, accounting is shown to involve not only specific methods of counting and numerical calculation, but also wider information and data processing practices, including note-taking and the keeping, organising, and use of notebooks, files, and archives, as well as reading, writing, and transferring different kinds of tabular and narrative representations. Information practices are shown to produce cost calculations for medical treatments (and indeed the very notion of 'units' of medical care), tables of figures about patients, vital and other medical statistics, an accounting of the charges imposed by insurance companies and the rates they set, and the classification of information and data about patients. The sources range from practitioners' notebooks to hospital ledgers, from files and visual tables to budgets, reports, charts, publications, and the records of meetings and debates.

In addition, in all chapters – directly or indirectly – calculative practices are related to health, medicine, and medical knowledge in a broader sense. Studies on the emergence of political arithmetic and the population sciences are included alongside those on the quantification of clinical medicine, the development of remedies, occupational health and insurance medicine, metabolism, and health management.

Finally, the volume combines various medical institutions like asylums (Chapter 7), different kinds of hospitals (Chapter 4, Chapter 5, Chapter 6), and private practices (Chapter 1, Chapter 2, Chapter 3), or more broadly health insurance organisations (Chapter 13), pharmaceutical companies, research institutes (Chapter 9, Chapter 10), and supranational public health institutions (Chapter 14). The volume and its structure is the result of a series of three intensive workshops. Especially at the last workshops, we discussed a variety of structures that stressed countries or regions, temporal clusters, accounting practices, and sources or dimensions of accounting. A mere chronological ordering would probably suggest that we assume a 'development' of accounting practices over time – which we do not. Given that we favour a broader understanding of accounting that comprises and combines different practices and paper technologies, and that we consider accounting to be entwined with monetary, moral, and epistemic dimensions, we abandoned these ideas as undermining such complex entanglements.

Instead, we opted for a classical institutional structure, presenting accounting and calculative practices in four different institutional settings, including the physician's practice (Keeping the books), the hospital (Household), medical research and production facilities (Production), and welfare institutions (Polity). All chapters deal with accounting and calculative practices in their various medical meanings and effects. All parts contain three to five chapters that span an extended period of time (at least two centuries) and that deal with accounting practices in at least three countries (and/or supranational organisations).

The first part 'Keeping the books' adopts a micro-perspective on bookkeeping and other paper technologies, accounting, and calculative practices undertaken by physicians in their medical practices, more specifically bookkeeping in the medical practice of a physician in sixteenth-century Germany (Michael Stolberg, Chapter 1), in the medical market in and around eighteenth-century Geneva (Philip Rieder, Chapter 2), and in the complex system of patient accounts developed by the American diabetes specialist Elliot Joslin in the first half of the twentieth century (Oliver Falk, Chapter 3). The second part 'Household' examines accounting practices in larger health care institutions like the Charité hospital in Berlin in the long nineteenth century (Axel C. Hüntelmann, Chapter 4), the Leuven University Hospital in Belgium between the 1940s and 1960s (Joris Vandendriessche, Chapter 6), mental asylums in the nineteenth century (Theodore M. Porter, Chapter 7), and hospitals in England and France in the late nineteenth and early twentieth century (Barry Doyle, Chapter 5).

The third part 'Production' deals with calculative practices and the production of numbers in the broader health industry and valorisations in clinical research. Andrea Rusnock in Chapter 8 examines the accounting practices of vaccine production in Britain in the early nineteenth century, whereas Volker Hess and Jean-Paul Gaudillière in Chapter 9 show how clinical research changed from being based on relatively unspecified trial-and-error – 'without protocol, research plan, or study design' – in the 1950s into an 'industrialised' accounting practice in the 1980s. Laura Stark in Chapter 10 asks how financial contracts shaped epistemic possibilities. The fourth part on 'Polity' deals with accounting practices in societies/corporations like miners' associations (Chapter 12), military organisations (Chapter 11), insurance companies and friendly societies (Chapter 13), and supranational organisations (Chapter 14).

Dimensions of *Accounting for health*

If we understand accounting for health as an administrative, scientific, and social technique and practice, there are three fundamental dimensions to accounting: a financial, an epistemological, and a social/moral dimension. These dimensions are not discrete and accounting for health involves of all three of them. We consider the entanglement of these techniques and their corresponding dimensions as the essence of accounting for health. However, in each of the subsequent chapters, one dimension might be more relevant than the others, depending on the author's focus or sources.

How must we imagine this entanglement of techniques and dimensions of accounting for health?

While accounting generates figures and paper techniques and relies on the very formats it produces, accounting practices can be put to use in various ways. James Delbourgo and Staffan Müller-Wille have pointed out that early modern naturalists adopted recording techniques similar to double-entry ledgers and inventories that recorded the accumulation of capital, goods, and labour in order to keep track of the collection, accumulation, and exchange of specimens.[64] Similarly, Anke te Heesen has shown how German naturalists used accounting techniques for purposes of recording and organising specimens.[65] These scholars have emphasised the vital role of these techniques in the process of knowledge production, which illustrates that the boundaries between the administrative, financial, epistemological, and moral dimensions of accounting can be fluid, superimposed on each other, interdependent, and sometimes distinct.

The link between accounting's monetary and moral dimension is sometimes obvious. As Amanda Berry, George C. Gosling, and Barry Doyle[66] have shown, many British hospitals derived the largest portion of their income from monetary donations (and from rental properties that had been donated to the hospital) by wealthy individuals and middle-class donors. With reference to Marcel Mauss and his economy of give and take, donations and gifts are always linked with intentions and expectations.[67] In return, and depending on the amount contributed, donors and their family members could receive medical treatment at the hospital (and/or recommend treatment of others), similar to a system of subscriptions. Donors could also be appointed honorary members of the hospital board.

Another example of the monetary and moral entanglement of accounting relates to a divine economy wherein donations (to hospitals) compensated for earthly misconduct and balanced one's own account in heaven.[68] Michael Stolberg's analysis in Chapter 1 of Jacob Finzel demonstrates how this early modern physician kept his ledger not only to provide an overview of his patients' visits or of his income, expenses, and donations, but also to justify his own work and himself before God. In addition, Stolberg's example illustrates that accounting books were used not just to note patients' payments, but also to list their treatment.

The moral and social aspects of accounting become evident in Helene Castenbrandt's Chapter 13 about a Swedish women's health insurance fund in the first half of the twentieth century. She shows how closely economic and organisational considerations were combined with practices of social and moral control. Members of the insurance fund had not only to pay their fees at the obligatory monthly meeting, but also to endure 'sick visits' if they claimed benefits. These visits were an important tool to ensure that fund members would avail themselves of benefits only according to the rules. Furthermore, the visits allowed members' illnesses to be monitored and investigated.

The epistemic dimension of accounting becomes evident in the chapters of Oliver Falk (Chapter 3) and Volker Hess and Jean-Paul Gaudillière (Chapter 9). They argue that legitimate scientific outcomes relied essentially on calculative practices governing both the administration of the flow of information in experimental settings and clinical trials, and the transformation of that information into numerical data, i.e. statistical and empirical research results. In other words, such results required sophisticated techniques of bookkeeping, recording, calculating, listing, or tabulating. Oliver Falk in Chapter 3 illustrates how the American diabetes specialist Elliott Joslin developed a complex system of patient accounts, comprised of ledgers, notebooks, and account books, that served as a repository of data for Joslin's systematic diabetes research and his dealings with life insurance companies.

Medical knowledge also includes knowledge or know-how about making a living (Chapter 1, Chapter 2), organising a medical practice, or funding and managing a hospital (Chapter 4, Chapter 5, Chapter 6). It involves knowledge about the number of patients cured in order to evaluate the success of a treatment (either to promote one's own remedies or elicit donations) (Chapter 3, Chapter 7) or knowledge about the number of wounded or unwounded (healthy?) soldiers (Chapter 11). Financial accounting provides information about medical cost structures and future income or expenses; it serves as a tool to inform decisions about health plans, medical treatment schemes, or to prioritise research agendas. Axel C. Hüntelmann in Chapter 4 shows how practical knowledge, the know-how of managing and financing a hospital, provides the basis for a discipline known as 'hospital economics'.

These examples show that accounting for health was and is more than the mere tallying of income or the collection and administration of money. It also becomes clear that medical knowledge is not limited to research on the aetiology of diseases or the development of new therapeutics, the treatment of patients or bedside practices. Medical knowledge also comprises a specific expertise or knowledge, such as how to keep the note-, case-, or account-books, how to keep records and organise knowledge about patients, how to finance and manage a medical practice, or how to manage a hospital – as Joris Vandendriessche shows in his Chapter 6 on the Leuven University Hospital.

The complexity of these questions is illustrated in Andrew Mendelsohn's Chapter 12 on mining brotherhoods in early modern German countries. In Mendelsohn's case history, the members of the brotherhood were obliged to deposit a certain amount of their income into a box. In case of occupational illness, invalidity, or death (due to their work), the miners or their families received financial aid or a pension drawn from the collected money. But what does 'occupational' mean? In dealing with a typical economic problem (i.e. the allocation and fair distribution of limited resources), questions arose about the afflictions of the miners who were applying for a pension. Was the disease or invalidity actually caused by their work? How, in this case, were the symptoms and their work correlated? How were they defined and classified and what compensation did the miners deserve? In general, examples like brotherhoods and mutual health insurances therefore point to the entangled dimensions of calculative practices and accounting. Questions of resource allocation needed clear definitions, distinctions, and classifications. Who was entitled to a claim? Who could be treated? Who was already sick and who still healthy? Which diseases were treated and which were not? Or to return to our example of the poor box, how were 'poor' or 'poor sick' defined and who had the jurisdiction and authority to apply the definitions? Finally, all three dimensions are condensed in Laura Stark's Chapter 10. She describes how two retired teachers, who worked as local accountants in their Mennonite church, decided to perform their regular voluntary service as witnesses to 'the teachings of Jesus' at the Clinical Center of the US

National Institutes of Health in Bethesda, where they served as 'normal control' research subjects and, as unit leaders, kept the local accounts. Stark analyses 'how they were accounting and being accounted for – by NIH budget offices, clinical researchers, the Mennonite church, and themselves'. The dimensions of accounting for health become clear not only in the broad use of the term 'accounting' or 'to account', but also in the use of similar terms such as 'benefit', which is used here in the sense of financial profit, therapeutic benefit and social (sickness) benefit.

These examples illustrate that accounting for health is characterised by different, albeit related and historically contingent, social and cultural practices and techniques. The production of numbers was, as Ian Hacking argues for population statistics, only a surface effect. 'Behind it lay new technologies for classifying and enumerating, and new bureaucracies with the authority and continuity to deploy the technology.'[69] Against this backdrop, we assert that calculative practices and considerations, as well as administrative techniques like bookkeeping and accounting, have been an essential part of medicine for centuries – linked not only to organisational and economic issues, but also used as an important research tool to address knowledge-generating interests and problems.

Calculative practices are not simply incidental to health care. In an essential way they shape health, medicine, and medical knowledge. This also applies to the present, as health care today seems caught between too much and not enough. On the one hand, there are swollen national health budgets, massive hospital and medical technology costs, big pharma, and an ever-growing market of medical products and services. On the other hand, lack of access to health care is a global problem, as is the political challenge of resource allocation, the ethical dilemmas of 'rationing', and the search for ways to reduce costs, to achieve a more equal distribution of care, and to improve the efficiency of the government's regulation of markets.

These challenges refer back to the historicity of accounting, economic, calculative, and administrative practices in medicine. Nowadays, physicians in the (Western) industrial world complain about the commodification of health, the economisation of medicine, and the administrative burdens that limit the growth of medical knowledge and its benefits and that prevent them from doing 'real' medicine, i.e. curing the sick. This seems to imply that once upon a time practising medicine was free of economic interests and unencumbered by accounting or administrative practices. But it has hardly been noticed in current debates that similar patterns and problems have existed in health and medicine for centuries – not only in the modern sense of accounting as economic efficiency, but especially in a more traditional sense of good medical practice. Moreover, the perceived patterns, problems, and solutions under discussion have all been enabled by various forms of accounting – both in the narrower sense of bookkeeping methods and in the broader sense of economic, political, and moral monitoring, calculating, and decision-making. These, in turn, appear to have shaped medical knowledge and practice in ways still poorly understood. By focusing on the links and entangled relationships between medicine and accounting – i.e. on the practices and values of economic and medical knowing and on the links between administrative techniques, calculative practices, and medical knowledge – this volume addresses the crucial question of how calculative practices and administrative techniques have influenced and generated medical knowledge and vice versa.

Our aim is not to show the different accounting practices in every chapter. Nor are the financial, moral, or epistemic dimensions of accounting balanced in every chapter. Some emphasise accounting's financial aspects, others the epistemic aspects of calculative practices, and still others the moral and social dimensions. An overview of all the chapters shows the broad variety and entanglement of calculative and managerial practices and technologies, the different settings in which accounting takes place, and the effects of accounting practices on and in relation to health, medicine, and medical knowledge. In summation, this volume shows how accounting practices were adjusted, adapted, and transformed over time, depending on certain social settings, aims and purposes, and that those practices have played a decisive role in medicine for over 500 years.

Acknowledgements

This volume and chapter emerged from a broader project on paper technologies entitled 'Ways of Writing: How Physicians Know 1550–1950', funded by the European Research Council. The chapters have been discussed at an international conference, funded by the Thyssen

Foundation and the Center for Interdisciplinary Research at Bielefeld University, and we would like to thank the Center and the Thyssen Foundation, and our commentators Lars Behrisch, Martin Gorsky, Anne Hardy, Heinrich Hartmann, Johannes Kassar, Martin Lengwiler, Harro Maas, Staffan Müller-Wille, Ruth Schilling, Jakob Tanner, Hendrik Vollmer, David Cantor, as well as two unknown peer reviewers for Manchester University Press. Additionally, we would like to thank Alexa Geisthövel, Alix Cooper, Jan Geisbüsch, and Eric J. Engstrom for their insightful comments at various stages in the development of this book.

Notes

1 *The Newcastle Literary Magazine and Northern Chronicle*, No. 1 (1824), p. 21.
2 In the Cambridge Advanced Learners Dictionary & Thesaurus, *Cambridge Dictionaries Online* 2013, accounting is defined as the 'skill of keeping records of the money a person or organization earns and spends'. In *Merriam-Webster* (Online-Dictionary 2013), accounting is defined as a 'system of recording and summarizing business and financial transactions and analysing, verifying, and reporting the results'.
3 See, for instance, the discussion about cure rates in insane asylums and the related 'accounts in health and in money' in T.M. Porter's Chapter 7 in this volume.
4 In general, these studies have criticised actual economic processes in which (good) medical practice has been compromised by economic constraints. By adopting this normative perspective and dealing almost entirely with current developments in public health as they relate to the rising costs of medicine, these studies have overlooked the ways in which medical and economic practices have been deeply intertwined for centuries.
5 See, for instance, the contributions in V. Berridge and K. Loughlin (eds), *Medicine, the Market and the Mass Media. Producing Health in the Twentieth Century* (London: Routledge, 2005); T. Ueyama, *Health in the Marketplace: Professionalism, Therapeutic Desires, and Medical Commodification in Late-Victorian London* (Palo Alto: Society for the Promotion of Science and Scholarship, 2010).
6 A. Mennicken and H. Vollmer, 'Einleitung: Fundstellen von Zahlenforschung', in A. Mennicken and H. Vollmer (eds), *Zahlenwerk. Kalkulation, Organisation und Gesellschaft* (Wiesbaden: Verlag für Sozialwissenschaft, 2007), pp. 9–17, especially p. 10.

7. H. Vollmer, 'Bookkeeping, accounting, calculative practice: The sociological suspense of calculation', *Critical Perspectives on Accounting* 3 (2003), 353–81.
8. U. Vormbusch, *Die Herrschaft der Zahlen. Zur Kalkulation des Sozialen in der kapitalistischen Moderne* (Frankfurt: Campus, 2012), p. 32; also A.A. Rusnock, *Vital Accounts. Quantifying Health and Population in Eighteenth-Century England and France* (Cambridge: Cambridge University Press, 2002).
9. For instance, Rusnock, *Vital Accounts* or the contributions in G. Jorland, A. Opinel, and G. Weisz (eds), *Body Counts. Medical Quantification in Historical and Sociological Perspective* (Montréal: McGill-Queen's University Press, 2005). A few very intriguing studies in the history of quantification deal with risk calculation and life insurance, but they focus on insurance, not medical practice; for instance, G. Clark, *Betting on Lives. The Culture of Life Insurance in England, 1695–1775* (Manchester: Manchester University Press, 1999).
10. See, for instance, G. Cheyne, *An Essay of Health and Long Life* (London: Printed for George Strahan, 1725).
11. P. Sarasin, *Reizbare Maschinen. Eine Geschichte des Körpers 1765–1914* (Frankfurt: Suhrkamp, 2001); and the contributions in P. Sarasin and J. Tanner (eds), *Physiologie und industrielle Gesellschaft. Studien zur Verwissenschaftlichung des Körpers im 19. und 20. Jahrhundert* (Frankfurt: Suhrkamp, 1998); and Jorland et al. (eds), *Body Counts*.
12. T.M. Porter, *Trust in Numbers. The Pursuit of Objectivity in Science and Public Life* (Princeton: Princeton University Press, 1995).
13. L. Behrisch, 'Political economy and statistics in the late Ancien Régime', in W. Steinmetz, I. Gilcher-Holtey, and H.-G. Haupt (eds), *Writing Political History Today* (Frankfurt: Campus, 2013), pp. 175–90, especially p. 175.
14. J. Gleeson-White, *Double Entry. How the Merchants of Venice Created Modern Finance* (London: W.W. Norton & Company, 2013); J. Soll, *The Reckoning. Financial Accountability and the Making and Breaking of Nations* (New York: Basic Books, 2014).
15. J.R. Edwards and S.P. Walker (eds), *The Routledge Companion to Accounting History* (London: Routledge, 2009).
16. See the contributions in Edwards and Walker, *Companion to Accounting History*; G.J. Previts (ed.), *A Global History of Accounting, Financial Reporting and Public Policy*, 3 vols. (Bingley: Emerald, 2010–11); Y. Levant and O. de la Villarmois (eds), *French Accounting History. New Contributions* (London: Routledge, 2012); T. Boyns and J.R. Edwards (eds), *A History of Management Accounting. The British Experience* (New York: Routledge, 2013).

17 R.E. Connor, *Woman, Accounting, and Narrative. Keeping Books in Eighteenth-Century England* (London: Routledge, 2004).
18 To name but a few of the groundbreaking studies: A.G. Hopwood, 'The archaeology of accounting systems', *Accounting, Organizations and Society* 12 (1987), 207–34; P. Miller, 'On the interrelation between accounting and the state', *Accounting, Organizations and Society* 15 (1990), 315–38; P. Miller and T. O'Leary, 'Accounting and the construction of the governable person', *Accounting, Organizations and Society* 12 (1987), 235–65; M. Power (ed.), *Accounting and Science. Natural Inquiry and Commercial Reason* (Cambridge: Cambridge University Press, 1994); M. Power, *The Audit Society. Rituals of Verification* (Oxford: Oxford University Press, 1999).
19 A.M. Preston, 'The birth of clinical accounting: A study of the emergence and transformations of discourses on costs and practices of accounting in U.S. hospitals', *Accounting, Organizations and Society* 17 (1992), 63–100; see also Miller, 'Interrelation between accounting and the state'.
20 Preston, 'Birth of clinical accounting', 63.
21 Vormbusch, *Herrschaft der Zahlen*, p. 17.
22 P. Miller, 'Kalkulierende Subjekte', in *Ökonomie der Subjektivität – Subjektivität der Ökonomie*, ed. by Arbeitsgruppe SubArO (Berlin: Edition Sigma, 2005), pp. 19–33.
23 What follows is only a very cursory account of the numerous studies that have been published. For a more complete review of the literature, see F. Gebreiter and W.J. Jackson, 'Fertile ground: The history of accounting in hospitals', *Accounting History Review* 25 (2015), 177–82; and N. Robson, 'A Contextual History of Accounting in UK Hospitals, 1880–1974' (Diss. Phil., Cardiff University, 2006), chap. 3.
24 See the contributions in M. Gorsky and Sally Sheard (eds), *Financing Medicine. The British Experience since 1750* (London: Routledge, 2006); A. Labisch and Reinhard Spree (eds), *Krankenhaus-Report 19. Jahrhundert. Krankenhausträger, Krankenhausfinanzierung, Krankenhauspatienten* (Frankfurt: Campus, 2001).
25 See the contributions in Labisch and Spree (eds), *Krankenhaus-Report*; U. Frevert, *Krankheit als politisches Problem 1770–1880. Soziale Unterschichten in Preußen zwischen medizinischer Polizei und staatlicher Sozialversicherung* (Göttingen: Vandenhoeck & Ruprecht, 1984); E. Brinkschulte, *Krankenhaus und Krankenkassen. Soziale und ökonomische Faktoren der Entstehung des modernen Krankenhauses im frühen 19. Jahrhundert. Die Beispiele Würzburg und Bamberg* (Husum: Matthiesen, 1998).
26 Compare M. Gorsky and S. Sheard, 'Introduction', in Gorsky and Sheard (eds), *Financing Medicine*, pp. 1–19, especially p. 2.

27 For the evolving contributory schemes in twentieth-century British hospitals, see M. Gorsky, J. Mohan, and T. Willis, *Mutualism and Health Care. British Hospital Contributory Schemes in the Twentieth Century* (Manchester: Manchester University Press, 2006); B. Doyle, *The Politics of Hospital Provision in Early Twentieth-Century Britain* (London: Pickering & Chatto, 2014); and G.C. Gosling, *Payment and Philanthropy in British Healthcare, 1918–48* (Manchester: Manchester University Press, 2017).
28 See N. Robson, 'From voluntary to state control and the emergence of the department in UK hospital accounting', *Accounting, Business and Financial History* 13 (2003), 99–123; N. Robson, *Contextual History of Accounting*; A. Holden, W. Funnell, and D. Oldroyed 'Accounting and the moral economy of illness in Victorian England, the Newcastle Infirmary', *Accounting, Auditing and Accountability Journal* 22 (2009), 525–52.
29 See Gebreiter and Jackson, 'Fertile ground', 177.
30 See Preston, 'Birth of clinical accounting'.
31 For France, see the dissertation of J.-P. Domin, 'Une histoire économique de l'hôpital (XIXe–XXe siècles): Une analyse rétrospective du développement hospitalier' (Paris: Assoc. pour l'Étude de l'Histoire de la Sécurité Sociale, 2008). For a comparison between France and British hospital accounting (and further literature), see also Barry Doyle's Chapter 5 in this volume.
32 Compare Labisch and Spree (eds), *Krankenhaus-Report*. On German health insurance, compare Frevert, *Krankheit als politisches Problem*; and on early forms of friendly societies in Würzburg and Bamberg see Brinkschulte, *Krankenhaus und Krankenkassen*.
33 See A. Berry, '"Balancing the books". Funding provincial hospitals in eighteenth-century England', *Accounting, Business & Financial History* 7 (1997), 1–30; Robson, 'From voluntary to state control'.
34 Compare P. Quattrone, 'Accounting for God: Accounting and accountability practices in the Society of Jesus (Italy XVI–XVII centuries)', *Accounting, Organizations and Society* 29 (2004), 647–83; P. Quattrone, 'Books to be practiced: Memory, the power of the visual and the success of accounting', *Accounting, Organizations and Society* 34 (2009), 85–118.
35 Compare Holden et al., 'Accounting and the moral economy'.
36 Compare E. Bracci, L. Maran, and E. Vagnoni, 'Saint Anna's Hospital in Ferrara, Italy: Accounting and organizational change during the devolution', *Accounting History* 15 (2010), 463–504.
37 For the gift economy, see M. Mauss, *Die Gabe. Form und Funktion des Austauschs in archaischen Gesellschaften* (Frankfurt: Suhrkamp, 1990 [FE 1923/1924]); A. Caillé, *Anthropologie der Gabe* (Frankfurt: Campus, 2008); F. Adloff and S. Mau (eds), *Vom Geben und Nehmen. Zur Soziologie*

der Reziprozität (Frankfurt: Campus, 2005); and especially the chapter on philanthropy by F. Adloff and S. Sigmund.
38 See Berry, 'Balancing the books'; and also on charitable funding Bronwyn Croxson and Jonathan Reinarz's chapter in Gorsky and Sheard (eds), *Financing Medicine*.
39 See Holden et al., 'Accounting and the moral economy'. On the concept of moral economy (beyond E.P. Thompson), see L. Daston, 'The moral economy of science', *Osiris* 10 (1995), 2–24.
40 See Quattrone, 'Accounting for God'; Quattrone, 'Books to be practiced'; and Bracci et al., 'Saint Anna's Hospital'.
41 J. Aho, *Confession and Bookkeeping. The Religious, Moral, and Rhetorical Roots of Modern Accounting* (Albany: State University of New York Press, 2005); D. Groh, *Göttliche Weltökonomie. Perspektiven der wissenschaftlichen Revolution vom 15. bis zum 17. Jahrhundert* (Berlin: Suhrkamp, 2010).
42 Aho, *Confession and Bookkeeping*, pp. XIII–XIV. Hanseatic and Italian merchants often created an extra account for God as a co-owner or joint owner of the company. The money booked to this account – as a share of profits – was donated to the church or to charity. In this sense, double-entry bookkeeping meant that for every gift received (as profit) a portion had to be given to the community. However, this double-entry bookkeeping was driven by the ulterior motive of ensuring success by making God a co-owner of the enterprise.
43 B. Pohl-Resl, *Rechnen mit der Ewigkeit. Das Wiener Bürgerspital im Mittelalter* (Munich: Oldenbourg, 1996); M.T. Sneider, 'The treasury of the poor: Hospital finance in sixteenth- and seventeenth-century Bologna', in J. Henderson, P. Horden, and A. Pastore (eds), *The Impact of Hospitals 300–2000* (Frankfurt: Peter Lang, 2007), pp. 93–116; M. Garbellotti, 'Assets of the poor, assets of the city: The management of hospital resources in Verona between the sixteenth and eighteenth centuries', in Henderson et al. (eds), *Impact of Hospitals*, pp. 117–34; F. Dross, 'Their daily bread: Managing hospital finances in early modern Germany', in L. Abreu and S. Sheard (eds), *Hospital Life. Theory and Practice from the Medieval to the Modern* (Frankfurt: Peter Lang, 2013), pp. 49–66.
44 As shown in the case of the account books of the Datini-di Berto trading company by F.-J. Arlinghaus, *Zwischen Notiz und Bilanz. Zur Eigendynamik des Schriftgebrauchs in der kaufmännischen Buchführung am Beispiel der Datini/di Berto-Handelsgesellschaft in Avignon (1367–1373)* (Frankfurt: Peter Lang, 2000).
45 B. Kafka, 'Paperwork. The state of the discipline', *Book History* 12 (2009), 340–53.

46 C. Vismann, *Files. Law and Media Technology* (Stanford: Stanford University Press, 2008); A. te Heesen, 'Accounting for the natural world. Double-entry bookkeeping in the field', in L. Schiebinger and C. Swan (eds), *Colonial Botany. Science, Commerce and Politics in the Early Modern World* (Philadelphia: University of Pennsylvania Press, 2005), pp. 237–51; A. te Heesen, 'The notebook: A paper-technology', in B. Latour and P. Weibel (eds), *Making Things Public. Atmospheres of Democracy* (Cambridge: MIT Press, 2005), pp. 582–9; V. Hess and J.A. Mendelsohn, 'Paper technology und Wissensgeschichte', *NTM. Zeitschrift für Geschichte der Wissenschaften, Technik und Medizin* 21 (2013), 1–10; and L. Gitelman, *Paper Knowledge. Toward a Media History of Documents* (Durham, NC: Duke University Press, 2014).
47 Edwards and Walker (eds), *Companion to Accounting History*.
48 M. Power and R. Laughlin, 'Critical theory and accounting', in M. Alvesson and H. Willmott (eds), *Critical Management Studies* (London: Sage, 1992), pp. 113–35; Aho, *Confession and Bookkeeping*, Preface.
49 Vollmer, 'Bookkeeping, accounting, calculative practice'.
50 Vormbusch, *Herrschaft der Zahlen*.
51 Compare M. Power, 'Counting, control and calculation: Reflections on measuring and measurement', *Human Relations* 57 (2004), 765–83.
52 See the classic study of V.A. Zelizer, *Pricing the Priceless Child. The Changing Social Value of Children* (Princeton: Princeton University Press, 1985).
53 'Report of the Committee on Terminology, Midyear 1940', *Accounting Research Bulletin* No. 7/November 1940, 51–61, quotations at 55.
54 It is only recently that a number of publications have 'recovered' the hidden social meanings of accounting, see Quattrone, 'Accounting for God'; Quattrone, 'Books to be practiced'; Aho, *Confession and Bookkeeping*; Soll, *Reckoning*.
55 B. Latour, *We Have Never Been Modern* (Cambridge, MA: Harvard University Press, 1993).
56 Porter, *Trust in Numbers*.
57 For an expanded meaning of accountability, see for instance the contributions in R. Munro and J. Mouritsen (eds), *Accountability. Power, Ethos and the Technologies of Managing* (London: Thompson Business Press, 1996).
58 In a broader sense, the *Oxford English Dictionary* defines accounting as 'giving a satisfactory explanation' or serving as 'justification for conduct'. This definition also includes 'giving an account of [something]' or 'being accountable for', see s.v. 'accounting' in the OED, Online-Version.
59 This approach is exemplified in A. te Heesen's 'Accounting for the natural world' in which she describes the dual bookkeeping used by the natural

scientist Daniel Gottlieb Messerschmidt during his expedition in Siberia in the early eighteenth century.
60 K. Knorr Cetina, 'Culture in global knowledge societies. Knowledge cultures and epistemic cultures', *Interdisciplinary Science Reviews* 32 (2007), 361–75.
61 H. Blumenberg, *Die Legitimität der Neuzeit* (Frankfurt: Suhrkamp, 1966), p. 344.
62 Vismann, *Files*, p. 209.
63 H. Willmott, 'Thinking accountability: accounting for the disciplined production of self', in Munro and Mouritsen (eds), *Accountability*, pp. 23–39.
64 J. Delbourgo and S. Müller-Wille, 'Introduction', *ISIS* 103 (2012), 710–15.
65 Te Heesen, 'Accounting for the natural world'.
66 See Berry, 'Balancing the books'; Doyle, *Politics of Hospital Provision*; Gosling, *Payment and Philanthropy*; and Barry Doyle's Chapter 5 in this volume.
67 For the give and take within gift economies, which are especially important in transplantation medicine and medical philanthropy, see Mauss, *Gabe*; Caillé, *Anthropologie der Gabe*; and the contributions in Adloff and Mau (eds), *Vom Geben und Nehmen*. For the multiple 'meanings of payment' in modern health care and philanthropy in interwar Britain, see Gosling, *Payment and Philanthropy*, pp. 157–94.
68 Several studies describe accounting practices in religious organisations (especially early modern hospitals) that relied mainly on donations (or on interest and rents from donated capital or land); see, for instance, S. Moggi, V. Filippi, C. Leardini, and G. Rossi, 'Accountability for a place in heaven. A stakeholders' portrait in Verona's confraternities', *Accounting History* 21 (2016), 236–62. On donors' motives, see Pohl-Resl, *Rechnen mit der Ewigkeit*.
69 I. Hacking, *The Taming of Chance* (Cambridge: Cambridge University Press, 1990), pp. 2–3.

Part I
Keeping the books

1
Accounting, religion, and the economics of medical care in sixteenth-century Germany: Hiob Finzel's *Rationarium praxeos medicae*, 1565–89

Michael Stolberg

In the sixteenth century, with growing numbers of *doctores medicinae* graduating from the universities, learned physicians became major representatives of a new group of urban professionals whose economic fortunes rested almost entirely on their academic training and the skills they had acquired. Their prosperity and indeed their livelihood depended on their success as practitioners – all the more so, since many of them set up their 'business' in places to which they had come as strangers, attracted by a salary as town physicians. Yet we know very little, at this point, about the economic aspects of learned medical practice in sixteenth-century Europe and even less about how physicians dealt with them. How did physicians fare financially? How high were their fees and how did they vary according to the patient's economic and social status? To what degree did their income depend on what they received from a small elite of upper-class patients? How important, compared to the payments they received from their patients, were their salaries as town physicians or personal physicians to individual families or institutions such as monasteries? Last but not least, what do we know about their accounting practices? How did they make sure that they received what was due to them?

A major reason for our ignorance in these matters is a lack of adequate sources. Physicians' letters, contracts, and occasional autobiographical writings offer only fragmentary evidence on such matters.[1] In this chapter, I will approach the questions outlined above through a detailed analysis of the only extensive practice journal and account book that is known to have survived from the hands of a learned medical doctor in the sixteenth century and that medical historians (as well as the various biographers of its author) have ignored. From 1565 until shortly before his death in 1589, Hiob Finzel (c. 1526–89), a physician in Weimar, Eisenach, and finally in Zwickau, recorded more than 10,000 consultations in three heavy folio volumes.[2] They contain a wealth of information about not only the diagnostic and therapeutic practices of a learned physician, but also his patients and his interactions with them.[3] As the title under which it has come down to us, *Rationarium praxeos medicae*, correctly indicates, bookkeeping was a major reason for Finzel maintaining this journal. At the time, *Rationes* was a familiar term for 'accounts' and 'rationarium' must be translated as 'account book' here.[4]

In what follows, I will provide a brief sketch of Finzel's biography, and describe my source and the way in which Finzel recorded the payments he received. In the following section, I will highlight the striking religious elements and connotations of his *Rationarium* and will place them into the context of his strong Protestant faith. My chapter will conclude with an analysis of the economics of Finzel's practice and of the relative importance of the payments he received from patients of different social and economic status.

Hiob Finzel

Hiob Finzel, or Iobus Fincelius as he latinised his name, was born around 1526 in Weimar, where his father Conrad acquired citizenship in 1525.[5] Little is known about his family background. According to an *epicedion* for his sister Anna, she excelled in weaving fabrics and eventually lived at the court of Anna of Saxony. This might indicate that the family was in the cloth-making business, but more likely must be read to mean in general terms that she – and Hiob – came from a well-to-do family (that could also pay for Hiob's studies).[6] He studied at the liberal arts faculty in Wittenberg[7] and after his graduation, in 1549, we find him lecturing on natural history in the *Gymnasium academicum* in Jena, where he eventually served as a professor when the *Gymnasium* became a university in 1558.⁸ Finzel initially sought to establish himself as a humanist scholar and poet. He translated the elegies of the Greek poet Tyrtaios and published various poems of his own. From 1556 to 1562, the first edition of his famous *Wunderzeichen* was published,⁹ a collection of stories of miracles and portents, which Finzel, a devout Protestant, presented as divine warnings that humankind must change its ways.¹⁰ This is the work for which Hiob Finzel is well known among historians of German literature and popular culture; it includes stories like that of the pied piper of Hameln that have remained famous to this day.¹¹

But by the time the last volume of the *Wunderzeichen* appeared, Finzel had already turned to medicine. In December 1562, he received his medical doctorate in Jena. In the spring of 1564, he accepted the position of a town physician in Weimar for three years, with an annual salary of 100 *gulden* (fl) and a *malter* of grain.¹² In addition to that, he was appointed, in December 1566, as personal physician to the Saxon duke Johann Friedrich, 'from home', i.e. without the obligation to reside permanently at court, with an annual salary of 50 fl and another *malter* of grain.¹³ Finzel's professional future seemed secured. But Finzel became involved in the controversy between Duke Johann Friedrich and the Saxon Elector Johann Wilhelm. He was imprisoned for several weeks and his contract was not renewed. He was without a salaried position for two years, until May 1569, when he started working as a resident physician at the court in Eisenach.¹⁴ Finally, in 1571, he was appointed as town physician in Zwickau, with a salary of 60 fl and two piles of firewood per year (worth another 6 fl). In return, he promised to serve the town and its citizens in health matters, to perform an annual visitation of the local pharmacies, and to advise patients in the hospitals and sick-houses out of 'Christian charity', i.e. presumably for free.¹⁵ He was not allowed to leave the town over night without the mayor's permission.

Zwickau was a fairly prosperous town with a strong tradition in cloth production and some sizeable mining activities in the area. At least for much of the time there was a second town physician, but competition from other learned physicians seems to have been limited.¹⁶ Finzel was to remain in Zwickau until his death, in 1589.¹⁷ He had found his place, professionally, economically, and as a *pater familias* with a growing family.

Finzel's *Rationarium praxeos medicae*

Finzel's *Rationarium praxeos medicae* comprises some 1,500 pages in three heavy folio volumes. The entries start in April 1565 when he was still a town physician in Weimar, and they end in the spring of 1589, shortly before his death. Finzel's did not use an *album*, i.e. a book with empty pages, but wrote on little fascicles or individual sheets of paper instead. They were almost certainly bound into three volumes only after his death. There are no empty pages at the end, the three volumes have an almost identical binding taken from a dissolved liturgical manuscript, and some of the records for the last years are bound in the wrong order.

The entries are all in Finzel's distinctive hand. During the first couple of years, they are dated only sporadically. From 1572, Finzel marked the beginning of every new month. As a rule, each entry seems to have corresponded to a single consultation. Even when patients consulted him only a couple of days later, Finzel made a new entry, and occasionally two entries in succession for the same patient with headings like 'idem' or 'derselbe', i.e. 'the same patient'. The length of the various entries and the amount of information Finzel recorded vary considerably (see Figure 1.1). A complete entry comprises: first, the name of the patient viz., in the case of wives, children or servants, usually that of the husband, father or employer; second, the breadwinner's profession or, in the case of noble patients, the title; third, the place of residence; fourth, the diagnosis; fifth, the medicines Finzel prescribed; and sixth, the payment he received.

As Axel Hüntelmann and Oliver Falk have outlined in their Introduction, the contributors to this volume were invited to understand 'accounting' in a broad sense, as referring not only to money and goods but also to other objects and phenomena, including countable physiological and pathological parameters. Recording the diagnosis and his prescriptions in a journal allowed the physician to quickly retrieve the necessary information when a patient returned. But, in principle, it could also serve as an important tool to assess the efficacy of his treatment and as a means to arrive, by analogy, at conclusions on how to treat other patients with similar diagnoses or similar symptoms. However, the majority of entries in Finzel's journal do not provide any information about the patient's symptoms and on the effects of Finzel's

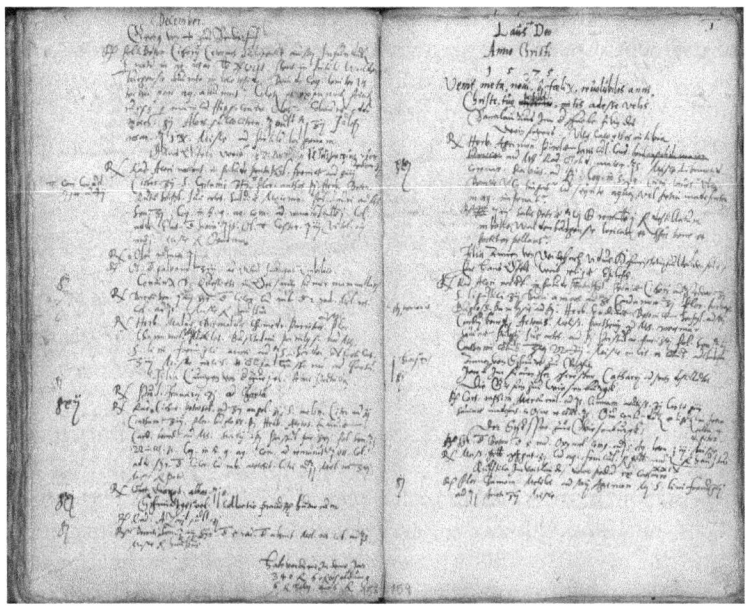

1.1 Double page from Hiob Finzel's *Rationarium*.

treatment. In most cases, the more strictly medical information is limited to a diagnostic term and/or Finzel's prescription – and even this information is often missing. In marked contrast, for example, to the extensive notes of his contemporary, the Bohemian physician Georg Handsch,[18] Finzel clearly did not use his *Rationarium* as a tool for the systematic creation of new medical knowledge nor as means to improve his therapeutic outcomes.

Instead, the primary purpose of Finzel's *Rationarium* was financial accounting. He calculated his annual earnings at the end of most years. In addition, we frequently find figures after a certain number of pages, where Finzel added up his earnings since January of that year. Finzel went to some lengths in order to arrive at precise annual figures. If necessary, he converted the value of the payments for individual consultations – many were in *taler* and *groschen* (gr) – into *gulden* (fl) and *kreuzer*. Likewise, he calculated the value in *gulden* and *kreuzer* of the animals, foodstuffs, or other objects that he sometimes received instead of or in addition to monetary payments.

In order to arrive at precise figures, Finzel very consistently entered the payments he received for individual consultations – and frequently this is all we find, in fact, apart from the name or some other identifying information, like 'baker from Schneeberge'.[19] At first glance, there are some gaps: in about 20 to 25 per cent of entries for individual consultations, information on payment is missing. Many of these consultations were by patients from the upper classes, however, who sought Finzel's advice repeatedly. Here we tend to find more occasional entries, citing relatively large amounts of money, presumably lump payments for several consultations with the patient and possibly also with other members of his or her family. In exceptional cases, Finzel even recorded a 'salary' he received at regular intervals. Wolf von Weisbach, for example, gave him 7 *taler* as a 'half-year salary'[20] and from Jörg Albrecht von Witzleben he got 30 fl, i.e. about 23 *taler* per year.[21] Heinrich von Enda, a captain in Glauchau who frequently consulted him for his *podagra*, paid him 10 *taler* for half a year.[22] There are only a few entries for consultations with artisans and country folks, with no information about the payment. These patients likely received free treatment – perhaps in return for some favor or work they did for Finzel – or they quite simply never paid.

According to his own calculations, over the course of sixteen years from 1573 to 1588, Finzel earned a total of 6,960 fl or, on average, 435 fl per year, including his salary of 60 fl and some rare gratifications (see Figure 1.2).[23] In Eisenach, he had made 262 fl viz. 258 fl per year (including his salary of 100 fl).[24] By way of comparison, the annual salary that the famous botanist and humanist physician Leonhard Fuchs received as a professor in Tübingen amounted to 200 fl and some additional benefits, and when Fuchs envisaged the prestigious position of a royal physician to Christian III of Denmark, he hoped to receive 700 to 800 fl per year.[25]

Finzel's earnings put the importance of his salary as a town physician into perspective. His salary was quite typical for a town physician at the

73	74	75	76	77	78	79	80	81	82	83	84	85	86	87	88
403	406	501	477	504	506	566	481	481	363	363	413	469	415	319	293

1.2 Finzel's annual income 1573–88 in *gulden*.

time. Many of his colleagues in other places were paid between 50 to 100 fl per year for their services.[26] Clearly, we must not mistake these salaries for the physician's income. Finzel's figures show that, during his Zwickau years, his salary as a town physician constituted only about 10 to 15 per cent of his total earnings.

The religious context of Finzel's *Rationarium*

In the light of the paramount role of economic considerations in health care today, it may not seem surprising to the modern reader that a sixteenth-century town physician, whose livelihood largely depended on the fees he received from his patients, would seek to keep track of them the way Finzel did. But upon closer analysis, things are not quite so straightforward.

To start with, Finzel was remarkably sloppy. Recording the payments he had received in the margins, next to the entries for the corresponding consultation, would have allowed him to identify the patients who had already paid and to track those who had not. This is what we find in the (later) practice journals of other medical practitioners, some of whom carefully crossed out entries for patients, apparently because they had paid their fees, or marked in other ways, like 'he has paid', that they had received a payment.[27] Finzel, by contrast, often simply entered the figures somewhere near the consultation in question. As a result, when brief entries for consultations with several different patients follow in direct succession, some recording no payment, it is frequently not clear to which patient the figures in the margins refer.

Finzel may have relied on his memory when it came to linking payments and patients correctly. However, a major rationale for keeping notebooks or account books was that they served as 'forgetting machines'.[28] They freed the writer from having to remember such details. And it would hardly have taken Finzel much additional time if he had bothered to write the sums he received exactly next to the name of the corresponding patient. This strongly suggests that the primary reason for entering the fees was not that he wanted to be able to identify patients who still owed him money. His rationale was a different one: he needed these figures above all in order to keep track of his annual earnings. Which leads us to a more general question: why would someone like Finzel want to keep an account book in the first place?

In modern English usage, 'accounting' has two quite distinct meanings. It can refer to keeping track of income or earnings and expenses. But 'accounting' can also be used in the sense of 'to account for something': describing and justifying what had been done, with goods and money in particular, or explaining and indeed legitimising certain actions or events. In this sense, the financial accounts that we find in the annual reports of companies today also serve to 'account' for the way in which those who are 'accountable', namely management, are running the company in question. As the 'new' history of accounting has shown, the two meanings were historically much more closely linked than today, and – more surprisingly for the modern reader – both were in turn closely intertwined with religious ideas about the Judgement Day.[29]

The purpose of bookkeeping, according to Grahame Thompson's historical analysis, 'was largely rhetorical – that is, to justify an activity about which there existed in medieval Christian Europe a considerable suspicion, namely commerce itself'.[30] James Aho, who originally developed this argument in the 1980s,[31] has laid out these connections in greater detail in his book on *Confession and Bookkeeping*.[32] The very historical roots of double-entry bookkeeping and its rapid dissemination in the late Middle Ages, Aho argues, are to be found in the desire and need of Northern Italian merchants to 'account' for their profits in a moral, religious, and financial sense. In his words, double-entry bookkeeping 'arose from a sense of indebtedness on the part of late medieval merchants toward creator, church, and commune'. In a culture which condemned usury and ranked avarice among the deadly sins, and in which even the mere pursuit of profit for its own sake was, at best, morally ambiguous, the merchants, according to Aho, 'felt compelled to certify in writing that for everything they earned something of equal value had been returned, and that for everything meted out something else was deserved.'[33] In certain respects, the ledgers in which the merchants carefully synthesised the data and figures on individual transactions from their more casual journals thus resembled the 'little books', the diaries which some medieval sinners kept as a tool of self-reflection and as a basis for confession: 'As the personal account of their spiritual development was to the medieval poet and mystic, the financial account was to their more worldly counterparts, the urban merchant and the rural estate manager.'[34] Indeed, in many ways accounting was a kind of confession, and medieval confessionals, in turn, likened the (oral) confession, which became the rule in 1215, to the manorial account that the steward of a rural estate read to the bailiff.

The religious connotations of pre-modern accounting found their most concrete expression in the prominent role of religious tropes and symbols that can be found in account books. Guides to accounting declared it as imperative to invoke first and foremost God. 'And here is specially above all things to be noted,' Hugh Oldcastle advised the readers of his *A briefe instruction and maner how to keep bookes of accompts*, for example, 'that you take God always before your eyes, daily remembering first of all to serve him, knowing that your prayers unto almightie God, never letteth your labour nor journey, etc.' Therefore 'upon the first cleane leafe of paper on the right hande of this book, as also upon that first cleane leafe of the Inventorie, and Journall ought to be written first. In the name of God, Amen. With the date of our lord, the day of the monethes, and the title of every booke, declaring the name and effect thereof.'[35] In the same sense, Luca Pacioli in his *Tractatus de computis et scripturis* (first published in 1494), the most successful and influential of these guidebooks, had already admonished his readers that business must always be conducted in the 'sweet name of Jesus' and recommended that the merchant start every ledger writing 'In the name of God' or at least sign the pages with a cross.[36] This is precisely what we find not only in the sample pages offered by such guidebooks but also in surviving copies of merchant ledgers.[37]

How can these findings help us make better sense of Finzel's *Rationarium*? At first glance, the world of merchants may seem far removed from that of the learned physician. Upon closer analysis, however, physicians faced a moral dilemma that was at least as serious as that of profiting from trading goods: they made their living from other people's suffering. They earned their livelihood – and sometimes acquired quite considerable affluence – by doing something that was, from a Christian perspective, a charitable obligation. Jesus himself had set the example: it was the duty of any pious Christian to help the sick and needy. Indeed, as Michael Boudewijns discussed in his *Ventilabrum medico-theologicum*, physicians might even be accused of simony: after all, it was God who ultimately cured the patients, but the physicians took the money.[38]

Seen from this perspective, early modern physicians had at least as much reason to worry about the moral ambiguities of their work and their earnings as the merchants. What could be more reprehensible than making profit from the pain and sufferings of other people? What were physicians actually praying for, when they recited the Lord's Prayer and asked for their 'daily bread', if not for people to get sick?[39]

Medical writers struggled with this dilemma. They frequently pointed to passages in the Bible and *Jesus Sirach (Ecclesiastes)* in particular, which demanded that the physician be honoured, because God had given medicine and the physician to humankind.[40] Moreover, they sought to distance physicians from artisans and merchants who offered services or goods for a payment that was equivalent in value. The physician, as Roderigo da Castro and other writers on the duties and rights of the physician underscored, did not receive a certain, fixed payment (*'praemium certum'*). He only took what patients paid him as a token of their gratitude,[41] a *'honorarium'*, as Michael Boudewijns and Friedrich Hoffmann later explained, not a *'servile sostrum'*.[42] The physicians deserved it too: according to Roderigo da Castro, physicians could rightly call those patients sordid, avaricious, and indeed godless (*'scelestos'*) who did not reward the physician who had cured them.[43]

A certain unease remains palpable, however. The physician's intentions must not be directed toward money, Gabriele da Zerbi warned his readers, quoting the Persian physician Haly Abbas. He should expect his rewards from God.[44] The physician should accept without shame or regret what he was given, Hoffmann advised his readers, but he should not barter.[45] The good physician had to be very careful, da Castro admonished his readers, not to show that he coveted his patients' possessions, some piece of clothing, books, a horse, or household items, let alone attempt to purchase them. Patients might see this as a request or indeed as an attempt to extort things from them.[46] Even da Castro conceded that some physicians might be suspected of avarice, adding that 'most of the physicians' – interestingly he did not claim that this was true for all of them – who were perceived as greedy, worked to re-establish their patients' health, sometimes even at their own expense.[47]

In the light of the religious connotations of premodern accounting in general and of the moral dilemma of physicians profiting from other people's suffering, some striking elements in Finzel's *Rationarium* acquire a more precise meaning (see Figure 1.3). At times, it almost seems as if he had read what accounting guides advised merchants to do – or as if he were familiar with these elements thanks to his own

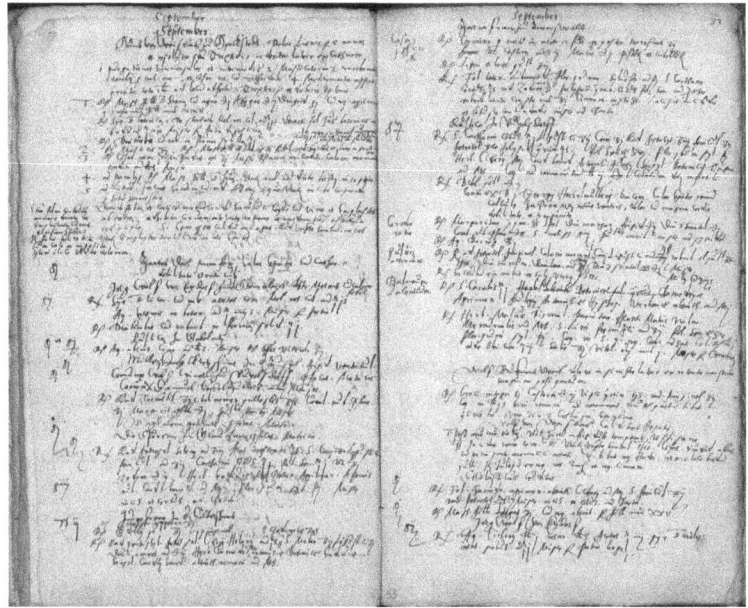

1.3 Double page from Hiob Finzel's *Rationarium*.

family background; unfortunately, as we have seen, his father's profession is not known.

Just as Pacioli and others recommended, Finzel placed a little cross on the top of most pages of his journal that marked the beginning of a new year – and only on these pages. It was often small and inconspicuous, more like a modern 'plus' sign but, considering the routine use of the cross in merchants' account books and its exclusive use, by Finzel, on the first page devoted to a new year, we must undoubtedly understand it as a Christian symbol. In some years, the cross is followed, again as the guides to accounting would have it, by a 'Year of the Lord', an '*Annus Christi*'. In other years, Finzel only wrote '*Annus* 1576' or just the year itself, in Arabic numbers, as a heading. Frequently he added a '*Laus Deo*' ('Praise to the Lord'), however, and most strikingly, he usually marked the end of a year and the beginning of a new one with a pious poem or even two. The wording was rarely the same but many of these poetic prayers referred in some way to the progress or rather the yearly cycle of time[48] and asked God or Jesus for an auspicious new year.[49]

Frequently, he was even more specific. He prayed for a good year for his family and himself, for a 'happy marriage' (*'coniugium foelix'*) and especially in his later years for bread (*'furni fructus'*), for a good life (*'commoda vitae'*; *'commoda multa'*), or indeed for a prosperous year (*'Illa sit ut nobis prospera. Christe iuva'*).

Just as the conventions of bookkeeping would have it, Finzel thus gave his accounting – and his lucrative practice with it – a religious note and situated it within the Christian cosmos.[50] Yet there are elements that point beyond the Catholic tradition, as represented by the Franciscan Pacioli's influential guidebook, and which make Finzel's *Rationarium* a more specifically Protestant undertaking. Not only do we sometimes find him raving against the Pope and the (Catholic) kings of France and Spain as 'servants of the Devil'.[51] Finzel's entries also make his practice and his earnings appear in a different, distinctly positive light. He not only explicitly asked God for a 'happy' and indeed a 'prosperous' year. He also praised God for his financial success[52] and even in the middle of a year, amid entries for patients and payments, we find him thanking God.[53] The rhetoric, the message could hardly be clearer. He owed his earnings to God. His income did not indicate potential sinfulness but God's benevolence. His practice was pleasing to God and his success showed that God was with him.

Only a general comparison of Catholic and Protestant accounting practices – and of the place of religious elements in them – would permit more wide-ranging conclusions at this point. Certainly, the religious elements in Finzel's account book would seem to illustrate Max Weber's famous claim, however, that the Protestant faith dignified work and helped turn affluence into a sign of divine benevolence and indeed salvation.[54] Finzel was inevitably sinful, like any human being, but his earnings, his *Rationarium* suggests, were nothing to be ashamed of and by no means sinful. Quite to the contrary, they showed that he was one of the 'pious' who could hope for God's protection.[55] Two poetic prayers, both of which mark tellingly not the beginning but the end of a financially quite successful year, are particularly explicit in this respect because they link the ideas of general sinfulness and gratitude. Having calculated his earnings in 1579, which added up to the considerable sum of 566 fl and 2 gr, Finzel appended a poem. Under the heading '*In novum annum* 1580', he appealed to Christ, the Saviour, who washes 'our crimes' away with his blood (*'Christe salus hominum, patris omnipotentis imago/Crimina confuso nostra cruore luis*'), but he also thanked Christ with all his heart.[56] Similarly, after his entry for the last consultation in 1585, Finzel wrote in German: 'In this year 1585, I have earned 403 fl. 19 g. Town council 66 fl. Summa 469 fol. 19g.'. And right underneath he added a poetic prayer in Latin: 'Praise and glory be to God in all eternity/Who is the triune and the one/truthful, just and merciful God/who forgives our crimes/and gives us new life.'[57] Finzel's *Rationarium*, we can conclude from all this, was not simply a bookkeeping device. It was also to a considerable extent a means of communing with God, of justifying his earnings, and, indeed, of giving them religious meaning.

Serving the rich and the poor

We might be tempted to consider all this to be mere rhetoric, as a lame excuse for making a good living from the suffering of other people. But Finzel's *Rationarium* holds a further surprise in store: Finzel came remarkably close to the idea of the charitable Christian physician. It has often been assumed that learned physicians in the early modern period treated only, or at least primarily, a small minority of upper-class patients who sought their advice and could afford to pay for it. But Finzel's journal conveys a very different picture. In the years from 1573 until 1588 he recorded 8,096 consultations. Since we find on average only about 1.3 consultations per patient – he saw many patients only once – this amounts to more than 6,000 different patients.[58] Now, Zwickau was a medium sized town with less than 10,000 inhabitants.[59] Even though Finzel also treated many patients from nearby communities of unknown size, the sheer number of different patients indicates that at one time or another a substantial portion of the population – and not only the rich – asked Finzel for advice and paid him for his services. This conclusion is corroborated by the many entries that include references to patients' status or profession or, in the case of women and children, to that of the male breadwinner. About 8 per cent came from noble families, but more than 92 per cent did not. For about 2,000 of these remaining patients, Finzel recorded the profession of the patient (viz. that of the husband, father or, more rarely, employer) or other indicators of social status and economic background. Among them, we find mayors, town councillors, and administrative officials as well as members of the literate elite, like teachers and pastors. However, we also find hundreds of millers, butchers, tailors, shoemakers, blacksmiths, and other craftsmen, in addition to 683 patients who were simply recorded as 'country folk' (*'rusticus'*, *'rustica'*).

Finzel's contract as a town physician did not stipulate the free treatment of patients, except for those patients for whom the town would have had to pay.[60] There can be no doubt then: people from many or indeed all walks of life sought Finzel's advice and could afford his services. Finzel's detailed figures on the payments he received make clear that this was indeed the case. For many patients he noted 'g 1', i.e. 1 gr, and the large majority did not pay more than 3 gr for a consultation (see Figures 1.1 and 1.3).[61] Prices and monetary values are notoriously difficult to compare over time, but Finzel's own assessment of the monetary value of different edibles that patients gave him, as well as other contemporary sources, can help us gauge their worth. According to Finzel's calculations, a hare was the equivalent of 7 to 8 gr, and that of a big cheese 9 gr. According to other contemporary sources, around 1560 in the area around Hamburg and Lübeck, a chicken cost 1 gr, 10 eggs a bit less than that, and a pound of butter 1.5 gr. In 1580 in Mecklenburg, one chicken was 1.5 gr, a goose cost a bit more than 3 gr; a journeyman in carpentry got 4 gr. a day, a thresher 1.5 gr and food.[62] Certainly, prices and salaries in Zwickau may have been slightly different and for small farmers and simple craftsmen the physician's fee (plus the cost of the remedies Finzel prescribed) may well have been a major consideration when it came to deciding whether they should consult a learned physician or rather resort to the less expensive services of a barber-surgeon or an unlicensed healer. But Finzel's fees were far from prohibitive.

Patients who could afford to do so frequently paid much more than just a few *groschen*. For dozens of patients, Finzel recorded between one and five *gulden* or *taler* as payment – the *gulden* being worth slightly less than the *taler*[63] – i.e. between about 20 and 100 gr. Such patients might also reward the medical treatment of their maidens and servants with similar generosity.[64] Exceptionally, particularly high-ranking patients paid even more.[65] Katharina, the wife of the Margrave of Brandenburg, gave Finzel 20 fl and Anna von Zedwitz paid him 30 *taler* and only a few weeks later another 12 fl.[66]

As these huge differences suggest, the payments Finzel received from his patients must not be taken to reflect a standard 'price' of his services.

Nor is there evidence suggesting that Finzel either demanded these amounts or indeed billed his patients accordingly. Rather, Finzel's more affluent patients seem to have taken it for granted that they were to pay much more than an ordinary farmer or artisan. Presumably, it would have offended their own sense of honour and social prestige if they had not rewarded his efforts in a way that reflected their financial and social status. Another striking feature in Finzel's journal points in the same direction. As mentioned above, Finzel quite frequently also recorded various non-monetary 'payments', usually edibles of some kind: cheese, butter, hares, geese, a lamb, different kinds of birds, the leg of a deer, boar's meat, fish, or, more rarely, a certain quantity of grain, beer, or wine. One might assume that the practice of rewarding physicians with goods rather than money was an archaic one and could be found primarily among ordinary people and in particular among farmers. Just the opposite is true, however: we find such non-monetary rewards virtually without exception only among the upper classes. As mentioned above, Finzel, when he calculated his annual earnings, frequently also added the monetary value in *groschen*. From his high-ranking patients' point of view, however, these were probably gifts rather than fees and a way of underscoring their own social status. It is hardly a coincidence that wild animals were particularly common non-monetary rewards. Hunting – and certainly hunting larger animals like deer and boars – was usually the privilege of the nobility. In turn, the 'big cheeses' sometimes given to Finzel – with a value of up to 16 gr – may well have been what noble families received from farmers over whom they ruled and thus again signalled their dominant social status.

Due to the variety of coins that Finzel recorded and their (possibly changing) relative value in Zwickau at the time, it is impossible to arrive at exact figures on the relative importance of different groups of patients for his income. But a rough and cursory study of individual sample years is instructive. In 1573, income from his practice (excluding his salary) amounted to roughly 337 fl. Some 220 fl (about 65 per cent) came from the 7.5 per cent of consultations (60 out of 794) for which he received at least 1 fl. In other words, the bulk of his consultations (92.5 per cent) – and presumably his workload – were with patients of more modest financial means. These consultations earned him only half of what he received for the far smaller number of consultations with the more affluent minority of his patients. Over the years, his practices seem to have focused even more on this minority. By 1586, 55 of 245, or some 22 per cent of all consultations were with patients who paid at least 1 fl. And their payments accounted for 307 or almost 90 per cent of the 349 fl he made from his practice in that year. Moreover, many more patients than in 1573 paid between 10 and 20 gr. Nevertheless, throughout his time in Zwickau, he never stopped treating patients for only one or two *groschen*.

Conclusion

Finzel's *Rationarium* offers unique insights into the practice and economics of an 'ordinary' sixteenth-century town physician. As a closer look at the way in which Finzel recorded his earning and 'commented' on them has made clear, however, our modern understanding of bookkeeping does not do justice to the multi-layered meaning of his *Rationarium*. This was far more than just a practical device, a paper tool that helped Finzel run his practice. Indeed, Finzel did not even use it for what would seem to be its most obvious purpose today, namely tracking outstanding payments. Finzel's *Rationarium*, as I have tried to show in this chapter, was part of his communion with God. The religious elements and the pious poems he entered at the turn of every year, frequently right next to his calculation of annual earnings, were not a mere decorative veneer. They point to the very core of this undertaking. Finzel's *Rationarium* documents the profound belief of a devout sixteenth-century Protestant physician that he was quite literally accountable to God for his practice and, above all, for the annual profits he derived from it.

As we have also seen, Finzel could account for his earnings with some confidence. His response to the moral dilemma that physicians owed their livelihood and indeed their prosperity to other people's suffering, was not merely rhetorical. Finzel earned well and his practice was lucrative, but a major part of his income came from a limited group of wealthier citizens and aristocrats. The number of consultations with poorer patients did diminish over the years (which was not necessarily Finzel's fault). However, throughout his life he continued to serve many patients of very limited financial means, patients who hardly contributed anything to his income. In this sense, his *Rationarium* showed that he was faithful to the ideal of the pious, charitable Christian physician who helped the poor. At the same time, he could take comfort in the fact that the considerable earnings that he nevertheless accrued every year showed that God listened to his prayers and that he walked in His light.

Notes

1 See T. Walter, 'Ärztehaushalte im 16. Jahrhundert. Einkünfte, Status und Praktiken der Repräsentation', *Medizin, Geschichte und Gesellschaft* 27 (2008), 31–73.
2 Ratschulbibliothek Zwickau, Zwickau (RSBZ), MS QQQQ1a, QQQQ1, and QQQQ1b.
3 See M. Stolberg, 'A sixteenth century physician and his patients: The practice journal of Hiob Finzel, 1565–89', *Social History of Medicine* 31 (2018): https://DOI.org/10.1093/shm/hkx063; on practice journals as a genre of medical note-taking, see M. Stolberg, 'Medical note-taking in the sixteenth and seventeenth centuries', in A. Cevolini (ed.), *Forgetting Machines: Knowledge Management Evolution in Early Modern Europe* (Leiden: Brill, 2016), pp. 243–64.
4 The title was probably added by an early modern archivist.
5 In the registry of new citizens in Weimar the spelling varies: we find 'Funtzschel', 'Funczel', or 'Fundschel', compare W. Huschke, *Die Neubürger der Stadt Weimar, 1520–1620* (Neustadt: Degener, 1973), and in the latest known record (ibid., p. 63) 'Conradt Funtschel'; blending the Latin and German versions of his name, German scholars have later often called him 'Hiob Fincel' but I know of no contemporary who used this rather strange hybrid form.
6 See H. Finzel, *Epicedion honestae puellae Anna Finceliae Vinariensis pie defunctae in Pomerania* (Jena: Rödinger, 1556).
7 See K.E. Förstemann (ed.), *Album Academiae Vitebergensis: ab a[nno] Ch[risti] MDII usque ad a[nnum] MDLX* (Leipzig: Tauchnitz, 1841), p. 218, 'Hiob Funtzschel'; and A. Beier, *Syllabus rectorum, et professorum Jenae* (Jena: Typis Casparis Freyschmidii, 1659), pp. 896, 968.
8 Ibid., p. 968.
9 See H. Finzel, *Wunderzeichen*, 3 vols (Nuremberg: Johann vom Berg and Ulrich Neuber, 1552–62).
10 The literature on Finzel's *Wunderzeichen* is quite extensive. For good overviews, see H. Schilling, 'Job Fincel und die Zeichen der Endzeit', in

W. Brückner (ed.), *Volkserzählung und Reformation. Ein Handbuch zur Tradierung und Funktion von Erzählstoffen und Erzählliteratur im Protestantismus* (Berlin: Erich Schmidt, 1974), pp. 326–93; and B. Aewerdieck, *Register zu den Wunderzeichenbüchern Job Fincels* (Frankfurt: Lang, 2010), pp. 7–54 (introduction).

11 See Finzel, *Wunderzeichen*.
12 G.A. Wette, *Historische Nachrichten von der berühmten Residentz-Stadt Weimar* (Weimar: Hoffmann, 1737), p. 137. On early modern town physicians, see A. Russell (ed.), *The Town and State Physician in Europe from the Middle Ages to the Enlightenment* (Wolfenbüttel: Herzog-August-Bibliothek, 1981); R. Schilling, S. Schlegelmilch, and S. Splinter, 'Stadtarzt oder Arzt in der Stadt? Drei Ärzte der Frühen Neuzeit und ihr Verständnis des städtischen Amtes', *Medizinhistorisches Journal* 46 (2011), 99–133.
13 Thüringisches Hauptstaatsarchiv, Weimar, EGA, Reg. Rr pag. 1–316 Nr. 400, 1^{r-v}, 18 December 1566.
14 RSBZ, MS QQQQ1a, fol., p. 163.
15 At the time, there were three hospitals for the poor in Zwickau, compare E. Herzog, *Chronik der Kreisstadt Zwickau*, 2 vols (Zwickau: Zückler, 1839), vol. 2, p. 330.
16 Günther Grosche has collected some fragmentary evidence on learned physicians in local sources, see G. Grosche, *Zwickauer Medizingeschichte im 16. Jahrhundert*, unpublished typescript, Zwickau 2000 = RSBZ, 4° 71 -1, -2, and -3.
17 According to Herzog, *Chronik*, p. 319, Finzel died on 1 July 1589. Herzog probably still had access to the parish registers, which are no longer extant. In December 1589, Finzel's successor as town physician, Petrus Poach, received his first salary.
18 See M. Stolberg, 'Empiricism in sixteenth-century medical practice. The notebooks of Georg Handsch', *Early Science and Medicine* 18 (2013), 487–516.
19 Occasionally we also find entries with two figures for payments that both clearly refer to the same consultation, and sometimes Finzel even added an 'and' ['*et*'] between the figures. The most plausible explanation would seem that the patient in question did not pay the full sum all at once. There is no evidence that Finzel owed some of his income to the dispensation of medicines. We do find entries where Finzel resorted to terms like '*dedi*' ('I gave'), rather than using the standard format of a prescription, as he usually did, starting with the sign for 'recipe' and ending with the 'signa', the German words that the pharmacist was to write on the medicine before giving it to the patient. This suggests that Finzel sometimes gave medicines that he had at hand. Even in these cases, he recorded, as a rule, only one

figure for the consultation and no extra fee for the medicines and the payment he received for these consultations tended to be in the same range as for those in which he only wrote out a prescription.
20 RSBZ, MS QQQQ1a, fol. 385, 'halb Jar Besoldung'; ibid., MS QQQQ1, fol. 39.
21 Ibid., fol. 42, 'Jar Besoldung'.
22 Ibid., fol. 39, 'halbe Jar Besoldung'.
23 My figures are based on Finzel's own calculations; we do not know the precise value of the different coins he received. Finzel did not record his annual earnings for 1580, 1582, and 1583 and my figures are derived from the sums that Finzel calculated towards the end of these years to which I have added, with a tolerable margin of error, the payments he received over the remaining weeks. For the years after 1584, some fascicles and individual leaves of paper were bound in the wrong order. The old pagination and Finzel's ongoing calculations of his accumulated earnings for the individual year make it possible to reconstruct the original order quite reliably, however. In 1582, his income included an additional gratification of 30 fl from the town council for his book on the plague, see RSBZ, MS QQQQ1b, fol. 339, October 1582; and A. Drechsel, 'Das Gesundheitswesen der Stadt Zwickau von den Anfängen bis zum Ausgang des 17. Jahrhunderts' (Medical Dissertation, University Leipzig, 2003, p. 89). In 1588, his salary was again 90 fl instead of 60 fl, which may reflect another gratification.
24 RSBZ, MS QQQQ1a, fol. 236 and fol. 247.
25 See Walter, 'Ärztehaushalte', 36–7.
26 Ibid., p. 57 (footnote).
27 A good eighteenth-century example is MS B78751 in the Stadsarchief in Antwerp; the unidentified author, who worked primarily as a surgeon and man-midwife, recorded his fees and crossed out most of his entries, clearly because the patient had paid. See also the contributions in M. Dinges, K.-P. Jankrift, S. Schlegelmilch, and M. Stolberg (eds), *Medical Practice (1600–1900). Physicians and their Patients* (Leiden: Brill, 2016).
28 See Cevolini (ed.), *Forgetting Machines*.
29 Over the last three decades, the historiography of accounting has greatly expanded its scope. Traditional studies that focused on the technicalities and the improvement of accounting techniques have been supplemented by studies on the cultural and social history of accounting and on its intrinsically ideological and political nature, see the Introduction to this volume; and P. Miller, T. Hopper, and R. Laughlin, 'The new accounting history: An introduction', *Accounting, Organizations and Society* 16 (1991), 395–403. The links, more specifically, between accounting and theology

were the topic of a special issue of the *Accounting, Auditing & Accountability Journal* in 2004 (320–497).
30 See G. Thompson, 'Is accounting rhetorical? Methodology, Luca Pacioli and printing', *Accounting, Organizations and Society* 16 (1991), 572–99.
31 See J. Aho, 'Rhetoric and the invention of double entry bookkeeping', *Rhetorica* (1985), Winter Issue, 21–43.
32 See J. Aho, *Confession and Bookkeeping. The Religious, Moral, and Rhetorical Roots of Modern Accounting* (Albany: State University of New York Press, 2005). My thanks to Erica Charters, who pointed out Aho's book to me.
33 Ibid., pp. XIII–XIV.
34 Ibid., p. 28.
35 See H. Oldcastle, *A briefe instruction and maner hovv to keepe bookes of accompts after the order of debitor and creditor: as well for proper accompts partible, &c. By the three bookes named the memoriall iournall & leager, and of other necessaries appertaining to a good and diligent marchant*, ed. John Mellis (London: John Windet, 1588), chapters 4 and 6 (no page numbers).
36 See L. Pacioli, *Trattato di partita doppia: Venezia 1494* (Venice: Albrizzi, 1994).
37 See Aho, *Confession*.
38 See M. Boudewijns, *Ventilabrum medico-theologicum*. (Antwerp: Cornelius Woons, 1666), p. 266.
39 See F. Hoffmann, *Medicus politicus sive regulae prudentiae secundum quas medicus juvenis studia sua & vitae rationem dirigere debet, si famam sibi felicemque praxin & cito acquirere & conservare cupit* (Leiden: Bonk, 1738), p. 177.
40 An early example is E. Cordus, *Von der Kunst auch Missbrauch und Trug des Harnsehens* (Magdeburg: sine loco, 1536), frontispiece.
41 See R. da Castro, *Medicus-politicus: sive de officiis medico-politicis tractatus* (Hamburg: Hertelius, 1614), p. 187.
42 See Boudewijns, *Ventilabrum*, p. 268; Hoffmann, *Medicus politicus*, p. 241.
43 See Castro, *Medicus-politicus*, p. 187.
44 See G. Zerbi, *De cautelis medicorum* (Venice: de Pensis, c. 1495), chapter on *De mercede medici accipienda* (no page numbers).
45 See Hoffmann, *Medicus politicus*, pp. 239–40.
46 See Castro, *Medicus-politicus*, p. 191.
47 Ibid., p. 187.
48 For example, 'Exactae redeunt metae revolubilis anni'.
49 For example, 'Sit precor auspicium foelix venientis ut anni'; 'Auspicijs novus annus eat foelicibus opto'.
50 For an illuminating case study on the links between economic accounting and 'accounting for sins' in the Society of Jesus during the

Counter-Reformation, see P. Quattrone, 'Accounting for God: Accounting and accountability practices in the Society of Jesus (Italy, XVI–XVII centuries)', *Accounting, Organizations and Society* 29 (2004), 647–83.
51 'Unica Christe salus hominum/Divinaque pios ipse tuere manu/Tolle hostes contra Christe trophoea [sic] tuos/Bella parant etenim latius funesta Dialis/Et sathanae servi Gallus. Iberus atrox.' My thanks to Sabine Schlegelmilch for pointing out that 'Dialis', the highest priest of Jupiter, could refer not only to the priests of pagan gods but, in Protestant writing, also to the Pope.
52 For example, RSBZ, MS QQQQ1b, fol. 176.
53 RSBZ, MS QQQQ1b, fol. 278, 'Nos Dei gratia', August 1581.
54 See M. Weber, *The Protestant Ethic and the Spirit of Capitalism* (New York: Charles Scribner's Sons, 1958).
55 RSBZ, MS QQQQ1b, fol. 239: 'Divinaque pios ipse tuere manu'.
56 RSBZ, MS QQQQ1b, fol. 176.
57 RSBZ, MS QQQQ1b, fol. 520: 'DEO sit laus et gloria in sempiterna saecula/Qui trinus est et unus est/Verax, iustus, miserans DEUS/ Nobis remittens crimina/Donansque vitam nos novam.'
58 See Stolberg, 'A sixteenth century physician' for more detailed figures and for a discussion of the methodological issues involved.
59 See H. Bräuer, *Wider den Rat. Der Zwickauer Konflikt 1516/17* (Leipzig: Leipziger Universitätsverlag, 1999), p. 34 estimates the population to have been around 7,300 in 1530; the figure for the mid-sixteenth century cited in H. Berthold, K. Hahn, and A. Schultze, *Die Zwickauer Stadtrechtsreformation 1539/69* (Leipzig: Hirzel, 1935), p. 2, is 7,677.
60 Finzel recorded twenty-one patients as 'poor' or as hospital inmates and presumably treated them for free, as part of his duties as a town physician.
61 In this period there is no evidence for Zwickau or Saxony of a "Tax-Ordnung", i.e. an official list of the fees a physician could ask and which later, in other regions, usually established maximum fees for patients of different economic status.
62 See H. Voigtlaender, *Löhne und Preise in vier Jahrtausenden* (Speyer: Numismatische Gesellschaft Speyer, 1994).
63 Finzel seems to have taken a *taler* to be worth about 1.15 fl, but I have not been able to identify a precise and consistent ratio, perhaps due to changes over time.
64 Finzel received a golden coin ('*Goltgulden*'), for example, for treating the servant ('*Knecht*') of Jörg Marschall, cf. RSBZ, MS QQQQ1a, fol. 47.
65 RSBZ, Ms QQQQ1b, fol. 77.
66 RSBZ, Ms QQQQ1a, fol. 299 and fol. 310.

2

'Making a living': Accounting and the medical market in and around Geneva, 1760–1820[1]

Philip Rieder

In October 1812, the Genevese physician Louis Odier (1748–1817) wrote to Jean-Pierre Maunoir (1768–1861) after it had come to his knowledge that his friend and colleague was to travel with a Mr Fazy, a former patient of Odier's. 'I am happy to hear', Odier wrote, that 'he is better' and he asked his friend to send greetings. But above all, he was curious to learn why Fazy no longer required his services: 'if you get the chance, and without compromising me, you could find out why he left me for [Pierre] Butini, I would be curious to know. I had healed him very promptly from dysentery and was quite surprised some time afterwards to learn that he had changed physician.'[2]

The request highlights the situation of competing physicians in Geneva in the late eighteenth and early nineteenth century. Physicians cared for patients, but they also cared for knowledge about their patients. Understanding patients' motivations enlightened their apprehension of the demand for medical commodities and services, reinforced their position on the medical market, and could thus enhance or consolidate their income. Odier's request also conveys the idea that the medical market was not a neutral locus of display for medical commodities and services, but a complex social system in which alliances, collaborations, and strategies were necessary. Professional and public discourses alternatively presented the physician as reduced to poverty due to low fees or as making a mint of money out of other peoples' miseries. In truth, we know little about money in medicine and, more generally, the economics of medical practice prior to the twentieth century. Putting the economics of medical practice at the forefront and questioning, as Anne Digby has for the British context,[3] how practitioners made or failed to make a living, can help reveal the dynamics of an otherwise apparently erratic market.

Beginning with the account books of three medical practitioners, this chapter investigates another marketplace – or more precisely, a section of the medical market and medical practice in and around Geneva. By studying these three healers' accounting practices and related sources, it is possible to reconstruct the role accounting and economics played in their practices and thus to gain an understanding of their roles in the regional medical market.

Three practitioners in and around Geneva

Few practitioners' accounts prior to 1700 have survived, but more are available after that date.[4] Among them are the ledgers started between 1766 and 1776 by three medical practitioners active in the region to the west of Lake Geneva. Keeping accounts was certainly an administrative necessity for practitioners intent on monitoring income and tracking their patients' outstanding debts for medical services. Most physicians complained that many bills weren't paid and that patients who did pay, were slow to do so.[5] Gaspard Vieusseux (1746–1814), a physician who set up his Geneva practice in 1771, wrote shortly afterwards to complain: '*God damn all the patients* not only don't they pay well, but some *don't pay at all when after being cured,* and would you believe it, a *shabby* ¼ écu is considered to be a lot?'[6]

The account books of all three practitioners not only provide data on relationships between practitioners and their patients, the medical market, and the competitive relationships among practitioners, but also allow insights into the social and professional status of practitioners. Although active in the same region, all three practitioners worked in quite distinct political and medical settings with specific social and professional profiles. The oldest, Catherin Pichollet (1711–88), was a country practitioner who had been admitted as a surgeon on 10 December 1738 by the College of Surgeons of Turin, before establishing a village practice a few kilometres to the south-west of Geneva (1764–85).[7] His ledger covers the year 1766. The entries record medical activities carried out in Catholic villages close to Geneva (Bernex, Confignon,

Aire-la-ville, and St-Julien) where there was no competition and very little control of medical practices.[8] References to other volumes suggest that Pichollet kept a volume for each year.

Somewhat younger and further up the social ladder was Joseph Despine (1737–1830). Despine came from a well-established bourgeois background; his father was a notary in Chambéry. He graduated as a physician in Turin[9] and studied childbirth in Paris.[10] In the 1760s and early 1770s, he travelled to the medical capitals of Europe, studied thermal cures and inoculation, and wrote medical reports in favour of reforms. In 1772, when he started his ledger, he had married into an affluent family and settled in Annecy – a town in Savoy which boasted some 4,000 to 5,000 inhabitants.[11] He practised medicine both in town and in the rural surroundings. Savoy was then part of the Kingdom of Sardinia with no medical guild. Physicians were spread out in a number of relatively small localities.[12] In 1783, he was appointed emeritus physician to King Victor-Amédée III of Savoy for having inoculated the royal children. A further title of doctor and director of the royal baths of Aix-les-Bains bestowed upon him in 1787 confirmed his expertise in thermal cures and compelled him to maintain a practice there during the bathing season.[13] His account book starts with his first patients in Annecy (1772) and runs until 1823 with regular entries between 1772 and 1815.[14] It covers his years as honoured physician of the realm of Sardinia, his loss both of favour and of his privileged status at the baths after the occupation of Savoy by the French in 1792, and his subsequent rehabilitation when he was reinstated as director to the royal baths and promoted to 'vice-protomédecin' (1816).[15]

The third and youngest medical practitioner, Louis Odier, was born in Geneva and travelled to Edinburgh for his medical training. His social status placed him between Despine and Pichollet: as the son of a rich merchant, he knew that he would inherit some money, but also that this would be insufficient to pay his household costs. He was understandably distressed when he realised that physicians were relatively badly paid in his hometown.[16] In 1774, when he started his accounts, he was 24 years old and setting out in practice.[17] Geneva was then an important town and boasted some 20,000 inhabitants and over ten physicians. During the following fifty odd years he practised in the town and its immediate vicinity. He managed to occupy prominent medical and political positions under three political regimes. During the French

Three practitioners

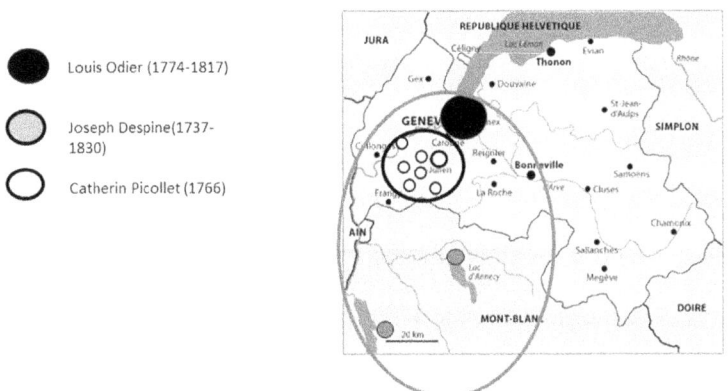

2.1 Three practitioners in and around Geneva.

period (1798–1813), he was promoted to honorary professor of medicine and became a member of the Jury d'instruction. Odier's first ledger runs from 1774 until January 1794.[18] The subsequent interruption of his accounts until 1800 was due to the political and economic turmoil of the times. He held a second series of accounts (from April 1800 until February 1802)[19] and a third series (from January 1804 until December 1810).[20] All ledgers share the same structure (Figure 2.1).

Organic accounts

The purpose of each account book varies from author to author. Joseph Despine's ledger is described by its author as a 'Book of accounts both of visits which I have made and what is due to me for practicing medicine.'[21] The organisation is chronological, although there are some exceptions and evidence that Despine was not always systematic in his entries. Calendar months are regularly noted in the margins and each item includes one or more medical services described in a small paragraph. It is likely that the entries were made either when a bill was issued or treatment ended. The first pages cover amounts owed by patients treated in Annecy: an address is given, the number of visits is specified, but no travel expenses are billed. Occasionally locations outside the town and a charge for the trip are mentioned. Patients were billed for each visit, sometimes for one or two, elsewhere for ten, twenty, or even more visits. A canon named Perran paid 37 livres for sixty visits made between September 1773 and April 1774.[22] A nominal index placed at the beginning of the ledger offers a quick access to all entries concerning any one patient. When sums were paid, the author barred the entry. This mode of recordkeeping enabled the physician to add services performed at a later date to any item: in the summer of 1774, Despine recorded a sum of 8 livres owed by M. Favre Diaconis for six visits in July to which he added six visits made the previous year. The entry was not barred before 1780 when he added 'plus 2 [visits] in March 1780 throat ache', a service for which he charged 1 livre and 10 sols. This, like many other items, was never recorded as having been paid. In his accounts, Despine does occasionally indicate his diagnosis. Marechal Ranquin, for instance, was charged for twenty visits when he suffered from a malignant fever in February 1772. Other diseases mentioned include measles, fevers, smallpox, rheumatism, jaundice, and wasting disease. Despine took care of women after giving birth,[23] but he did not explicitly mention obstetrical work.[24] In 1775, the physician reduced the details included in each entry, limiting information to the patient's name, a date, and the number of visits: 'Mrs Charlet, in July 1775 3 vis[its] and a consultation 4 [livres]' is a typical example. Entries continue to include trips, visits, and consultations. Entries resume in 1777, in a yet more rational form: short entries are followed by large spaces which the physician later filled, when relevant, with services provided to the same family at a later date.[25] At times, Despine was absent for long periods. From April until August 1778, for instance, he was in Turin presenting inoculation techniques, a source of medical income which is not mentioned in the extant ledger (Figure 2.2).

The nature of Despine's ledger changes over the years as entries for services provided in villages outside Annecy progressively predominate, a transition confirmed in 1784 when a second column appears to the right of the name list in the index, signalling the appropriate location. The list reveals that, after 1785, he only rarely included patients living in Annecy in the ledger. Moreover, there is no trace of his activity

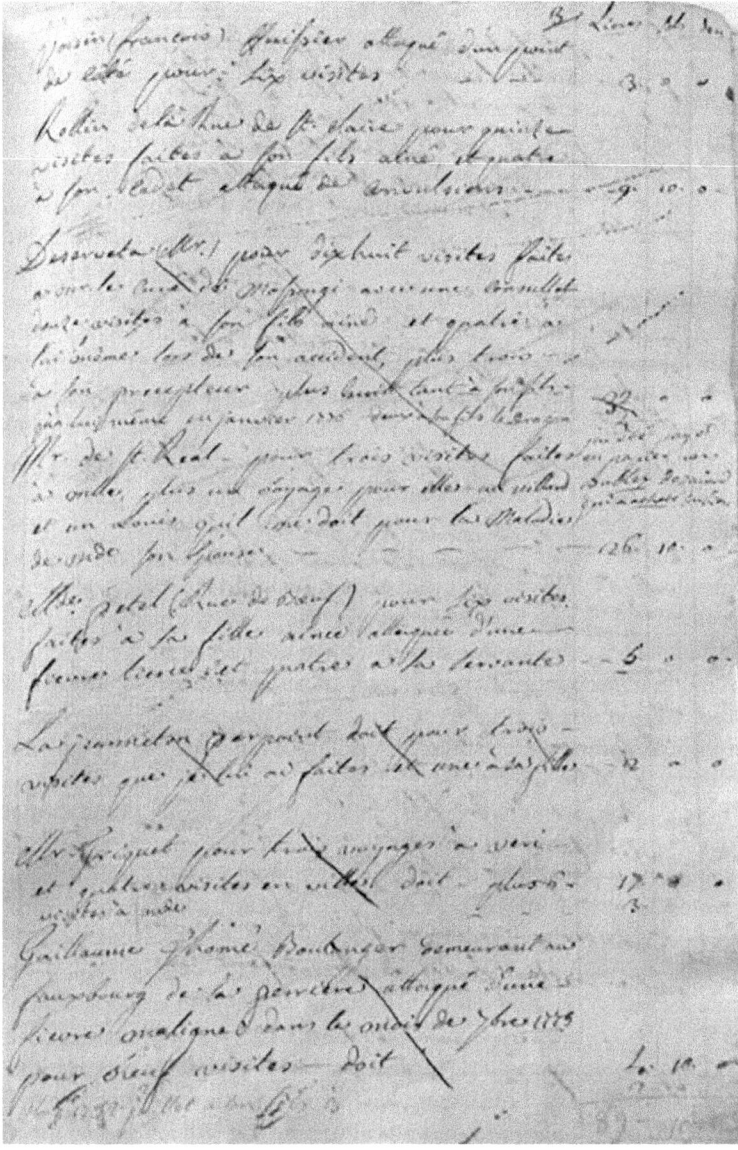

2.2 Page of Joseph Despine's ledger.

as physician of the baths following his regular establishment in Aix-les-Bains for the summer season as from 1783.[26] By 1795, most of the items listed in the ledger concern visits to patients living in distant localities and this pattern prevails in the following years. The physician regularly rode out to patients living within a radius of 20 km from his home, but was prepared to travel up to 80 km to visit specific patients. In October 1795, for instance, only four activities are recorded.[27] On each occasion, the physician travelled to a different village for a single patient: on the 4th, he travelled to Epagny; five days later he took a trip to Les Molasses, the next day he went to Vieugy, and on the 25th of the same month he found his way to Novel. Apart from Novel, which was only slightly more than 1 km away from Annecy, all locations were between 6 and 10 km from Annecy.[28] This was common, but the physician regularly ventured further afield. On 22 August 1799, he travelled from Aix-les-bains to Marcellaz (74 km) for a consultation with a colleague (Dr Brunier) and then returned to Annecy (44 km), charging 22 livres and 15 sols.[29] He rarely saw these patients more than once, or at most a couple of times.

Catherin Pichollet's ledger also focuses on medical activity beyond the village of Chilly, where he was born, died, and most probably practised.[30] He may well have had a separate ledger for his home practice.[31] Pichollet's accounts are structurally similar to Despine's as both authors used their accounts to detail services and commodities for which payment was due. Formally, the items they registered were comparable to contemporary medical bills: for instance, a bill signed by the surgeon Albert in 1763 included the same elements (diagnosis, trip, medicines) at comparable prices to those listed in Pichollet's book in 1766.[32] That said, comparing both ledgers also reveals many differences in treating clientele and providing medical services. Pichollet regularly visited the same villages where he provided primary care and a variety of medical services and commodities.

Such detailed information is absent from Odier's ledger, which was constructed quite differently. Odier was fresh from medical school in 1774 when he started what was then an all-purpose medical and financial notebook, including data on his first patients, his fortune, his investments, and his expenses. This information, although spread out over more than a decade, ends after nine pages and a simple list of payments received for medical services follows. It is introduced by a solemn statement: 'I was received as a medical doctor at Edinburgh on

12 September 1770 and admitted to Geneva's Faculty on 28 October 1773. Since then, here is the note of payments I have received for my visits.'[33] The partnership established with Daniel de la Roche late in 1773 may explain why he started the series: the partners had undertaken to share their profits and Odier needed to note down the precise amount he earned each year.[34] Systematic records of payments received were thus necessary. In the list itself, the information on services provided by Odier is typically limited to the number of visits for which a payment was received, although other paid services are also itemised, such as written or oral consultations, inoculations, legal reports, and on one occasion, medical data provided to an insurance company.

In short, whereas Odier's ledger enabled its author to keep track of his medical income, Pichollet and Despine's books were more practical and enabled both practitioners to prepare bills and to keep track of incoming payments. All three systems convey information about the practitioners' activities.

Accounting practices and medical services

To understand the role accounting played in each healer's practice, a more detailed analysis is necessary. Pichollet and Despine used indexes to identify debtors and the precise amounts owed by each patient or family. In these indexes, few patients have more than one or two entries, and the fact that the indexes were up to date suggests that most patients living out of town only called on the practitioner in times of crisis. Pichollet added a topographical index, which was probably useful to remind him of patients he had in each village, possibly making it easier for him to follow up on patients' health and to collect payments as he made his rounds. In short, Despine and Pichollet appear to have devised their bookkeeping to answer practical problems, to record money owed to them, and to write up bills. Other patients may well have paid straight away and were therefore never mentioned in either of the account books, although it must be said that Pichollet does detail, for no apparent reason, some services given free of charge.[35]

One striking element in Pichollet's practice is that he did not systematically set a price for his services. At times he may have set no precise amount until he had negotiated with his patient. In the case of the Megevend brothers residing in Beaumont, for instance, no sum is mentioned as due for the medical services they received between 18 April and 2 June 1766 – six trips, one phlebotomy, and six pharmaceutical preparations – despite the fact that Pichollet had already prepared a space in which to insert the total amount. In this case, 'payé' was written before and after their names to indicate that they had paid, but not how much.[36] More often, the amounts quoted in his book cannot be equated with money received: Pichollet occasionally jotted down details of the final arrangements made with patients or their families, sometimes years later. Such arrangements could include substantial discounts, as in the case of Claude Pillet, a cordwainer established in Chables. Pillet owed Pichollet 4 livres and 14 sols for treatment given to his wife between May and July 1766. When Pillet paid in August of the following year, Pichollet reduced the debt by 4 sols.[37]

Despine certainly expected at times to be paid immediately, namely for small amounts. In June 1813, for instance, he mentioned a bill of 1 franc and 10 centimes owed by Martine Pethou for a consultation and a prescription. He added a comment: 'her son went off without paying me, pretending to go to get some change'.[38] This is a rare piece of information about possible attitudes about payments and confirms that non-payment justified an entry in the ledger.[39] Other traces suggest that the ledger was used to record bills that were due or even overdue. In 1774, Despine noted that 'Mr Cugniez of Sarraval owes me for part of a trip that I undertook specially to see him: 9 livres 10 sols. I only received 17 livres of the 24 livres which I expected – without counting the rental of a horse which cost me 2 livres and 10 sols.'[40] Any indication that the physician had already received partial payment is not documented: the ledger does not indicate all amounts charged by or paid to the physician, but does list the bills due. In this respect, the index is necessary for the physician to check how much each patient owed him.

Like other ledgers, those of Despine and Pichollet offer no precise overview of how much patients actually paid and provide only a vague idea of the practitioner's medical income.[41] The sum owed to Pichollet by a certain Antoine Guilliot, for instance, is only partially mentioned on the far right of the ledger's first page (see Figure 2.3). On the left, the practitioner added 'paid' to items such as a temperating powder and an enema. This suggests that he received immediate payment for a remedy, but not for nursing and counselling services. This is one of

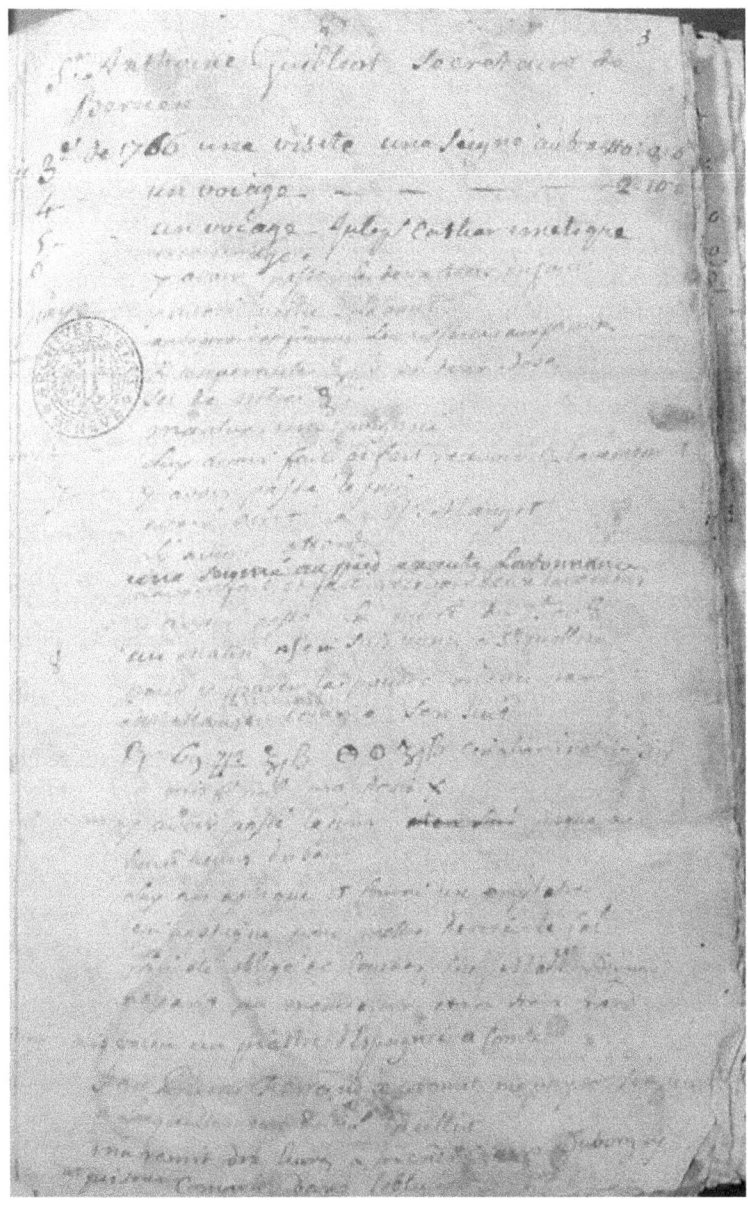

2.3 First page of Catherin Pichollet's ledger.

many signs that payments for medical commodities were deemed more pressing than medical counsel. Many other items on the same page – covering 8 and 9 January 1766 – were not priced. The last lines concern payment. A first entry refers to a negotiated agreement. 'Jean Pierre Ferrand promised to pay me 6 livres' and finally 'gave me 10 livres'.[42] In fact, trouble collecting on bills is recurrent. The wife of a carpenter in Confignon, Claude Dunand, was sick in September 1766. Picollet visited her six times within a month and billed her husband 8 livres 5 sols. Below he added that he had received ¼ of a measure of wheat on 18 September. Thirteen years later, on 14 September 1779, Picollet comments 'The son [...] promised to pay the bill' and again below 'promised to pay in all 8 livres'.[43] Despine was confronted with similar problems. He also received payment in kind, such as 'a calf hyde to make a pair of boots' from a tanner living in Alby.[44] Payments in naturalia or services were possible, if not common.

Interestingly, Louis Odier did not draw up an index for the entries of his accounts. In his ledger, entries are chronological, giving the date of each payment (Figure 2.4). He was able to follow the evolution of his income, and actually added up his monthly and yearly payments to a precise total for each year. For his first years (1775–92), he even filled in a table comparing his income from year to year.[45]

His concerns were more worldly that those of Hiob Finzel, who summarised his annual income to justify his probity before God.[46] Odier analysed the progression of his medical income to evaluate his material and symbolic success on earth: financial success meant professional progress. In the summer 1787, he felt blue after realising that he was doing less well than previously:

> I have noticed that [Charles] Dunant makes every day more progress at my expense. I heard that he had acquired the practice of Lullin the councillor who formerly appeared to trust me entirely. It sorrows me, all the more as money is not coming in. For the entire month of June, I only received 183 louis courants 4 sols and 9 deniers. I am more than 300 louis courant behind what I had earned at this time last year. It worries me for the future and it would sadden me to lose the trust that I have gained.[47]

Keeping track of incoming payments was a way of counting new patients, but also taking stock of the loss of influential clients. In

J'ai été reçu Docteur en médecine à Edinburgh le 12° Sept. 1770. † aggrégé à la Faculté de Geneve le 28° Oct. 1773. Depuis lors, voici la note de l'argent que j'ai reçu pour le payement de mes visites.

1774.		£.	s.	d.
Janv.– Mars. De Mr. Batal.		1.	10.	—
Mr. Dolfous		6.	—	—
Mlle Gourdon		1.	—	—
Mad. Pictet.		21.	16.	—
Mr. Poitevin		2.	—	—
Mr. Parolaz.		3.	13.	—
Mr. Rocca		16.	—	6.
Mr. Vaerli		3.	13.	—
		55.	12.	6.
Avril – Juin. De Mr. Claparède		3.	—	—
Mr. Cavet.		—	18.	—
Mr. Julien		7.	5.	3.
Mr. Lamande		7.	5.	3.
Mr. Moré		3.	13.	—
Mr. Petit		4.	10.	—
Md. Brandoin		29.	—	—
Mr. Rainfe		1.	—	—
Mr. Verli		7.	5.	3.
		63.	3.	10.

2.4 Page of Louis Odier's ledger/Livre de comptes de Louis Odier.

Geneva, an affluent citizen with political influence such as Pierre Lullin (1712–89)[48] was a desirable patient: when ill, he could afford to call on a physician regularly and pay him decently; as a politician he could facilitate lucrative assignments; and as a member of the elite, he could enhance a physician's reputation in the most desirable social context. The reason why Odier lost Lullin was not clear to him. He certainly understood why he lost the d'Hauteville account some years later. As the family's physician, he had diagnosed their six-month-old son with measles in February 1813, but no spots surfaced and he changed his prognosis.[49] He later predicted that the baby would improve rapidly, but this did not happen and the family called in a second physician, Pierre Butini (1759–1838), later to replace Odier as the family's physician.[50] Physicians were competing for solvent patients and some patients were willing to change physicians. The social economy revealed by these two examples was at the core of medical practice. Accounting enabled Odier to evaluate his progress, but also to recognise his failures and to identify possible causes.

Value of health and units of value

The visit was the traditional unit of value for medical practice in and around Geneva. A typical visit cost approximately the same amount as a day's work by an unqualified labourer.[51] The term 'visit' covered both house calls to the patient as well as consultations at the physician's own home. Nonetheless, in Odier's eyes the system was far from perfect and he strove to find new ways of enhancing the value of his medical services. As a student in Edinburgh, he was inspired by the higher value of physicians' visits in Great Britain. He planned to raise the price of visits in Geneva for well-off patients and to treat the poor free of charge.[52] His future wife Suzanne Baux was at first enthusiastic, but after some thought she reconsidered:

> People in this country are at least as proud as the English. Were you to announce that you intended to treat the poor free of charge, they would prefer to die without medicines rather than consult you. As for the rich, who know the price of money more than in any other part of the world as they have almost all earned it thanks to their own sweat and blood, they would be shocked by the extraordinary price that you would attach to your knowledge and to their health; they would do out of miserliness

what the others would do out of pride, and you would find yourself abandoned.[53]

The pending catastrophe was enough to put off a young physician! Odier did not insist and soon explored other schemes. He imagined charging for visiting days, a means of being free to see his patient as many times as required, but the system was never implemented.[54] A second project, which he did implement, involved sharing annual income with his partner Daniel de la Roche. The partner who had earned less was to pay back the difference over the following ten years.[55] In another scheme, Odier tried to set up a system of subscriptions, only to abandon it when less than 5 per cent of his patients agreed to take part. Finally, he adopted the common practice of billing for each visit.[56] A visit was ideally a short encounter with a patient a few minutes walk from the physician's home, but some visits involved far more: a sum of 58 livres and 2 sols was recorded in Odier's accounts for two visits made to Louis-François Guiguer in Prangins. The payment was handsome, something like ten times more than what Odier would expect for two normal visits, but Prangins was 30 km away from Geneva and one visit included a trip in the middle of the night and an overnight stay.

Visits were not a stable measure of the physician's activity. Odier himself wrote an essay on medical billing, claiming that patients should be charged more if they took up more of the physician's time.[57] Despine and Pichollet adapted their fees to accommodate similar situations. Despine adapted his price depending on the inconvenience incurred. Mrs de Monthoux, for instance, ran up a hefty bill in 1774, including ninety visits covering the months from June to December. The physician added to the list 'visits often lasted more than half an hour and I made some of them after supper – costing 20 sols per visit'. He also included in the same bill 26 livres to cover the cost of a two-day trip to Aix-les-Bains, the rental of a horse, and the letter he had written to Mr Cabanis.[58] Despine, like Pichollet and Odier, adjusted his prices according to his patient's status. Mrs de Montoux was charged double the usual price for a less affluent patient. Despine also routinely jotted down specific circumstances: weather and getting wet were the most common. The direct effect of such information is not clear, but probably helped the physician to justify his bill. An emergency could also justify an extra charge: in June 1797, Despine was called to a patient living in

Marlens, some 30 km away, whom he had treated episodically since 1780. He commented in the relevant entry that 'they came to fetch me from two different locations' and that he had immediately interrupted what he had been doing.[59] The urgency presumably justified an extraordinary bill of 40 livres and 16 sols.

In addition to medical counsel, Despine, Odier, and Pichollet also provided medicines which were either given to patients during the visits or sent to them at a later date. Odier occasionally provided his patients with remedies, but this was a service and he did not expect to make a profit. Despine charged patients for specific remedies, such as for twelve bottles containing carbon dioxide to M. Paget, the provost of the Cathedral in Annecy in February 1773 – a 'modern' remedy delivered to a member of the town's elite. The bill for 30 livres was one of the most expensive bills that year. At times, Despine simply sent remedies to his patients for specific ailments and billed them accordingly. His ledger shows that, at least for common remedies, he billed the price he had paid and thus forfeited a profit.[60] Unlike Britain, where many physicians apparently practised as pharmacists, physicians in the Geneva region did not expect to make a profit on the medicines they provided.[61] Pichollet is described as an apothecary in some documents and may well have made money selling his own compound medicines, as did other village surgeons.[62] In fact, he is the practitioner who offered and billed the greatest variety of services and products. These included remedies identified in precise pharmaceutical formulas, writing to a town physician, waiting for the arrival of the physician, and nursing the patients overnight. Trips to his patients were also a lucrative source of revenue and he occasionally only billed for the trip. For instance, visits to Gabriel Bernard's wife on three separate occasions in January 1766 were each charged 10 sols. An interesting aspect of Pichollet's activity as a surgeon is that he regularly wrote to Geneva for help, calling in a physician for patients in critical situation and, by doing so, acknowledging the limits of his own competence.

For all three practitioners, extracting payment was a problem. Pichollet and Despine negotiated regularly with patients and patients' families. Odier opted for a more original path. He stopped sending bills: '[t]here are no doubt a great number of patients who do not pay me. Some pay me badly; but a great number of others pay me incomparably better than they would have had I sent them a bill and, all things considered, I think I have gained more than I have lost with this method.'[63] Whether they sent bills or not, both Odier and Despine did not earn enough money as physicians to live in the genteel fashion their status and rank required. They both had other sources of income. Odier inherited money from his father, invested heavily in life annuity schemes, and subsequently lost it. His practice was later subsidised by his wife who ran a boarding-house and then a wholesale fabric business. Despine had fewer financial worries. He had married well, administered his wife's estate, worked for the King of Sardinia, and developed a practice at the baths of Aix-les-Bains.[64] As an artisan, Pichollet probably had fewer expenses. He most certainly practised both as a surgeon and an apothecary. It is quite possible that, like a counterpart in Angoulême, part of his livelihood came from farming.[65] That said, there is very little information available on his finances and none on his expenses.

Accounting and medical knowledge

The accounts kept by Pichollet and Despine give some idea of the nature of their practices and the complexity of the medical market. But little can be said about their theoretical understanding of their patients's diseases because their ledgers offer scant information about exact medical situations or details on diagnosis and follow up. Odier's accounts are both less detailed and more systematic. As a medical student in Edinburgh, he had been taught how to take casenotes and how to organise his records, and in his private practice he adapted these techniques to practical requirements.[66]

On the first pages of the booklet that was later to serve as a ledger, he jotted down his first case histories. Each case was allocated one page and organised into four sections – state of health, chronology of symptoms, prescribed remedies, and physician's comments – just as he had been taught in Edinburgh.[67] Facing a large number of patients in private practice, he rapidly abandoned using individual sheets of paper and modified the way he took case histories. For each month, Odier kept a clinical notebook in which he jotted down details about his patients' disease and treatment, and he drew up an index which enabled him to keep track of how many visits each patient owed him (Figure 2.5). For

2.5 Page of Odier's clinical pocket books.

each day of the week, Odier included a one-page overview in which he recorded both the indications for each patient and the details of the remedies he prescribed. The nominal index for each month showed the number of visits received by each patient.[68]

Odier could therefore work out precisely how many visits were owed him.[69] The pocket book illustrates how a specific paper technology, acquired during his medical training, was transformed to suit the needs of a medical practitioner: in his practice, information about visits and treatments were important both as memory aids and to keep track of the money he was owed. As a practitioner, Odier expected payment from his patients regardless of their calling or circumstances. Despite consciously avoiding a condescending attitude when treating the poor early in his career,[70] he did not treat poorer patients quite in the same way he did richer ones. While aristocrats or bourgeois patients were always named, poorer patients were often not identified as individuals in his ledger but instead described by their occupation: a 'servant' or 'a locksmith', for instance. Poor patients paid less than others, something between one half and a quarter of what would have been expected from an affluent patient. The 'peasant' who paid him 13 sols for a visit on 19 March 1783 is a good example. But considered as a group, poorer patients had an important impact on Odier's practice as they accounted for 50 per cent of the payments made (sums below 10 louis courant). In short, a big slice of the practitioner's time was spent treating this particular group, despite it only counting for 10 per cent of his medical income.[71] Although poorer social groups took a considerable amount of his time, Odier did not treat individual poorer patients over long periods and at best met them a couple of times. He did not know them very well and considered them an altogether different clientele. In his later years, Odier treated hardly any poorer patients and distanced himself from indigent patients, suggesting that they had particular diseases and suffered differently.

When treating those hailing from his own or a more affluent social group, he paid considerably more attention.[72] He visited them consistently and studied the evolution of their illnesses over time. Odier became a specialist of diseases of the well-to-do. His medical observations and knowledge were drawn from a small group of families and were valid, in his eyes at least, in that particular environment.[73] Most of the affluent patients he saw regularly were acquaintances and friends.

Accounting practices, medical practice, and the medical market

Examining the account books held by three medical practitioners in the late eighteenth and early nineteenth century offers insights into both their medical practices and the broader workings of the medical market.[74] Beyond the obvious competition for lucrative patients, healers' profiles were also complementary and collaboration with other healers was essential. The account books were responses to specific needs and thus served different purposes. By recording amounts due and indexing patients' names in ledgers, Despine and Pichollet essentially created an overview of amounts due. Their habit of indexing locations presumably helped them to plan their trips and answer calls, but also to collect money owed. For this purpose, it was necessary neither to record all amounts, nor to be systematic about the content of the entries. Odier's accounting was more systematic. By recording all incoming money, he aimed to gain an overview of his annual income. Moreover, comparing his annual income with that of previous years enabled him to evaluate his success as a medical practitioner. Such a professional perspective contrasts markedly with that of Hiob Finzel, who summarised his income in order to justify his work in the eyes of God. The contrast between Finzel's accounts in the sixteenth century and the contents of all three account books considered here is all the stronger because, like other private documents stemming from Catholics or Protestants in the region, they contain no religious references.[75] Moreover, whereas mainly religious motives led Finzel to treat some patients for free, two centuries later in Geneva free treatment was more often provided for professional and social reasons. This confirms the distinction that others have observed between medical and religious matters in French-speaking culture in the late Ancien Régime.[76]

Financial issues were a central preoccupation of practitioners. That two out of three ledgers were penned by physicians is remarkable; doctor's ledgers are rare.[77] The fact that both physicians came from non-medical backgrounds, specifically from groups where earning a living or keeping accounts was the norm, is a possible explanation. This fact reinforces Margaret Pelling's contention about the importance of considering medical practitioners' activities on their own terms and in relation to other occupations.[78] Odier's commercial background might also explain the diversity of financial arrangements he imagined.[79] The evolving practice of keeping ledgers at the time may thus not only be a consequence of idiosyncratic conservation, but also of the growing attraction of medical practice as an occupation for upwardly mobile social groups. As mentioned above, both Despine and Odier had other sources of income, and this was probably also the case for Pichollet.[80] This income stemmed either from their medical entrepreneurship or their family situation and involved administering farms and estates, investing money, or marketing expertise. In short, Odier and Despine were elite physicians and certainly among the best paid of their generation. Their yearly incomes would have seemed handsome to many contemporary patients. The fact that they required alternative sources of income was largely due to their status and their need to mix with their rich patients.

Extant data suggest that physicians were not necessarily the highest earners. Louis Odier, who had studied at prominent universities and inherited a small fortune, left his widow some 60,000 francs. His friend and the son of a humble weaver, the surgeon Louis Jurine, who was trained only as an apprentice, died leaving some 600,000 francs to his heirs.[81] The emphasis that practitioners, and more specifically physicians, placed on being paid was not necessarily a sign of avarice. This is all the more obvious as all three healers treated at least occasionally poor patients for free.[82] In short, the medical market was a market in which both symbolic and financial rewards were at stake. Setting and accepting the appropriate payment was an important issue in medical ethics;[83] the relevant social practices tended to shape the scope of the practitioners' activities.

All in all, and despite treating poor patients and facing many difficulties in their practices, it may well be, as suggested by Irvine Loudon for Britain, that the cohort of these three practitioners was a lucky one: they were active in a 'golden age' of growing demand for medical services.[84] Theirs was a transitional generation,[85] dealing with growing requests from patients capable of paying and, at the same time, striving to ensure higher compensation for the medical services. Assessing medical practices in their own right is therefore essential and allows one to highlight links with other social practices (trades) and to reveal the nature of 'professional' postures. Pichollet, Despine, and Odier did not simply play a specific professional role; they adapted their practices to the demand.

The entries in the account books of Pichollet, Despine, and Odier convey medical, financial, and socio-economic information. As medical instruments, they enabled practitioners to record patients' names and the medical services provided, to follow up medications and to link different medical interventions in time, to evaluate money owed, to revise commercial strategies, to compare income at different moments in time, and thus to evaluate success.

The account books also confirm the importance of place, social practices, and customs in the organisation of the medical marketplace. Physicians billed their time and travel expenses, despite being intent on charging only for their counsel. Moreover, although they occasionally provided medicines for their patients, this was not necessarily a lucrative service, or at least not directly so.

Notes

1 Research for this chapter was supported by a research grant funded by the Fonds National Suisse de la Recherche Scientifique (subsidy number 100016–144565/1). Quotations from French sources have been translated into English.
2 Musée d'histoire des sciences (henceforth: MHS), Z 3, Louis Odier à Jean-Pierre Maunoir, Genève, 2 October 1812.
3 A. Digby, *Making a Medical Living. Doctors and Patients in the English Market for Medicine, 1720–1911* (Cambridge: Cambridge University Press, 1994).
4 For a sixteenth-century example, see Chapter 1 by M. Stolberg about the physician Hiob Finzel. The account books described here for the eighteenth and nineteenth centuries are rare in the Geneva region and, to date, no earlier examples have been found.
5 See L. Odier, 'Mémoire sur les honoraires des médecins', in P. Rieder and M. Louis-Courvoisier (eds), *Les Honoraires médicaux et autres mémoires d'éthique médicale* (Paris: Classiques Gallimard, 2011), p. 113. For other examples: J.-P. Goubert, *Médecins d'hier, médecins d'aujourd'hui: le cas du docteur Lavergne (1756–1831)* (Paris: Publisud, 1992), p. 217; P. Treuttel, 'Un médecin de Fontenay-le-Comte au début du XVIIIe siècle', *Annales de Bretagne et des Pays de l'Ouest*, vol. xx (1983) 19–33; W.F. Daems, *Johann Anton Grass von Portein: 1684–1770: Arzt, Chirurg, Zahnarzt, Harndiagnostiker, Pharmazeut, Viehdoktor und Dorfpolitiker: Ein Beitrag zur Kultur- und Medizingeschichte des Domleschgs und Heinzenbergs im 18. Jahrhundert* (Chur: Terra Grischuna Buchverlag, 1985), pp. 133–4; and Digby, *Making a Medical Living*, pp. 155–8.

Accounting and the medical market, Geneva, 1760–1820   77

6 The words in italics are in English in the original manuscript. Bibliothèque de Genève (henceforth: BGE), MS fr 4163, Gaspard Vieussieux to Louis Odier, Genève, 7 June 1771.
7 Archives d'Etat de Genève (henceforth: AEG), Manuscrit historique 201, pp. 50, 85, 88.
8 See J.-M. Duverney, 'La Médecine en Savoie au XVIIIe siècle d'après l'activité du docteur Joseph Despine' (Medical Dissertation, Université Joseph Fourier, 1990), pp. 20–2; L. Gautier, *La Médecine à Genève jusqu'à la fin du 18e siècle* (Genève: Société d'Histoire et d'Archéologie de Genève, 1906).
9 He graduated on 25 April 1761. Archives départementales de Savoie (henceforth: ADS), Fonds Despine, 45 J art. 55.
10 See the certificate he received in 1768: ADS, 45 J art. 55.
11 Despine's wife's dowery was valued at 48,000 livre piémontais in July 1773. At the turn of the century, his properties were estimated to be worth 200,000 livres (4,100 livres of income). This was considerably more than his own mother's dowery (2,000 livres piémontais). On his family and marriage, see Duverney, *La Médecine en Savoie*, pp. 1–5, 23. ADHS 45 J art. 66, copie de lettre du 7 Ventôse an 4. Many other physicians in France and Britain acquired property thanks to their wives or by investing their profits, see among others L. Brockliss, *Calvet's Web: Enlightenment and the Republic of Letters in Eighteenth-Century France* (Oxford: Oxford University Press, 2002), pp. 58–62; Goubert, *Médecins d'hier*, pp. 224–7; I. Loudon, *Medical Care and the General Practitioner (1750–1850)* (Oxford: Oxford University Press, 1986), pp. 106–8.
12 The licensing and practice of surgeons and apothecaries was governed by a protomédicat appointed by the Sarde administration, see J. Nicolas, *La Savoie au 18e siècle: noblesse et bourgeoisie* (Paris: Maloine, 1978), pp. 84–5.
13 The original acts are available: ADS, Fonds Despine, 45 J. 55. Victor Amé of Savoy signed his patent as doctor of the baths on 22 February 1787.
14 The last pages list debts due for the period between 1815 and 1823. ADS, Fonds Despine, 11 J 106 (henceforth: Despine).
15 He lost his privilege as director of the baths in 1798 (and was excluded from activities there in 1805). In 1815, he was reappointed as physician to the baths, see Avis signed by Desmaison on 6 Fructidor year 13 (24 August 1805), ADS, 45 J 64. On 13 March 1816, he was awarded an official patent as vice-protomédecin. ADS, Fonds Despine, 45 J art. 63.
16 The obvious reference was then Great Britain. On the situation in Geneva, see P. Rieder, 'The physician Louis Odier and the medical market in Geneva (1774–1817)', *Gesnerus* 69 (2012), 54–75.
17 BGE, MS fr 5647/9.

18 Ibid.
19 MHS, Z 92/2 *Diarium clinicum*, starting in April 1800.
20 BGE, MS fr 5647/10.
21 Despine, title page.
22 Despine, fol. 3v.
23 For instance, in February 1773, he reported six visits to Mme de Seissel 'following her delivery', see Despine, fol. 4.
24 Some 'visits' to women were more expensive than others, suggesting a specific service, possibly related to childbirth. According to Jean-Marc Duverney, less than 3 per cent were obstetrical or gynaecological cases, see Duverney, *La Médecine en Savoie*, p. 60.
25 See e.g. Despine, fol. 14v.
26 Fashionable baths attracted a rich clientele to spas throughout Europe. For Britain and France, see Digby, *Making a Medical Living*, pp. 187–8; and P. Cosma-Muller 'Entre science et commerce: Les eaux minérales en France à la fin de l'Ancien Régime', in J.-P. Goubert (ed.), *La Médicalisation de la société française, 1770–1830* (Waterloo: Historical Reflections Press, 1982), pp. 249–62.
27 A hefty price when compared to the 1 livre and 10 sols paid for a simple visit in town during the same period.
28 Despine, fol. 35.
29 Despine, fol. 34.
30 Information found on https://gw.geneanet.org [accessed 7 May 2018].
31 As did the contemporary country surgeon Thomas Hérier, see E.H. Lemay, 'Thomas Hérier, a country surgeon outside Anouglême at the end of the XVIIIth century: A contribution to social history', *Journal of Social History* 10 (1977) 524–37, esp. 524.
32 AEG, Villages Genevois, 4.13.2.
33 BGE, MS fr 5647/9, p. 10.
34 For this arrangement, see BGE, MS fr 5647/9, p. 11.
35 For instance, an entry citing three trips to treat the daughter of the widow of Cusin (Chables), including a pharmaceutical preparation (June 1766), is marked 'gratis'. AEG, Manuscrit historique 201 (henceforth: Pichollet) p. 65. For another case, see Pichollet, p. 61.
36 Pichollet, p. 46.
37 Pichollet, p. 59. There are many other cases (for instance, ibid., p. 62).
38 Despine, fol. 75v.
39 It was market day in Annecy and the physician could probably not wait around for him to come back, see Duverney, *La Médecine en Savoie*, p. 26.
40 Despine, fol. 6.

41 For another example, see Lemay, 'Thomas Hérier', p. 528.
42 Pichollet, p. 1.
43 Ibid.
44 On 9 September 1803, Despine records having written a letter to Mrs Meuguier about a large bill the family had owed him since 1775. He had already written a letter three years previously, see Despine, fol. 47v.
45 BGE, MS fr 5647/9, p. 30.
46 See Michael Stolberg's Chapter 1 in this book.
47 BGE, MS fr 4155, Louis Odier à Andrienne Odier Lecointe, Genève, 2 July 1787.
48 Between 1782 and 1785, Lullin had been a good client, paying three bills for a total of 50 louis courrant and 10 sols, see Rieder, 'The physician Louis Odier', p. 67.
49 ACV, PP410 C6/3/52, pp. 9–10. See Jennifer Lê, 'La Figure de l'enfant dans la famille au sortir de l'Ancien Régime. Le journal d'une mère noble de la Suisse occidentale au début du XXe siècle' (Masters Thesis, Département d'histoire générale, Université de Genève, 2014).
50 Simagrée: probably in the sense of 'to no purpose', see ACV, PP410 C6/3/52, pp. 53–5.
51 Glasgow University special collection, MS Cullen 138, Louis Odier to William Cullen, 23 August 1772.
52 The idea is discussed at the time both by Benjamin Rush and Thomas Percival, see B. Rush, 'Appendix containing observations on the duties of a physician and the methods improving medicine', in B. Rush, *Medical Enquiries and Observations* (Philadelphia: Dobson, 1794), pp. 316–25, 330; and T. Percival, *Medical Ethics, or, A Code of Institutes and Precepts Adapted to the Professional Conduct of Physicians and Surgeons* (Manchester: S. Russel, 1803), pp. 39–40. See the letter written by Louis Odier to William Cullen, 23 August 1772, printed in Rieder and Louis-Courvoisier (eds), *Les Honoraires médicaux*, pp. 167–70. On the British model, see Digby, *Making a Medical Living*, pp. 185–7; Loudon, *Medical Care*, pp. 109–25.
53 BGE, MS fr 4151, Suzanne Baux to Louis Odier, 1 October 1772. See also the letter dated 22 July.
54 He planned to ask approximately five times the price of a single visit (120 sols).
55 BGE, MS fr 5647/9, p. 12v.
56 See L. Odier, 'Second mémoire sur les professions médicales', in Rieder and Louis-Courvoisier (eds), *Les Honoraires médicaux*, p. 89.
57 Odier, 'Mémoire sur les honoraires des médecins', pp. 109–10.
58 Despine, fol. 6v.
59 Marlens is 30 km away from Annecy, Despine, fol. 45.

60 '*Miguet Jeanne Marie de Sarraval pour remèdes que je lui ai envoyé pour son mal d'yeux le 28 avril 1775*' charged 3 livres. Despine, fol. 8v; Despine, fol. 38.
61 This was confirmed in a contemporary court case, see AEG. PC 3e série 810. On practices in England, see I. Waddington, *The Medical Profession in the Industrial Revolution* (Dublin: Gill and Macmillan, 1984), pp. 10–12.
62 In Avully, a few kilometers away from Bernex where Pichollet was active, the surgeon Charles Lescureur had a 'pharmacie room' at his home, with instruments and ingredients to prepare medicines, see P. Rieder, 'La figure de l'apothicaire (1500–1800)', in P. Rieder and F. Zanetti (ed.), *Materia Medica: savoirs et usages des médicaments aux époques médiévales et modernes* (Genève: Droz, 2018), pp. 209–55, esp. 213–14.
63 Odier, 'Mémoire sur les honoraires des médecins', p. 113. His daughter confirms this practice: BGE, MS fr 5657, Souvenirs sur la vie privée de Louis Odier par Amélie Odier, t. 2, 7e cahier, p. 28.
64 On Odier's income, see Rieder, 'The physician Louis Odier', pp. 60–2 and BGE, MS fr 5656, 10e cahier. On Despine's situation, see endnote 11. The situation in Britain was similar, see M. Pelling, 'Trade or profession? Medical practice in Early Modern England', in M. Pelling, *The Common Lot, Sickness, Medical Occupations and the Urban Poor in Early Modern England* (London: Longman, 1998), pp. 230–58, esp. pp. 256–7.
65 See Lemay, 'Thomas Hérier', p. 528.
66 Musée d'histoire des sciences, Z 62, Clinical cases, 10 vols. On these volumes, see P. Rieder, 'Writing to fellow physicians: literary genres and medical questions in Louis Odier's (1748–1817) correspondence', in S. Vasset (ed.), *Medicine and Narration in the Eighteenth Century* (Oxford: Voltaire Foundation, 2013), pp. 47–63.
67 See G.B. Risse, *Hospital Life in Enlightenment Scotland: Care and Teaching at the Royal Infirmary of Edinburgh* (Cambridge: Cambridge University Press 1986), pp. 258–9.
68 MHS, Z 92/2 Diarium clinicum, starting in April 1800.
69 See BGE, MS fr 5647/9, p. 42.
70 'I know from experience that the poor love the hand that eases [their suffering] without making them feel the weight of their obligations.' BGE, MS fr 4151, Louis Odier to Suzanne Baux, 21 November 1772.
71 There is a slight exaggeration here as some rich patients paid handsomely for each service and would thus figure among the group of poor.
72 There are many examples, see for instance, BGE, MS fr 4155, Louis Odier to Andrienne Odier Lecointe, 30 July 1787.
73 Odier was thus physician to many of the prominent families in Geneva, including the Saussure family.

74 These themes have been taken up in recent research on case books, see for instance P. Klaas, H. Steinke, and A. Unterkircher, 'Daily business: The organisation and finances of doctor's practices', in M. Dinges, K.P. Jankrift, S. Schlegelmilch, and M. Stolberg (eds), *Medical Practice, 1600–1900: Physicians and their Patients* (Leiden: Brill Rodopi, 2016), pp. 71–98.
75 In contrast with the German speaking world, see P. Rieder, 'Therapeutic post-mortems in and around eighteenth-century Geneva', in S. de Renzi, M. Besadola, and M. Conforti (eds), *Pathology in Practice: Diseases and Dissections in Early Modern Europe* (London: Routledge, 2017), pp. 188–203, esp. 189–90.
76 See M. Stolberg, *Experiencing Illness and the Sick Body in Early Modern Europe* (Basingstoke: Palgrave Macmillan, 2011), p. 35; and Rieder, 'Therapeutic post-mortems', p. 191.
77 English doctors rarely kept ledgers, see Digby, *Making a Medical Living*, p. 185.
78 Pelling, 'Trade or profession', p. 236 et seq.
79 Payment systems were numerous on the medical market.
80 Local physicians had trouble earning a living as practitioners in this period and the situation was similar in provincial English towns, see H. Marland, *Medicine and Society in Wakefield and Huddersfield 1780 to 1870* (Cambridge: Cambridge University Press, 1987), pp. 291–3.
81 AEG (Terassière), 'Enregistrement et timbre', vol. 2, *Table des successions acquittées (1816–1824)*.
82 On Pichollet, see above p. 76. For Despine and Odier, see Duverney, *La Médecine en Savoie*, pp. 131–22 and Odier, 'Mémoire sur les honoraires des médecins'.
83 See Digby, *Making a Medical Living*, p. 60.
84 See I. Loudon, 'The nature of provincial medical practice in eighteenth-century England', *Medical History* 29 (1985), 1–32, esp. 1.
85 See Digby, *Making a Medical Living*, p. 37.

3

Accounted bodies and counted cases: Elliott Joslin's diabetes research, 1898–1950

Oliver Falk

After a long drive in May 1924, 46-year-old salesman Mr Rainsford from Maine did not feel very well. An unusual weakness and fatigue had taken hold of him, coupled with great thirst and hunger and an uncomfortable need to urinate. Worried about his physical well-being, he went to see a general practitioner who, apparently attentive to the symptoms, ordered a urine sugar test. The test result resolved any doubts: Rainsford suffered from diabetes mellitus. We know nothing more about the beginnings of Rainsford's 'diabetic career'. It is certain, however, that he began treatment under the most renowned US diabetes specialist of the day, Elliott Proctor Joslin (1869–1962), about one year later in March 1925.[1] From their first encounter in Joslin's practice on Bay State Road in Boston, a 21-year-long doctor–patient relationship emerged that exemplifies how Joslin linked the individual treatment of every single patient to diabetes research using a system of medical recordkeeping that allowed him to compare, aggregate, and statistically analyse patient data. Every patient treated by Joslin was not just someone to whom he sought to deliver the best possible treatment, but also party to his declared goal of 'victory over diabetes'. Every patient counted – literally!

Since the beginning of Joslin's interest in diabetes as a young student in 1893, he believed that its highly uncertain aetiology, classification, treatment, and prognosis was attributable to unsystematic data that rarely included more than autopsy logs and bedside observations.[2] Challenged by the outcomes of his first diabetic patients, he began systematically registering his patients in large ledgers, the so-called black books, and would continue to do so for the next six decades.[3] By the time of his death in 1962, Joslin had recorded around 50,000 diabetes cases in eight volumes of ledgers. For each of these entries, a patient file was created and filled with medical records, test results, charts, dietary prescriptions, follow-up information, and correspondences with his patients. This remarkable collection reflected Joslin's precise and well-ordered file keeping, which was meant to facilitate an 'intelligent management' of diabetes cases and thus ensure the proper treatment of diabetic patients by 'eliminating some of the annoying sources of errors.'[4] According to Joslin, these errors arose from an insufficient and inefficient recordkeeping practice that not only endangered the already fragile well-being of diabetic patients, but also made a thorough scientific evaluation impossible. Patient data were 'often printed or written down in four or five different places, and the labor of uniting them is so great that it is seldom attempted. Any accurate study of a case is thus extremely difficult.'[5] Joslin's goal was therefore to counteract this problem by standardising his patient records in a way that could be described as efficient medical accounting.

Unlike the other contributions in this Part, this chapter does not deal with accounting practices in a classical sense, i.e. as a financial or moral reckoning of income and expenses in a private practice (see Rieder's Chapter 2 and/or Stolberg's Chapter 1), but instead highlights the accounting and similar calculative practices used in treatment and research. Because accounting can be defined as a 'systematic process of identifying, recording, measuring, classifying, verifying, summarizing, interpreting and communicating financial information'[6] and in view of Michael Powers's statement that accounting isn't necessarily subordinate to economics,[7] Joslin's efforts to systematise his medical records combined more or less all of these aspects and can, therefore, count as (medical) accounting. Moreover, the calculative and accounting aspects in this chapter are related to the specificities of diabetes as a metabolic disorder and its underlying therapeutic rationalities. Diabetes therapy was and still is a calculative practice that incorporates techniques for measuring, calculating, and balancing the elements (for example, nutrients like fats, carbohydrates, or proteins) entering the organism and those leaving it, the relationship between those elements and the body's energy exchanges, and finally the effects of different states of nourishment, rest, exercise, age, health, and disease.[8]

But because diabetes was intrinsically linked to the complexities of human metabolism, it seemed almost impossible to establish a therapeutic standard or reliable prognoses. Thus, Joslin stated that 'there is no one symptom always present and indeed there are many diabetics who have no symptoms at all'.[9] How then could the infinite variety of diabetes and the associated impossibility of reliable prognoses be addressed and translated into a therapeutic standard? Joslin's answer was: 'One cannot standardize treatment. Each case must be individualized.'[10] Individualising cases meant actively involving patients in their treatment using techniques of self-measurement and self-control, making them into 'accountants' of their bodies.

Drawing on documents in the Joslin Diabetes Center,[11] as well as on Joslin's published manuals, textbooks, and early seminal articles, I shall, first, show how Joslin's patient registration system evolved and how these systematised patient files were used to compare cases and evaluate new therapies. I will then show how Joslin believed that addressing diabetes as a socio-medical problem required the cooperation of physicians, government authorities, life insurance companies, and patients themselves. Finally, I intend to focus on Joslin's relationship with his patients and how the qualitative and quantitative information he gathered could be used in therapy and research.

Comparing cases

Although Joslin's first entry dates back to 1893, it was not until 1908[12] that he systematised his notes, which had previously only 'consisted of simple and terse notes jotted onto index cards.'[13] A crucial catalyst for this change was his trip to Europe in 1907, which took him to Berlin, Munich, Vienna, and Strasbourg. There he met a number of mainly German clinicians studying diabetes. In particular, the meeting with Bernhard Naunyn (1839–1925) in Strasbourg shaped Joslin's further therapeutic thinking and recordkeeping techniques. In his memoirs, Naunyn recalled that Joslin asked him if he could come to Strasbourg to learn about his diabetes treatment. Naunyn agreed and seemed to be impressed of the young zealous American: 'He came directly from Boston to Strasbourg' Naunyn remembered and 'stayed little more than three weeks, but by using my extensive material and with his great eagerness he became familiar with my ideas and maxims in short time.'[14]

In Strasbourg, Joslin became convinced of the advantages of early and strict dietary treatment as well as of a file management system. That system now became the hallmark of his practice: no longer would he simply adapt new therapeutic approaches, but instead investigate their efficiency using his own cases. Accordingly, a few years later Joslin claimed that 'whenever I see the enthusiastic report of a new drug or remedy employed in the treatment of diabetes, certain cases of my own [...] come to mind. First of all I critically examine the data relating to the new methods, and then compare the results with the cases, which I have had under my eyes for years.'[15]

Exactly what this meant for Joslin can be seen in two articles published in 1913 and 1915, shortly after his European visits. They represent Joslin's first attempts to promote a case-based approach to compare the efficiency of past and present treatment methods. The 1913 article set out his idea of *diabetic standard cases*, which were designed to make his own treatment methods comparable to other therapeutic approaches. Since treatment with a new remedy usually lasted only a few weeks, rarely months, and almost never for years, Joslin selected cases of long duration, 'extending respectively over fifteen, twenty, thirteen, seven, twelve, three and eleven months, nineteen, and six years'.[16] Moreover, he selected eight cases of different age, sex, and severity, and subjected them to the same dietary regime of 100–150 grams of carbohydrates, which were gradually lowered until the sugar disappeared from their urine.[17] For each of the cases, he drew up detailed charts and tables that joined all the main test results, such as the urine volume in cubic centimetres and its sugar content in per cent and total grams, the amount of diacetic acid, the exact carbohydrate intake, and the patient's weight. The aim of this first systematic observation and evaluation was to describe the disease's further course through varying degrees of severity under a strict dietary regime and thus to draw more general conclusions about the efficiency of different therapeutic approaches.

However, Joslin's first attempt produced little information, as he was able to compare only a small number of cases and at that time had only incomplete data on the patients and the previous course of their illnesses and treatments. Joslin was well aware of these flaws, but he was convinced that 'each physician should have his own standard diabetic cases. This will enable him to compare the results of his past and present methods of treatment, and show him when to relinquish his own methods in favour of those of other men. Such comparisons unconsciously lead to better records of cases, and stimulate to better work.'[18]

Shortly thereafter, Joslin wrote another article in which he dealt with the results of the so-called starvation diet of the American physician Frederick Allen.[19] From 1914 onward, Joslin adopted the Allen diet, which consisted mainly of extremely low levels of carbohydrates, protein, and fat.[20] Allen highlighted the advantages of sugar-free urine, accepting the simultaneous inanition of his patients. At a time when most diabetic patients survived for only a few months, it seemed a reasonable price to pay, although he admitted that 'it was no fun to starve a child to let him live.'[21] In the twelve months from May 1914 to May 1915, Joslin reviewed, investigated, and compared 211 cases of which fifty-five had fasted.[22] Of these fifty-five patients, six had died, which, according to Joslin's calculations, resulted in a mortality rate of 10.9 per cent compared to 14.7 per cent of his other cases (see Figure 3.1). Based on this lower mortality rate and despite the fact that his first use of the Allen diet was by no means successful[23] and had produced widely different results depending on the severity of the illness, Joslin was sure that prolonged fasting produced results 'far and away ahead of any method' and that 'thanks to Dr. Frederick M. Allen we no longer nurse diabetics – we treat them!'[24] In addition to enthusiastically endorsing Allen's fasting diet, this article also illustrates several adjustments that Joslin made to improve diabetes therapy. Not only did he now compare several dozen cases (instead of just eight), but for the first time he explicitly emphasised the value of involving patients in treatment. Thoroughly educating them, guiding them, and following-up on their treatment[25] would not only ensure therapeutic success, but also make information 'available for statistics'.[26]

Cooperating with life insurance companies

Therapeutic developments around the late 1910s and early 1920s inspired Joslin's belief that diabetes needed to be regarded as a public health issue and addressed from a more rigorously epidemiological perspective. Newer treatment methods and improved examination technologies had brought with them, as Joslin found in his own practice, rising numbers of diabetic patients. Although the reasons for this rise in case numbers were relatively clear,[27] the emerging socio-medical

Cases	Total	Treated	Dead		Alive	
			No.	Percent	No.	Percent
Total	211	211	31	14,7	180	85,3
Old cases before May 1914	75	75	11	14,7	64	85,3
New cases since May 1914	136	136	20	14,7	116	85,3
Fasted	55	55	6	10,9	49	89,1
Not fasted						

3.1 Cases under observation 1 May 1914 to 1 May 1915.

consequences were incalculable. How could this 'growing army of diabetics'[28] be adequately addressed, especially since there were no reliable statistics on the total number of cases in the US or elsewhere? Accordingly, in 1921 Joslin expressed concern that the increase in case numbers over the last thirty years indicated that 'the outlook for the future would be startling'; the treatment of diabetes was a serious problem not only for the patients themselves but 'for the nation at large'.[29] Joslin concluded that one of the most urgent problems was to accurately estimate the total number of cases, since knowledge about them would determine the 'character of treatment'.[30] But this was by no means an easy task, especially since diabetes could be present even without symptoms. This was not only challenging in therapeutic terms, but also aggravated the profoundly difficult statistical recording of diabetes cases. Joslin therefore sought out partners who could help him address the problem, happening – not quite by chance – on the life insurance industry.

While re-evaluating his cases, Joslin found that seventy-six diagnoses had been reached at the behest of life insurance companies.[31] Furthermore, he found that the course of these cases was particularly favourable relative to many other cases. He attributed this to the early recognition of the disease, which would otherwise have been discovered only at the onset of the first symptoms and not of the disease itself. Since the 'Naunyn era', early recognition and subsequent rigorous therapeutic intervention had been recognised as a prerequisite for a favourable prognosis, but the question arose as to how to detect prodromal symptoms. To a certain extent, Joslin saw life insurance companies as being able to do this, especially since more and more of the US population was 'undergoing such examinations'.[32] 'The only way in which early diagnosis of diabetes will ever be made is to search for it. […] It is a hopeful sign that the insurance companies are offering to examine the urine of their policy holders gratis at frequent intervals. Everyone should have the urine examined upon his birthday.'[33]

However, Joslin not only envisioned the possibilities of earlier and therefore better therapeutic intervention, but also recognised the opportunity to collect more reliable data. Then as now, the slow and often unnoticed onset of diabetes was not just a therapeutic problem, but a statistical one as well when it came to accurately assessing the overall number of diabetics. Joslin hoped that by collaborating with insurance companies he would gain access to their statistical material for his own investigations, elicit the support of their statisticians in analysing his data, and explore the possibility of joint education campaigns.[34]

In the years that followed, Joslin intensified his informal cooperation with various life insurance companies, such as the New England Life Insurance Company[35] and the Metropolitan Life Insurance Company, and reached an official cooperation agreement with Met Life in 1931. In response to a letter from Joslin, Met Life's third Vice-President and statistician, Dr Louis Dublin, wrote that he was convinced 'that the diabetes problem is becoming more and more important and that in the next ten years, it is likely to take on a significance not much less than tuberculosis' and that his insurance company was glad to collaborate with Joslin's office.[36] Subsequently, the Insurance Welfare Committee also provided funding of 2,000 US-Dollars for the 'continuation of the several projects of mutual interest in the field of diabetes'.[37] In cooperation with Met Life, however, Joslin was less interested in financial support. A far more pressing problem for Joslin and many other contemporary biomedical researchers was the ever-increasing amount of data that could no longer be adequately analysed without deep knowledge of statistical methods. Or as the British geneticist and statistician Ronald Aylmer Fisher put it in his widely acclaimed book on *Statistical Methods for Research Workers* in 1925: 'Often analysis of large masses of data by statistical methods is necessary, and the biological worker is continually encountering advanced statistical problems the adequate solutions of which are not found in current statistical text-books.'[38]

According to a study commissioned in 2003 by Donald Barnett, Joslin too faced the problem of incorrectly conducted statistical calculations.[39] It is unclear whether Joslin was aware of this problem, or whether he simply did not want to be exposed to the 'great pains' of statistical case analysis.[40] In any case, from the 1930s onward, experts took over the statistical evaluation of his cases. This became particularly clear in the preface to the textbook's eighth edition in 1946, in which he thanked 'the Metropolitan Life Insurance Company through its Vice-President and Statistician, Dr. Louis Dublin […], the Massachusetts State Department of Health through Dr. Herbert Lombard, and the aid of officials of the U.S. Bureau of the Census' for their help in compiling the statistics.[41] Above all, however, Joslin was convinced that this eighth edition reflected Josiah Royce's principle of the 'fecundity of aggregation' because 'it represents the efforts and contribution of patients and doctors, of many, many clinicians throughout the world [and other] collaborators.'[42]

But patients themselves were the decisive factor in thorough and systematic data collection. Thanks to more effective therapeutic approaches based on recent findings in nutritional physiology (*Ernährungsphysiologie*), combined with improved measurement technologies that could be easily applied outside of laboratories by educated lay people, diabetic patients now became increasingly able to treat themselves and to control their prescribed therapies. Joslin was one of the keenest advocates of a medically controlled self-treatment of diabetics. He recognised the possibilities that arose from their active involvement in a therapeutic routine based on calculative practices, in which data on individual dietary intake and output, as well as other external factors affecting the impaired metabolism, could be collected regularly by patients themselves. Their participation would not only lead to more complete case histories and thus help to adjust therapeutic measures, but also facilitate in-depth research of the disease itself. In other words, it allowed him to observe the disease in everyday life.

'Go thou and do likewise' – Patients' contributions

In March 1920, 79-year-old Louisa Drumm came to Joslin's office with diabetes. After the usual examination and treatment suggestions, she was taught to examine her urine. She was then sent home and died of pneumonia a few days later. But in the meantime, she had examined the urine of ten other members of her household and discovered diabetes in a boy who then turned to Joslin for treatment and recounted this story.[43] This was exactly the sort of commitment that Joslin hoped to receive from his patients and from diabetics in general. As important as the collaboration between laboratories, clinics, life insurance, specialists, and general practitioners might be, Joslin believed that it was the diabetics themselves who would make the most important contributions to a 'victory over diabetes'. Joslin's rallying cry was therefore not just a rhetorical question, but also a moral call to action, '[c]an one not appropriately say to younger diabetic patients: "Go thou and do likewise"?'[44]

At least since the 1920s, Joslin had been convinced that diabetics should be their 'own nurse, the doctor's assistant and chemist'.[45] Given the steadily rising population of diabetics, the opportunities for further therapeutic improvements lay mainly outside of hospitals, namely in the homes of diabetics and the offices of their physicians. However, Joslin knew that the success of hospital treatment could not be transferred easily into private practice. The secret to the success of hospitals, he emphasised, 'lies in the close and continuous observation of the patient by the doctor. For success in home treatment, close and continuous observation of the patient by himself under the systematic guidance of a physician is just as essential.'[46] In order to guarantee this success, Joslin distinguished three groups of diabetics, emphasising their different treatment contexts according to the severity of the disease. The first group was comprised of diabetics who needed hospital care; the second included ambulatory cases who required initial treatment or an adjustment to their treatment and who could be housed in less expensive hospital beds, nursing homes, or even in families of trained diabetics; the third and largest group included patients who could be cared for by visiting the doctor's office, like Joslin's private practice.[47]

Office treatment

But successful treatment in doctors' offices required both patients' active cooperation as well as standardised recording and registration practices, which ensured the patients' safety as well as that their data was comparable, consolidated, and aggregated. Both of these aspects were inseparable for Joslin, as I shall demonstrate. He realised the epistemic possibility that arose from the socio-medical necessity of guided self-treatment, insofar as this gave way to 'diabetes field work'. However, this could only succeed if the patients were able to understand the necessity of their participation and thus, ideally, a regular exchange of information between doctor and patient could be established. 'The investigators and the patient considered themselves united in a partnership, having for its object the accumulation of knowledge for the benefit of all diabetics rather than for the given individual under investigation in particular.'[48]

In this sense, the accumulation of knowledge started with a thorough and standardised examination. Information about each single case would be gathered so that it could be compared with others, specifically with regard to anamnesis criteria; that is, the occurrence and course of the disease, the corresponding dispositions, i.e. heredity or possible risk factors, the results of the first physical examination, the further course of prescribed therapy, and so on. Joslin hoped that by comparing cases he could draw more general conclusions about the success of specific therapeutic approaches and at the same time investigate the disease and its course under specific conditions. In addition to the physical examination, Joslin's case recording included as much information about the living circumstances of his patients as possible. Especially the diabetic's first visit placed demands on all the resources of the doctor at his best:[49]

> He must learn the personal and family background of the patient and its relation to his constitution at the moment. There will be plenty of psychological problems to be met, but fascinating as these are and easy to elicit they must not divert the physician from acquiring a complete knowledge of the patients' physical status. […] During the first visit in the course of history taking and the physical and chemical examination

the endeavour is made to secure data, which will establish an absolute diagnosis.[50]

This first physical examination was accompanied by the patient's administrative registration, which was no less essential to Joslin's agenda. The registration forms, which were designed to make all information available at a glance, numbered patients consecutively. Their number did not change, regardless of whether a document was related to therapeutic or administrative concerns. All subsidiary records, such as laboratory or x-ray results, letters, prescriptions, follow-up information, or patients' account information, including billing information, included this specific number. 'Inasmuch as correct registration of the patient is essential to having proper records, it is recommended that every patient be registered. [...] This registration form should be numbered which will always be the number for that patient.'[51]

It is therefore no coincidence that we know so much about Mr Rainsford, patient number 4,465. When he entered Joslin's office on 27 March 1925, two men met who, although they could hardly have been more different, shared some sympathy for one other. On the one hand, Joslin was an ascetic physician, studded with puritanical earnestness and a zeal for work, who had taken a vow of temperance as a young boy, renouncing alcohol and excessive enjoyment or luxury and subordinating almost everything to his work. By contrast, Rainsford was a salesman who was on the road most of the year for various companies. By his own account, he had been a keen motorist since 1910, spending a lot of time in hotels, enjoying good food and alcohol, smoking at least a pack of Lucky Strikes every day, and paying for his lifestyle with a portly physique. By Joslin's medical reckoning, he must have been a 'perfect' candidate for diabetes because of his unhealthy lifestyle, bad habits, lack of exercise, and weight.[52]

Upon entering Joslin's practice on Bay State Road, was Mr Rainsford aware of the seriousness of his situation and of what would be expected of him? Probably not! If he had ever heard of diabetes before, then it was certainly because of the groundbreaking discovery that several Canadian researchers had made some three years earlier and for which they had received the Nobel Prize.[53] Wasn't there now an effective miracle cure for diabetes with this new drug insulin? And wasn't Joslin the most famous diabetes specialist on the East Coast, indeed the whole

US, with decades of experience treating this disease? So, wasn't there every reason to be optimistic about successfully addressing this ailment and continuing with normal life? Joslin, a man with a penchant for straight talk, might have responded to commonplace questions with: yes, but!

> *Yes*, 'the discovery of Insulin is a great boon [...].'[54] *But* 'Insulin does not cure diabetes.'[55]
>
> *Yes*, guidance by a physician is needed because if a patient 'tries to be his own doctor, he will come to grief'.[56] *But* 'there is no disease in which an understanding by the patient of the methods of treatment avails as much. Brain counts.'[57]
>
> *Yes*, a diabetic can live an almost normal and useful life *but* 'the treatment of a patient with diabetes lasts a long time. Consequently, the patient must be taught the nature of the disease and how to conquer it.'[58]

Joslin certainly didn't want to discourage his patients. Rather, this advice was an essential part of a patient's initial examination. For him, educating patients was a fundamental and revolutionary therapeutic approach and the best chance of surviving diabetes as long as possible without any symptoms or complications.[59] This included a profound knowledge about the disease itself and – even more importantly – practical skills for self-treatment like testing urine for sugar, computing and recording dietary summaries, knowing when and how to inject oneself with insulin (after 1922), and recognising the signs of too much or too little insulin. In his *Diabetic Manual for the Mutual Use of Doctor and Patient*, published in several editions since 1918, Joslin set out three principles that illustrate both his therapeutic beliefs and his underlying research agenda. Joslin was convinced that:

> [f]irst, every [...] patient can master his disease if he so wills, second, that his own length of days after his diabetes begins is in some degree a measure of the success he achieves, third, that he has an excellent chance by living long and well <u>to be an explorer of regions</u> of diabetes, <u>hitherto unknown</u>, and thus open up trails toward health and the cure of diabetes which others can more easily follow.[60]

However, Joslin's unknown regions could be reached only if patients stuck to the prescribed therapy, which included a variety of self-care routines. In this sense, Joslin's emphasis on patient responsibility was less concerned with a new understanding of the doctor–patient relationship that would empower diabetics to play a more active role in treatment. Rather, it expressed a growing understanding of the nature of the disease itself and the associated early twentieth-century therapeutic options.

Office efficacy

When patients visited Joslin's office, they were expected to provide important information about their urine and diet, the units of insulin they had administered, as well as any reactions to it or other complications that might have arisen. Joslin therefore strongly encouraged his patients to learn as much as possible about the disease, its treatment, and possible complications. Above all, a patient should know how:

1. to test urine for sugar
2. to record his diet
3. to explain the quantity of carbohydrate in it
4. to measure out his prescribed dose of insulin and to know when and where to inject it[61]
5. to describe what he is to do if sugar returns
6. to describe what he is to do if he feels sick
7. to describe an insulin reaction – symptoms, cause, prevention, and treatment
8. to state the danger of (a) too much insulin, and (b) its total omission
9. to care for his feet and explain the reason why
10. to fill out his identification card.[62]

Joslin's list was by no means arbitrary. It clearly presented a hierarchy of practices that his patients needed to learn. In addition to more general behavioural recommendations, testing urine sugar and correctly calculating the diet were the crucial practices entailed by therapeutic individualisation and knowledge-generating considerations. A precisely calculated and prescribed diet, as well as more subjective descriptions of a patient's general condition, could thus be related to each other, could if necessary facilitate further therapeutic systematisation, and could also help draw general conclusions for specific therapeutic approaches compared to other cases. This required not only a sufficient number of cases but also a uniform method of information extraction and data collection. Finally, each patient, including Rainsford, was instructed to keep his own notebook, or at least to note the diet, exercise, and, if prescribed, the units of insulin, as well as the Benedict test results. The therapeutic benefits were obvious. In other words, patients became accountants of their own body, controlling their intake and output and trying to keep everything in balance.

> It's a good plan to start a notebook at the first day of treatment. [...] The notebook should contain a statement as too whether sugar has been present or absent in the urine since the last report to the physician. Such data can be gathered on one page. [...] Furthermore, it is a great advantage [...] to keep a notebook, because gradually it becomes valuable for references, and his whole plan of treatment is systematized.[63]

Ideally, this notebook would serve as a personal manual for its patient and help the doctor evaluate the therapy. To ensure the greatest possible uniformity for information and data gathering, Joslin drew up guidelines for patients visiting his office. Even if the treatment itself could not be standardised, at least the examination could.

The first point dealt with 'Information obtained by examination of the Urine'[64] since knowledge about whether a patient's urine was sugar-free or not was essential in order to prescribe a diet or insulin. Patients were required to bring not only information but also a urine sample taken within the last 24 hours. To ensure the integrity of the sample, Joslin expected his patients 'to collect such a specimen [...], discard that voided at 7 A.M. and then save all urine passed up to and including that obtained at 7 the next morning. Take 60 cc. (2 ounces) of the thoroughly mixed twenty-four-hour quantity for examination. Record the twenty-four-hour amount of urine, the date, and the name of the bottle.'[65]

In addition, patients were encouraged to regularly check and record their urine content and communicate it to the doctor. A convenient method of reporting on urine samples was as shown in Figure 3.2.

Given the qualitative colour scale of this so-called Benedict's test,[66] quantifiable blood sugar concentrations could be estimated relatively accurately. For patients, this test served as a quick overview – like a traffic light – indicating dangerous or harmless sugar concentration; for

Date	Morning	Afternoon	Evening	Night
January 1	Red	Orange	Yellow	Green
January 2	R	Or	Y	G
January 3	Y	G	B	B
January 4	B	B	B	B

3.2 Reporting scheme for results of urine sugar tests.

physicians, it provided a relatively accurate depiction of the development of an individual's sugar concentration. Whereas a blue colour indicated no sugar, green tones signalled traces of sugar between 0.1–0.5 per cent, yellow to orange a concentration of 0.5–2 per cent, and red an alarming blood sugar concentration of over 2 per cent. The purpose of this examination routine was to learn what portion of the carbohydrates in the diet had been assimilated by the body by calculating the difference between the total quantity of sugar in the urine and the carbohydrates in the diet. It was therefore also important to record the quality and quantity of food eaten during the same period.

Joslin standardised the recording of urine test results using a 'urine test report card'.[67] Test results were to be recorded before breakfast, the noon meal, supper, and at bedtime. If possible, Joslin also had patients record their weight after fasting and, preferably undressed, on the morning of their visit.[68] This made it possible to correlate all the values with each other and to calculate the efficiency of the diet and, if necessary, adjust it. Joslin called this intelligent management, i.e. the 'frequent comparison between the diet, the urinary analysis and the weight of the patient'.[69] And this daily monitoring system provided the feedback necessary for therapeutic and prognostic adjustments.[70]

How this worked in daily practice can be shown using the example of Mr Rainsford. As a patient who dealt with the up and downs of daily life with diabetes in self-deprecating cartoons,[71] Rainsford's recordkeeping surely didn't match Joslin's idea of a systematic chart (see Figure 3.3). Nevertheless, it contained all the necessary information: the actual weight of 175 pounds, the foods eaten, and the Benedict test results. The calculation was based on the caloric content of the food eaten and it distinguished between the three major food groups (carbohydrates,

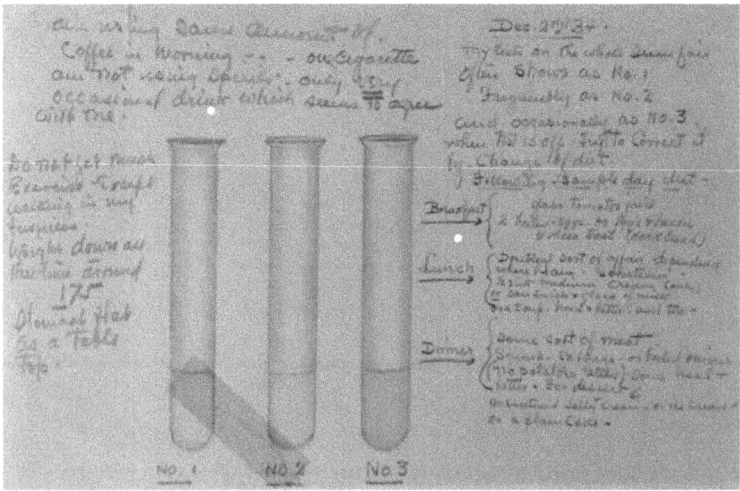

3.3 Drawing by Mr Rainsford showing the colours (no. 1 blue, no. 2 green, no. 3 light orange) of his urine sample in correlation with his daily diet. Copyright © Joslin Diabetes Center. All rights reserved. Reprinted with permission.

proteins, and fats) as specified by Max Rubner (1854–1932).[72] In the chapter on 'diabetic arithmetic', Joslin summarised this as follows:

  1 gram carbohydrate = 4 Calories
  1 gram protein   = 4 Calories
  1 gram fat   = 9 Calories.

In order to calculate the total amount of calories, the corresponding food groups would be determined and weighed. To ease the calculations for patients and physicians, so-called equivalency tables could be used (see Figure 3.4). In an easily understandable way, a certain number of grams of a common food (10, 15, or 30 g) were compared with the corresponding proportion of carbohydrates, protein, and fat, as well as with the calories of the food. 'Knowing the total quantity of each variety of food eaten by the patient during the day, by using table of food values,' Joslin explained, 'one can determine the amount of carbohydrates, protein and fat for each given food.'[73]

For example, if Rainsford had two boiled eggs, a slice of bacon, and two slices of toasted dark bread for breakfast, then he could calculate

TABLE 4.—THE QUANTITY OF CARBOHYDRATE, PROTEIN AND FAT AND THE CALORIC VALUE OF 30 GRAMS (1 OUNCE) OF FOODS IN COMMON USE.

30 grams (1 ounce) contain approximately:	Carbo-hydrate, grams.	Protein, grams.	Fat, grams.	Calories.
Vegetables, 5 per cent	1.0	0.5	0	6
Vegetables, 10 per cent	2.0	0.5	0	10
Potato	6.0	1.0	0	28
Bread	18.0	3.0	0	84
Uneeda Biscuits, 2	10.0	1.0	1	53
Oatmeal, dry weight	20.0	5.0	2	118
Shredded Wheat, 1	23.0	3.0	0	104
Milk	1.5	1.0	1	19
Meat, cooked, lean	0.0	8.0	5	77
Fish, fat-free	0.0	6.0	0	24
Chicken, cooked, lean	0.0	8.0	3	59
Egg, 1	0.0	6.0	6	78
Cheese	0.0	8.0	11	131
Bacon	0.0	5.0	15	155
Cream, 20 per cent	1.0	1.0	6	62
Cream, 40 per cent	1.0	1.0	12	116
Butter	0.0	0.0	25	225
Oil	0.0	0.0	30	270

3.4 Equivalency table for determining the quantities of carbohydrates, fats, and proteins and their caloric value in common foods.

the amount of carbohydrates (36 g), fat (19.6 g), protein (17.5 g), as well as the total number of ingested calories (401 cal). In this way, patients could control their own diet and physicians could extract useful therapeutic information. In addition, this form of monitoring enabled data to be collected not only during routine examinations, but anytime and anywhere, which was an invaluable advantage for laboratory and clinical examination routines.

Follow up

Joslin was also convinced that a 'physician must do everything in his power to keep in touch with his patients in regular intervals.'[74] He wanted to examine his patients at least every three, but usually every two months.[75] But that was not always easy because many of them lived and worked outside Boston and had to pay their travel expenses in addition to Joslin's fee.[76] Such economic burdens were especially acute during the Great Depression of the 1930s. Nevertheless, Joslin developed a follow-up method of bilateral exchange: on the one hand, physicians would inform patients by letter about test results and possible therapeutic adjustments; and on the other hand, patients could request from physicians information about their state of health. Joslin asked all his patients to write to him about their general condition, the amount of sugar in their urine, their weight, their exercise regime, and sometimes the dosage of insulin they had injected.[77] These bilateral exchanges helped Joslin underscore his therapeutic concern for each individual case and engender trust among his patients at a time when general information about diabetes and its therapy was largely unavailable to laymen. It therefore comes as no surprise that the letters Joslin received from his patients not only contained the information he wanted, but also frequently other questions and complaints about the private everyday concerns and needs of a diabetic's life.

Even after a patient died, Joslin tried to get all of the information he needed for his research. 'The follow-up of fatal cases is fundamental' Joslin stated, because 'this discloses what the enemy is and where the fight is fiercest.'[78] Thus, Joslin was convinced that 'a diabetic who dies without investigation of the ultimate cause has failed to render that service to his fellow men to which they are entitled.'[79] A letter dated 17 September 1946 to the Registrar of Vital Statistics in Dover-Foxtrot, Maine reveals that Rainsford did not fail in his service. Joslin wrote:

> Dear Sir,
> It has come to my attention that a former patient, Mr Guy L. Rainsford, died in May 1946. Would you be kind enough to tell me the date and the cause of death, in order to complete my records? Sincerely yours, EPJ

The response to this letter provided the information Joslin had requested. Mr Rainsford had died on 1 May 1946 of chronic nephritis due to diabetes mellitus and myocarditis hypertension.[80] This information was recorded onto standardised so-called post-treatment cards, which again at a glance made all the essential information available for later evaluations and closed the respective patient's file (Figure 3.5).

Joslin's professional diligence and empathy led him to take every individual patient seriously without losing sight of the big picture. In

3.5 Post-treatment history of patient no. 16158 (front and back side). These file cards brought together registration categories, examination results, and the cause of death onto a single card. Copyright © Joslin Diabetes Center. All rights reserved. Reprinted with permission.

1946, true to his therapeutic convictions, he surveyed the future course of diabetes research and therapy:

> Hitherto we have almost specialized in the follow-up of fatal cases, but from now onwards the purpose of tracing will be to protect the patients during life and to learn from their physical condition in the later years of their disease how treatment can be improved, rather than simply to record the lesson learned by their deaths. [...] The lives of these peoples must be preserved, but they must yield dividends of health for all. These patients are under constant supervision. Here is the opportunity for health examinations and health studies on a vast scale.[81]

Accounting for health

This chapter aimed to show how Joslin used calculative, accounting, and managerial practices for both therapeutic and scientific purposes. For him, therapy and research were not mutually exclusive. On the contrary, he was convinced that both were closely related. Research (especially laboratory research) without therapeutic ends was as meaningless as therapeutic measures that could not contribute to the process of generating medical knowledge. The prerequisite for this, however, was what Joslin called 'intelligent (case) management', meaning a systematic collection, aggregation, classifying, and evaluation of all available data – data that could be obtained and processed in cooperative collaboration between physicians, hospitals and out-patient clinics, life insurance companies, and not least patients. In a broad sense, Joslin was 'accounting for health' in two ways. On the one hand, he accounted for the individual patient body and its impaired metabolism by measuring and balancing energy input and output, thus controlling a physiological whole by means of calculative practices. And on the other hand, he accounted for thousands of patient records and their statistical processing and evaluation.

Unlike practitioners elsewhere (see Chapter 2), financial aspects played only a minor role for Joslin. He interpreted payments and donations as fiscal and moral support and as a sign of commitment in the fight against diabetes. His social status, his puritanism, and his utilitarian thinking shaped and characterised his medical practice, thus reflecting the therapeutic, epistemological, and not least moral dimensions of accounting practices and their medically productive as well as normative character.

Notes

1 See the medical certificate dated 29 September 1944, Joslin Diabetes Center Historical Archive (JDCHA), Box 20, Folder 6.
2 See, for example, his study with Reginald Fitz in 1898 on the medical records at Massachusetts General Hospital between 1824 and 1898. In over seventy years, only 172 cases were recorded, see R. Fitz and E. Joslin, *Diabetes Mellitus at the Massachusetts General Hospital from 1824 to 1898. A Study of the Medical Records* (Chicago: American Medical Association Press, 1898).
3 These included a total of seventeen columns which registered: 1) Patient number, 2) Date of the first visit, 3) Name and address, 4) Assumed date of the disease onset, 5) Diagnosis, 6) Duration, 7) Sex, 8) Marital status, 9) Race, 10) Heredity, 11) Familial disposal, 12) Aetiology (obesity, infections, other causes), 13) Physical conditions, 14) Type of onset (gradual or acute), 15) Hospital, 16) Cause of death, 17) Distinctive features.
4 E. Joslin and H. Goodall, 'A diabetic chart', *Boston Medical and Surgical Journal* 158 (1908), 248–51, here 248–9.
5 Ibid.
6 See the article 'Accounting', in www.businessdictionary.com/definition/accounting.html [accessed 15 July 2018].
7 M. Power, 'From science of accounts to financial accountability of science', *Science in Context* 7:3 (1994), 355–87, here 357.
8 See F.L. Holmes, *Between Biology and Medicine: The Formation of Intermediary Metabolism, four Lectures Delivered at the International Summer School in History of Science* (Berkeley: Office for History of Science and Technology, 1992), pp. 82–3.
9 E. Joslin, *A Diabetic Manual for the Mutual Use of Doctor and Patient* (Philadelphia: Lea & Febiger, 4th edn, 1929), p. 20.
10 E. Joslin, *The Treatment of Diabetes Mellitus* (Philadelphia: Lea & Febiger, 8th edn, 1946), pp. 339–40.
11 I am most grateful for the assistance of Matthew Brown and Dr Donald Barnett, who facilitated my archival research and shared his insights about the history of the Joslin Diabetes Center.
12 Joslin and Goodall, 'A diabetic chart'.
13 C. Feudtner, *Bittersweet: Diabetes, Insulin, and the Transformation of Illness* (Chapel Hill: University of North Carolina Press, 2003), p. 47.

14 B. Naunyn, *Erinnerungen, Gedanken und Meinungen* (Heidelberg: Springer, 1925), pp. 446–7.
15 E. Joslin, 'Diabetic Standards', *American Journal of the Medical Science* 145:4 (1913), 474–86.
16 Ibid., 475.
17 Ibid., 476.
18 Ibid., 475 [author's highlights].
19 E. Joslin, 'Present-day treatment and prognosis in diabetes', *American Journal of the Medical Science* 150:4 (1915), 485–96.
20 On Allen's diet in general, see F.M. Allen, 'Prolonged fasting in diabetes', *The American Journal of the Medical Sciences* 150:4 (1915), 480–5. For a historiographical review, see A. Mazur, 'Why were "starvation diets" promoted for diabetes in the pre-insulin period?' *Nutrition Journal* 10:23 (2011), doi: 10.1186/1475-2891-10-23.
21 E. Joslin, 'The diabetic', *The Canadian Medical Association Journal* 48:6 (1943), 488–97, here 491.
22 E. Joslin, 'Present-day treatment and prognosis in diabetes', *American Journal of the Medical Science* 150:4 (1915), 485–96, here 486.
23 E. Joslin, F.G. Brigham, and A.A. Hornor, 'An analysis of fourteen cases of diabetes mellitus unsuccessfully treated by fasting', *The Boston Medical and Surgical Journal* 174:12 (1916), 371–8.
24 Joslin, 'Present-day treatment and prognosis in diabetes', 486.
25 Ibid., 495.
26 Ibid., 486.
27 Three points were particularly crucial for Joslin: 1) greater accuracy of vital statistics, 2) more frequent urinary examinations, 3) general increase in duration of life, see E. Joslin's chapter on 'Increase in the incidence of diabetes mellitus', in Joslin, *The Treatment of Diabetes Mellitus* (2nd edn), pp. 19–28.
28 Estimates varied considerably between 100,000 and 1,000,000 diabetics in the US. Joslin assumed that the number was 'much nearer to 1,000,000 than to 100,000', in Joslin, *The Treatment of Diabetes Mellitus* (2nd edn), p. 25.
29 Ibid., preface.
30 Ibid., p. 28.
31 Ibid., p. 30.
32 Ibid.
33 See Joslin, *The Treatment of Diabetes Mellitus* (1st edn), pp. 673–84.
34 Originally, having diabetes was grounds for exclusion from life insurance policies. This changed gradually as the therapeutic prospects for diabetics improved. However, as one remark by Joslin underscores, this change was

coupled with high (moral) demands on the policy holder: '[t]rue is that rates will not be lowered until each diabetic does his best and lives longer. What I want is for an insurance company to tell my diabetics, when they take out insurance, it is true that we charge you an extra premium but if you will live beyond the standard number of years then the cost of your premium will be reduced.' See E. Joslin, 'Diabetes for the diabetics. Ninth Banting Memorial Lecture of the British Diabetic Association', *Diabetes* 5:2 (1956), 137–46, here 143.
35 'The medical director Dr Edwin Welles Dwight, has repeatedly aided me in my statistical studies.' Joslin, 'The prevention of diabetes mellitus', 81.
36 Letter from Louis Dublin, 3rd Vice President and Statistician to Joslin, JDCHA, Correspondences, Box 3, Folder 16, 5 November 1931.
37 Letter from Louis Dublin to Elliott Joslin, JDCHA, Correspondences, Box 3, Folder 16, 10 December 1933.
38 R.A. Fisher, *Statistical Methods for Research Workers* (Edinburgh: Oliver and Boyd, 1925), Preface.
39 R.E. Gleason, 'Biostatistical Evaluation of the Early Publications (1915–1923) of Dr. Elliott Joslin', Typoscript 2003 (JDCHA).
40 Joslin, *The Treatment of Diabetes Mellitus* (4th edn), Preface.
41 Joslin, *The Treatment of Diabetes Mellitus* (8th edn).
42 Ibid., p. 6.
43 Joslin, 'The prevention of diabetes mellitus', 84.
44 Ibid.
45 Joslin, *Diabetic Manual for the Mutual Use* (4th edn), p. 20.
46 Ibid., p. 24.
47 See Joslin, *The Treatment of Diabetes Mellitus* (8th edn), p. 328.
48 D.M. Barnett, *Elliott P. Joslin, MD: A Centennial Portrait* (Boston: Joslin Diabetes Center, 1998), p. 30.
49 Joslin, *The Treatment of Diabetes Mellitus* (8th edn), p. 328.
50 Ibid. [author's highlights].
51 JDCHA, Box 13.
52 Nowadays these traits are well known and no longer doubted as risk factors for diabetes, but at the time they were by no means generally accepted because the cause of diabetes was attributed primarily to heredity and not yet to behavioural or environmental factors. For Joslin, however, obesity was a decisive risk factor, see Joslin, *The Treatment of Diabetes Mellitus* (8th edn), p. 15.
53 See e.g. M. Bliss, *The Discovery of Insulin* (Chicago: University of Chicago Press, 25th anniversary edn, 2007), pp. 225–38.
54 Joslin, *Diabetic Manual for the Mutual Use* (4th edn), p. 18.

55 E. Joslin, 'The routine treatment of diabetes with insulin', *Journal of the American Medical Association* 80:22 (1923), 1581–83, here 1581.
56 Joslin, *Diabetic Manual for the Mutual Use* (4th edn), p. 20.
57 Ibid., p. 19.
58 Ibid., p. 33.
59 'The education of the diabetic is fundamental. It is so important that it is revolutionizing our approach to the treatment of diabetes.' See Joslin, *The Treatment of Diabetes Mellitus* (8th edn), p. 19.
60 Joslin, *Diabetic Manual for the Mutual Use* (4th edn) [author's highlights].
61 This depended on whether insulin was prescribed or not. A much larger proportion of diabetic patients was treated with dietary supplements – except for patients with juvenile (nowadays Type 1) diabetes – or, in the initial stages of treatment, only temporarily with insulin. Nevertheless, every diabetic had to learn how to administer insulin because it was their 'life insurance'. Compared to the first edition in 1918, the points cited here from the 1941 manual had barely changed.
62 This point had not been included in previous editions and aimed to ensure proper action in an emergency, either a life-threatening diabetic coma or hypoglycemia (low blood sugar), see Joslin, *Diabetic Manual for the Mutual Use* (7th edn), p. 41.
63 This section had remained virtually unchanged since the first edition in 1918, see Joslin, *Diabetic Manual for the Mutual Use* (1st edn), p. 45.
64 Joslin, *Diabetic Manual for the Mutual Use* (4th edn), p. 54.
65 Ibid.
66 On the development of the Benedict test, see S.R. Benedict, 'A reagent for the detection of reducing sugars', *Journal of Biological Chemistry* 5 (1909), 485–7.
67 Feudtner, *Bittersweet*, p. 95.
68 Joslin, *Diabetic Manual for the Mutual Use* (4th edn), p. 56.
69 Joslin, 'A diabetic chart', 248.
70 In this context, Feudtner points to the moral dimension of these daily practices and the implicit value-laden judgements about the patient's conduct, see Feudtner, *Bittersweet*, pp. 121–45.
71 On these unusual drawings, see Feudtner, *Bittersweet*, pp. 89–120.
72 M. Rubner, 'Calorimetrische Untersuchungen. II', *Zeitschrift für Biologie* 21 (1885), 337–410, here 377.
73 Joslin, *Diabetic Manual for the Mutual Use* (4th edn), p. 51.
74 Joslin, *The Treatment of Diabetes Mellitus* (8th edn), p. 351.
75 See the letter of 29 September 1944, JDCHA, Patient file no. 4456, Box 20, Folder 6.

76 See, for example, the letter of August 1935, Patient file no. 8877, JDCHA, Box 20, Folder 8: 'Dear Dr. White, I am writing you as regards your statement of June 8, 1935. At present I am out of work and cannot pay the bill for X-ray. Perhaps you know of some job in or about the hospital for which I am suitable. If so, I should appreciate any help you can give me in obtaining it. Sincerely B.P.'
77 See, for example, the letter of 28 December 1931, JDCHA, Patient file no. 4456, Box 20, Folder 6.
78 Joslin, *The Treatment of Diabetes Mellitus* (8th edn), p. 6.
79 Ibid., p. 20.
80 See letter of 17 September 1946, JDCHA, Patient file no. 4456, Box 20, Folder 6.
81 Joslin, *The Treatment of Diabetes Mellitus* (8th edn), p. 351.

Part II
Household

4

Economies of the hospital, 1790–1910

Axel C. Hüntelmann

The leading German physician Johann Theodor Eller (1689–1760) introduced his publication on *Useful medical and surgical notes about inner and exterior diseases observed at the Charité hospital in Berlin* with a short description of the hospital.[1] Upon publication in 1730, Eller had been one of two hospital directors and much of what we know about the hospital's early history derives from his book, which also includes an engraved illustration of the hospital building and surroundings (Figure 4.1).

Originally conceived as a pesthouse and a lazaret, the hospital was built outside the Berlin city wall in 1710, surrounded by open fields and a garden. In 1727, the Charité was rededicated as a municipal hospital and at the same time used as a military hospital for the Prussian army. Pictures from the 1730s and late 1760s show the main hospital building as a tetragon with each side measuring around 50 metres. The large courtyard housed the hospital's inspector and its housefather. A dining hall and kitchen were located on the left side of the main building and, in a gated area behind these facilities, we find stables and the brewery. At least until the end of the eighteenth century, the hospital was surrounded by meadows and fields, including gardens for growing vegetables, fruit, herbs, and cabbage.[2]

The ensemble of structures housing the stables, brewery, and later on a bakery, butchery, and kitchen, in addition to the fields and gardens, formed the so-called *Ökonomie*-buildings or simply the *Ökonomie*. The German term *Ökonomie* is derived from the Greek *oikos*, meaning the

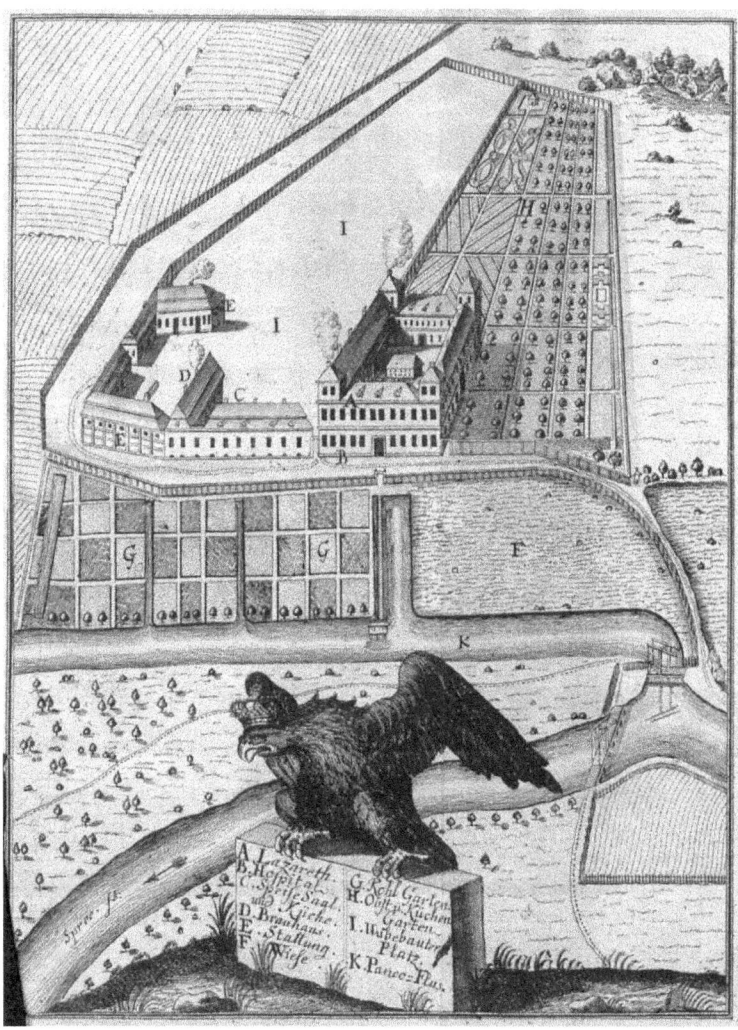

4.1 Royal Charité Hospital in Berlin, hospital and *Ökonomie* buildings, surrounded by fields and garden, around 1730.

'household'.[3] Whereas all these buildings surrounded the hospital, at its centre lived and worked the inspector, who oversaw the hospital.

In principle, the Charité was similar to other late medieval and early modern hospitals in Europe: its stables gave it the look of a country estate and the fact that it victualled the old and sick poor as well as invalids echoed hospitals associated with monasteries.[4] Indeed, invalids and the sick poor, so-called *Hospitaliten*, were housed separately from the curable sick, who received medicine and were treated by surgeons and physicians.[5] All inmates were provided with lodging and proper food, which was often, as Eller emphasised, more important for the sick poor than medicine.[6]

By the 1790s, the number of sick and infirm poor had increased and the lodging conditions in the hospital had worsened. There were public complaints about overcrowding, unhealthy housing conditions, insufficient and awful food;[7] and after the misappropriation of an enormous amount of money, it became obvious that the hospital's house- and bookkeeping was also in bad shape.[8] This period of time, the 1790s, is our starting point. Before then, the structure of the hospital as a household economy with production and consumption under one roof remained the same. With the erection of new buildings at the end of the century and their rearrangement in the 1830s, the nature of the hospital, as elsewhere in Europe, was being transformed from an asylum into a medical institution. In the 1790s, the hospital's accounting system had also been reorganised.

What does the Charité's cabbage garden have to do with medical knowledge and economy? And how are accounting, economy, and health interconnected beyond current discussions about economisation?

Bringing together health, medicine, and accounting, I will investigate the Charité hospital's various economies: its *Ökonomie* of functional entities like the kitchen, laundry, brewery; the bodily economy of its sick inmates; and the hospital's administrative economy that, after 1900, professionalised as 'hospital economics'. I argue that all of these different economies were linked together, and that health and accounting have long been deeply entangled with one another. At least since the eighteenth century, paperwork had been an indispensable precondition for all of these economies and involved extensive bookkeeping. I will demonstrate this by focusing especially on inmates' food and diet: in the hospital's *Ökonomie*, the production and supply of food was registered and balanced against consumption; daily consumption rates and diets were calculated for each person, monetised, and used to derive daily cost-rates and patient fees; annual budgeting and retrospective balancing were necessary because, as a royal institution, the Charité's budget comprised part of the Prussian government's budget.

Although this chapter benefits from a rich vein of literature on the history of accounting, and in particular on hospital accounting,[9] much of that literature focuses on British hospitals.[10] Furthermore, historians have tended to consider only financial accounts. In contrast, I will examine the hospital economy *in toto*. As such, this chapter complements existing literature on the history of the Charité hospital,[11] its administration,[12] as well as its dietary regimes and the management of its food supply.[13] I draw on archival records about accounting and budgeting, food supply, and the calculation of diets and patient fees.

I will first describe the arrangement of the Charité's physical plant and how the significance of the household *Ökonomie* diminished over the nineteenth century. I will then describe the hospital's administration and how it governed daily life, imposing managerial protocols and paperwork designed to ensure a constant flow of information. In subsequent sections, I will examine how this flow of information was needed to plan food supplies for more than a thousand people, to transform food requirements into monetary figures, and to recalculate expenditures. I will also describe the calculation of daily catering and cost-rates and thereafter summarise: how accounting pervaded and conjoined various hospital economies; how this entanglement changed over the nineteenth century and how accounting constituted the disciplines of hospital management and economics; and how accounting generated a specific kind of medical know-how and knowledge. My focus will be on the dietary and calculative schemes around 1800, 1850, and 1900.

The hospital *Ökonomie* – economy buildings and their accounts

As a royal hospital, founded and supported by the Prussian king, the Charité served several purposes. From 1727, it functioned as a military hospital as well as Berlin's main hospital. Throughout the eighteenth century, it was a teaching facility for military surgeons. After the establishment of the Friedrich Wilhelms University in 1810, it was increasingly used to teach medical students. Due to this mixed character, the Charité had not just various sources of income, but also various kinds of staff and patients.[14]

Initially, the hospital accommodated around 300 impoverished sick invalids[15] and provided beds for seventy patients.[16] After a third floor was added, the number of inmates nearly doubled by the end of the eighteenth century. Whereas the number of invalids remained constant, the number of curable sick rose to 400, among them impoverished residents, prostitutes with venereal diseases, unmarried pregnant women, wounded soldiers, and craftsmen who were part of guilds with a hospital subscription scheme. After Berlin's madhouse burned down in 1798, mentally ill patients were also housed in the Charité.[17] Hospital personnel included physicians and surgeons, especially military surgeons, medical students, a midwife, a priest, wardens, as well as kitchen, laundry, and cleaning staff. Around 1800, fifty physicians and officials as well as 200 staff (wardens and servants, stablemen, butchers, bakers, brewers, gardeners) worked and usually lived in the hospital. Patients and able-bodied inmates also worked in the kitchen and laundry, cultivated the garden, cleaned the wards, produced dressings, and delivered messages.[18] Altogether, some 1,200 people had to be provided for within an *Ökonomie* of buildings and a household community where production and consumption took place under the same roof.[19]

We know little about everyday life in this *Ökonomie*, but we can assume that it was much like that of other estates. Records show that every entity kept its own accounts listing income and expenses: a so-called 'fodder account' recorded the income from rye, straw, and hay; another account tallied the production of wine vinegar. The brewery's account recorded income in *Reichstaler* (Rthlr) for beer delivered to the Charité (3,612 and 1,123 Rthlr), the workhouse (2,110), the orphanage (104), the city's administration (362), as well as for direct sales of draff (234) and beer (566). This income was balanced against expenses of 4,851 Rthlr for five brewers, fuel, haulage, taxes and fees, barrels, and raw ingredients (barley, hops, and malt).[20] Another 'administrative' account showed income for haulage and the sale of livestock and milk, and a 'household' account recorded income for the sale of pelts, skins, tallow, and soap.[21] On land leased to the Charité in the 1740s, hospital inmates cultivated mulberries for a prospering silk industry in Berlin,[22] generating income from silk and spinning.[23] Although the hospital kept livestock and was located next to fields and gardens, these resources contributed only a small part of what was necessary to feed hundreds of people every day.

From the mid-1780s, the hospital and its physical plant underwent significant changes. Finished in 1800, a larger building with 750 beds for curable sick and 300 for invalids replaced the old hospital building, and from 1831 to 1835 a second hospital building was constructed. In subsequent decades, a mobile summer-camp hospital evolved into a separate hospital building, a smallpox quarantine station was built, and a lying-in hospital was added. Overall, this ensemble of buildings was scattered over a wide area and supported in the mid-1860s by a new large *Ökonomie*-building and a second kitchen, a separate laundry building, and an office building.[24] In December 1870, the hospital had 1,470 beds[25] for 13,603 patients per year and registered 428,000 catering days.[26]

The character of the hospital changed as well. Between the 1790s and the 1820s, the invalid and incurable sick were relocated to other institutions and the hospital's focus shifted from care to cure as the Charité increasingly became a medical institution. From the 1820s, more and more medical students were being trained at the Charité and in the mid-1850s it came to house Germany's first pathological institute. Parcels of land, formerly used to cultivate vegetables, were rededicated for the construction of new buildings or sold off.[27] And as the city of Berlin grew, it came to encompass the hospital complex.

Although in the eighteenth century the hospital cultivated its own vegetables and cereals, this covered only a portion of the hospital's overall needs. And so the hospital contracted with farmers and dairies around Berlin. As the farmland around the hospital diminished, these contracts became more important, whereas the focus of the household *Ökonomie* shifted to the organisation, acquisition, and preparation of food in the kitchen. This shift is manifested in the rededication of buildings: in the early 1840s, a 'modern', steam-operated laundry building was erected in place of the brewery and dairy; and the former kitchen gardens were rearranged into parkland to promote patients' convalescence.[28] Patients who now worked in the gardens did so for therapeutic reasons[29] and not to work off their hospital fees. From the mid-nineteenth century, the unity of production and consumption that had long characterised the hospital's household economy dissolved.

Rational management was deemed essential to provide for the hospital's growing population. Contemporary publications by hospital administrators[30] documented the reorganisation of hospitals according to functional principles, like the division of labour, and effused pride in them as modern, professionally managed institutions.

The order of the hospital (economy) – instructions and regulations

Drawing on his experience as the Charité's administrative director, Carl Heinrich Esse (1808–74) published a book in 1857 that became a milestone in the history of hospital management. Esse had begun his career in the military before becoming a civil administrator first in Szczecin and then in Berlin. From 1842, he soon advanced up the ranks from accountant to inspector and '*Rechnungsrat*' and in 1848 to '*Ober-Inspector*' charged with supervising the Charité and other health care institutions in Berlin. In 1851, Esse was appointed as the first administrative director,[31] who served alongside a medical director.

In his book on hospital management, Esse examined the optimal location for hospitals and their technical infrastructure: the arrangement and equipment of wards, sanitary facilities and baths, ventilation, lighting, heating, staff-rooms, the operating theatre, as well as kitchens and laundries. In addition, he described how hospital management could be enhanced using detailed staff instructions and established a clear hierarchy of power between different groups of workers.[32] The book also included examples of instructions for the kitchen inspector (*Ökonomie-Inspector*), the household manager (*Ökonomie-Hausverwalter*), the laundry inspector, and a detailed dietary regime and guidelines on monetary calculations for foodstuffs.[33]

According to these regulations, the household manager was responsible for order on the wards and in the garden, and for supervising servants, ward staff, and the porter, whereas the kitchen inspector was responsible for the cooking, kitchen staff, and food-stocks. All inspectors answered solely to the director's office. The main tasks and operations in the kitchen were regulated by instructions: the quality, amount, and provision of food were specified in detail. The daily deliveries of meat, milk, and bread were based on annual contracts; food like peas and other durable legumes could be purchased no more than one month in advance, whereas fresh vegetables had to be bought at the market at least twice a week.[34]

Esse also recommended that the kitchen inspector outline a dietary regime in advance that distinguished between the different classes of patients and staff.[35] After the menus were approved by the administrative director, the kitchen inspector calculated and ordered the necessary quantity of ingredients. In addition, hospital physicians and surgeons daily submitted special diets for individual patients.[36]

Hospital economy – the transformation of food into expenditures and the management of input and output

Esse's dietary regime drew on more than a century of experience. In his *Annotations*, Eller had already described the patients' dietary regime in 1730: in the morning, poor invalids received a 'proper breakfast' – some bread with salt – and weak inmates also received warm soup. At noon, the menu changed every day and included an appetiser and some meat and a garnish. For instance, on Monday porridge was served as an appetiser, followed by beef and carrots, and on Tuesday sausages were accompanied by baked apples. In the evening, inmates received various sorts of porridge and again some bread. On Sunday, fine meat with spices was served and in the evening broth. As beverages, hospital inmates received coffee in the morning and at 10 am and 4 pm the hospital brewery dispensed a quart of beer.[37]

During the eighteenth century, the menu became more differentiated. At least from the 1790s, detailed schedules were used to compute the quantities of food necessary per day and to project costs for the annual budget. These weekly and daily calculations, summarised in the annual foodstuff or consumption budget (*Victualien-Etat, Consumptions-Etat*), were the responsibility of the hospital's kitchen inspector who produced a weekly dietary schedule for every day of the week. This diet was divided into a schedule for '*Officianten*' and '*Deputanten*', which included physicians and hospital officials, and '*Domestiquen*', meaning servants and wardens. Extrapolating from the daily schedule yielded the total number of meals served and the amount of food needed. The meals were broken down into their component parts in a table called the meal 'Designation', meaning the distinction between different classes of meals (like those for physicians and servants) and between lunch and supper (Figure 4.2).

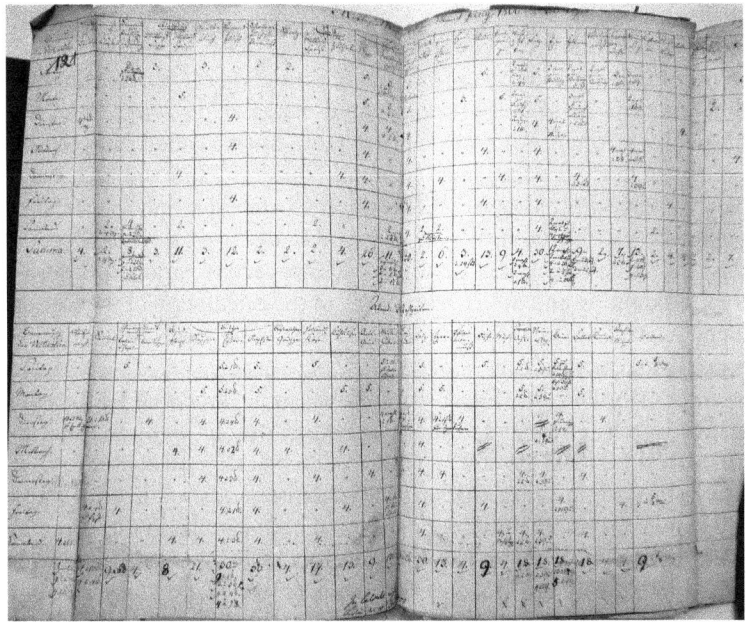

4.2 'Consumptions-Etat' – Designation of meals for '*Officianten*' and '*Deputanten*', June 1800.

For instance, for June 1800, the lunchtime meals for physicians and officials were calculated in a large table as follows: wheat flour for noodles (four units for Tuesday) and for dumplings (two units for Saturday); breadcrumbs for pudding (two units on Sunday), dumplings (two units for Saturday), and broth (two units on Saturday) etc. Further columns follow for each weekday and the necessary quantities for beef, mutton, pork, lard, butter, baked fruits, herring, rice, pearl barley, sugar, salt, eggs, plum jam, wine vinegar, kohlrabi, beans, spinach, raisins, and so on. There was a separate table for the different ingredients of evening meals.[38]

In calculating the quantity of the particular foodstuffs, administrators had to know how many people were being cared for in the hospital and how many staff members were entitled to board. In general, as the Charité evolved from a hospice to a medical institution, patients' length of stay declined and turnover rates rose, posing increased administrative challenges in calculating dietary schedules. Hence, lists of staff members were recorded in the accounts;[39] and by the 1830s, extensive tables[40] were compiled weekly on the number of patients in every department,[41] differentiated by sex, age, origin,[42] and status at discharge.[43] As the hospital was often overcrowded, the table distinguished between an estimated normal occupancy (*Normal Numerus*) and the real occupancy (*Wirklicher Numerus*).[44] This was important not only for calculating meals but also for justifying year-end budgetary overruns. Beyond this, the table listing the Charité's patients served various purposes, from accounting and police reporting[45] to the calculation of the weekly dietary schedule, and was only one of many other tables, like hospital mortality statistics.[46]

After compiling the 'Designation' tables in the foodstuff budget, the results were summarised and aggregated in various steps in order to calculate the overall monthly quantity of each basic food ingredient like wheat flour, for instance, that was the basis for noodles, dumplings, and other side dishes. The number of units of each garnish in the different 'Designation' tableaus for lunch and supper were aggregated and converted into the quantity of *Scheffel* (about a bushel) and *Metzen* (about a peck) of wheat flour. The calculations continued with further basic food ingredients like breadcrumbs, white bread, black bread, beef, and so on ad nauseam. The differentiation into groups like '*Deputanten*', servants, and physicians and other staff was necessary because each group received different rations: surgeons, for instance, got more black bread during the day than other officials.[47] The quantity of each kind of food ingredient for the different groups of staff and for patients were then merged into one account, summarised, and multiplied by the price in order to compute the overall cost. And finally, this amount was transferred into the overall budget: in the so-called Charité House budget we find expenditures for wheat flour amounting to 1,077 Rthlr, or for bread amounting to 6,081 Rthlr. Overall, budgeted expenditures[48] (and income) added up to 50,340 Rthlr with food (27,410 Rthlr) representing more than half of the overall expenditures.[49]

Clearing of accounts

Food was not only counted as an expenditure in the annual Charité House Budget (*Charité Haus Casse*). The hospital economy also produced food and generated revenue from sales of beer or hides. In addition, food and other staff boarding allowances [*Kostgelder*] were also counted as income in the economy's special budgets (for instance, the brewery or garden budget) and credited to another: as members of the Charité 'household', staff received a salary and additional allowances for food, candles, or heating.[50] The total amount paid in salary and allowances was debited as an expenditure, and the allowances of other budgets were credited as offsetting income. In the Charité's cameralistic accounting system, income and expenditures in different budgets offset one another, and finally, a total deficit in the Charité House Budget was transferred to and balanced in the so-called Charité Main Budget (*Charité Haupt Casse*). In the eighteenth and early nineteenth century, this main budget balanced general income from interest on capital, from other estates, and from state privileges or subsidies against the deficits of the different hospital budgets.[51]

Clearly, as these calculative practices and deeply entangled budgets suggest, the Charité hospital had a complex system of accounting at the beginning of the nineteenth century. The personnel responsible for this system included a supervisor or *Ober-Inspector*, *Oeconomie*-inspectors, two treasurers, three controllers, a calculator, a registrar, a clerk, two secretaries, and three office servants who were located near the entrance of the main hospital building. But the original information for the dates compiled and processed by these accountants were usually noted down and gathered by the medical and ward staff as part of their daily routine.

Paper technology and accounting of food and health in the 1850s

In principle, the management of the hospital economy and the procurement and preparation of food remained the same throughout the first half of the nineteenth century. Information continued to be gathered about the number of people served, the composition of their meals, and the quantities and costs of ingredients. At the turn of the century, tables were drawn up individually, either by hand or on simple pre-printed statistical forms. During the 1820s and 1830s, however, administrators introduced more forms, larger statistical tables, and weekly reports. The growing number and fluctuation of patients and staff, as well as the hospital's expanding physical plant, likely required more sophisticated administrative strategies. Furthermore, the Prussian reforms after 1806 resulted in significant changes in welfare and hospital administration.[52] In addition, the rise of statistical thinking,[53] growing awareness of accounting and (commercial) management techniques,[54] and an expanding bureaucracy[55] all likely influenced this development and vice versa.

The entire organisation of the Charité seems to have become structured around written instructions and standardised tables and forms designed to regulate workflow and ensure desired outcomes: the preparation of 1,200 meals twice a day. Furthermore, food had become part of a regime, a 'diet' that included regular food and dietary schedules as well as 'extra diets'. On their daily rounds, house physicians prescribed different kinds of diets, medicines, and treatments for each patient.[56] The *Unterarzt* (military surgeon)[57] noted these prescriptions on a treatment slip (*Kurzettel*) in each patient's case file. These surgeons also recorded ordinary and extraordinary diets for the next day in a special diet-book that was given to the senior warden.[58] In the afternoon, the surgeons also calculated the number of patients on the ward and filled out daily reports. Signed by the house physicians, these reports were handed over no later than 4:30 pm to the admissions office, where they were compiled into one single form.[59] The daily reports listed not just the number of patients on different wards, but also the number of physicians and clerks as well as wardens and servants.

As a blueprint for the scheduling of diets, Esse described the different tables and dietary variations *in extenso*. He suggested three classes of meals and within each class four specific diets in addition to extraordinary diets. The different meal classes mirrored the hospital's hierarchy: lower-class patients were catered 'third table', as were servants.[60] Second-class patients as well as ward staff and other hospital employees were catered 'second table' – whereby in both classes hospital staff received 'stronger' meals, i.e. larger portions.[61] Physicians and surgeons boarding at the hospital likely received the same food as patients served 'first table'.

The 'third table' was very basic – coffee in the morning, some vegetables and a piece of meat for lunch, for supper some soup, and throughout the day a pound of bread. Diet I included dark bread, diet II white bread, and diets III and IV were for patients in poor condition: instead of meat, soup or broth was served. At 'second table' more meat, better bread, and butter were served. In addition, at 'first table' patients also received soup or broth, vegetables, meat, salad, and fruit for lunch; and for dinner patients could chose between scrambled eggs, meat or fish, and side dishes. In addition to all three tables for diet III and IV, physicians could prescribe an extraordinary diet: grated potato, roast, vegetables, stewed fruits, and either wine (diet III and IV) or brandy (diet I and II). These extras were served mainly to strengthen third- and second-class patients and were primarily prescribed as a medical treatment.[62] Each patient's diet and extraordinary supplements, as prescribed by the physician and recorded during morning rounds, were also transmitted to the administration where they were summarised in a large spreadsheet for each 'table' (Figure 4.3).[63]

In his exemplary schedule, each meal had been broken down into single ingredients: for instance, for the preparation of broth served as a lunchtime appetiser at first table, he listed ¼ pound beef, ½ *loth* [about 7 grams] salt, 1½ *loth* [22 grams] pearl barley or noodles, or 2 *loth* [29 grams] rice, herbs and spices as required (Figure 4.4).[64]

In the 1850s, the Charité's former household *Ökonomie* had dwindled away to a kitchen that was located next to the main hospital

4.3 Normal diet schemes (*Hauptdiätverordnung*), compiled and accumulated for all patients.

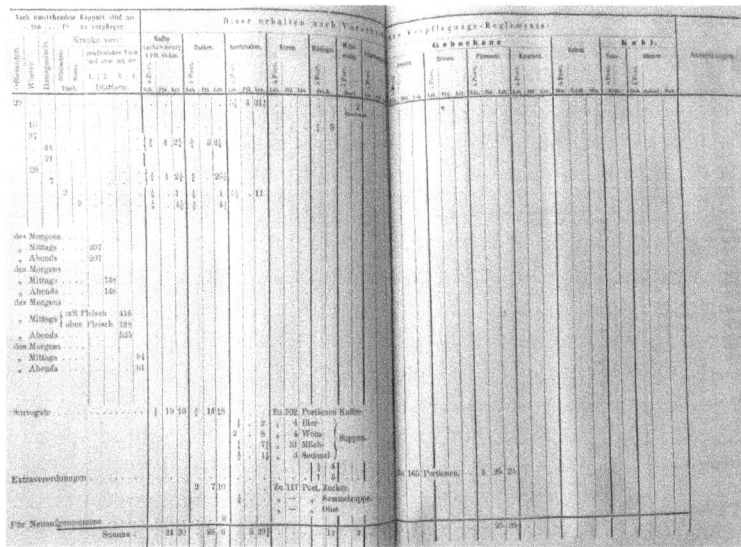

4.4 Form III breaking down the quantities of single ingredients (here i.e. coffee, sugar [...], herring, various baked fruits, cabbage) for the calculation of the daily diets.

building. Esse described the different parts of the kitchen, fireplaces, and storerooms, designed to ensure appropriate, i.e. rational and healthy food preparation.[65] Under the supervision of an inspector, female cooks and kitchen assistants prepared the food.[66] In subsequent decades, a new Ökonomie building was erected, including additional technical equipment like steam boilers. The introduction of gas and electricity in the kitchen and the ongoing mechanisation of cooking processes manifested themselves in the second edition of Esse's book.[67]

If food preparation was guided by paper technologies and calculative practices, this was even more the case for food consumption. Military surgeons recorded patients' names and prescribed diets for the next day in a so-called diet-book, which was then given to the kitchen.[68] Extraordinary diets were also recorded in patients' medical files, as was the output of their own bodily economy: amount of urine, the number of bowel movements and their characteristics, temperature fluctuations, and later on blood sugar levels – as Oliver Falk's Chapter 3 in this volume illustrates. And after meals, administrators computed the quantity of food that had been consumed in *Scheffel, Metzen,* or pounds and transferred the amount into Prussian *Thaler, Silbergroschen,* and *Pfennig*. But why was it necessary to account for every single *loth* and penny?

Accounting for health and the calculation of daily catering and cost-rates

In general, it was agreed that a responsible, i.e. economic management of resources and patients was a sine qua non of good medical practice. But patients' treatment had to be recorded in case files in order to follow up on the disease process and, if successful, account for the hospital's success[69] (and justify its expenditures). And financial accounting and cost calculations were necessary because the hospital was, as a royal institution, accountable to the Prussian state for every penny spent. The hospital administration had to draw up a budget for the following year (or years in the case of triennial budgets) and provide a full, year-end account of all expenses. Unlike British voluntary hospitals, patients or those responsible for them had to pay for medical treatment. Therefore, the Charité was also accountable to self-paying patients, health insurance companies, friendly societies with health insurance schemes, and municipal welfare authorities.

In the eighteenth century, the Charité received income from capital, state privileges, the hospital's own economy, and, to a smaller degree, from fees charged to patients and invalids. Around 1800, the income from state subsidies amounted to 25,000 Rthlr and from patient fees 9,173 Rthlr. In the late 1880s, the relationship had completely changed: subsidies from the Prussian state amounted to 256,955 Marks, whereas the income from patient fees added up to 889,000 Marks. Income from the Charité's own economy, as represented in various separate budgets in 1800, had become negligible,[70] whereas patient fees now provided the bulk of the hospital's revenue.[71]

In principle, eighteenth-century hospital care for the poor sick was free. Only people with venereal diseases or scabies, or prostitutes and those able to pay, had to pay. In the late 1730s, normal patients had to pay 8 *Groschen* (comparable to Shillings) per week, patients with venereal diseases, who were treated with costly sweating cures, paid 12 *Groschen* per week. Since the hospital fee was intended to cover expenditures for food, patients unable to pay worked off their debt in the hospital or the workhouse.[72] At the end of the eighteenth century, the cheapest daily catering rate (fourth class) amounted to 3 *Groschen*; servants or craftsmen who were members of guilds with health care schemes paid 4 *Groschen* and 3 pennies; middle (second) class patients paid 6 *Groschen* per day; and the best dietary scheme ran as high as 10 *Groschen* and 5 pennies per day.[73] Beside a monthly rate of 14 Rthlr for second-class patients or 25 Rthlr for first-class patients, the fee could rise to 50 Rthlr if a patient wanted extra candles, a single room, or additional servants.[74] In the aftermath of the Napoleonic Wars and the French occupation of Berlin, the hospital experienced an acute financial crisis.[75] Following the Prussian reforms that separated it from municipal poor relief, the Charité introduced hospital fees for all inmates, resulting in ongoing tensions with Berlin's municipal government, which now had to pay for the city's indigent sick.[76] Also, in addition to their board, patients had to pay separately for medical treatment, medicine, or extraordinary diets.

From 1846, uniform hospital tariffs had been introduced aiming at simplifying billing. The daily (catering) rate covered costs for administration, an ordinary (third-class) diet, lodging, linen, normal care, and basic medical treatment like baths, dressing, or an extraordinary diet. Patients who wished to have better food and their own room could pay higher rates.[77] In the 1870s, the tariffs again changed, but then remained more or less constant for decades. According to the tariff scales, patients from Berlin suffering from normal somatic diseases paid 2.5 and children 2 Marks per day. The rate for patients from Berlin with mental diseases amounted to 3 Marks, and for those who weren't residents of Berlin 4 Marks. The rate for patients with mental diseases was higher because their care was more time consuming and required more wardens. Second-class patients paid 6 and first-class patients 12 Marks per day.[78]

In addition to the daily catering rate, patients were charged separately for expensive remedies and treatments. At the end of the eighteenth century, accessorial costs arose for extra food, diets, and other services, whereas 100 years later more expensive remedies like anti-diphtheric serum or Salvarsan, and medical services like bacteriological diagnostics or x-rays, were invoiced separately and often paid by health insurance. From the 1910s, hospitals published booklets and price-lists

Economies of the hospital, 1790–1910 125

with medical services, especially as these services became more expensive.[79] Finally, the Charité also served municipal needs and was required to treat a portion of the city's sick and impoverished residents for free. In 1835, the Charité management and the municipal administration for poor relief negotiated that 100,000 catering days per year were free and all additional days had to be paid by the city. As a consequence, extensive administrative effort went into calculating daily rates for those patients and accounting for their number, length of stay, residency, and medical treatment.

Accounting and the calculation of our daily bread in the hospital economy

In the 1790s, the 'household' inspector was already able to calculate the amount of money spent on food and the different dietary classes per person and per day. But accounting at the hospital was not an end in itself. From the hospital's inception, accounts and expenses were inspected every year by the Royal Audit Chamber, item for item, invoice for invoice.[80] Food costs were verified using the consumption budget and patient numbers.[81] The attention that Prussian auditors paid to detail was designed to ensure retrospectively that resources (money, food) had been properly used and not misappropriated. But the same auditing and accounting practices also had prospective aims: the accuracy of past figures was needed to help plan for the future. Furthermore, auditing practices helped govern the hospital and generate data that could be used to justify administrators' actions.

In the 1890s, public complaints about the Charité hospital were widespread. Working-class people (and their advocates) complained about bad food, a strict, prison-like atmosphere on the wards, and the maltreatment of third-class patients by ward staff.[82] In addition, health insurance companies complained about high daily rates, and Prussian government ministries about rising expenditures. In light of these criticisms and because of a growing need for hospital beds in the expanding metropolis, the Prussian Crown embarked on a major overhaul of the Charité, seeking from administrators detailed information comparing the composition of daily catering and cure-rates over a five-year period.[83]

The Crown's inquiry, in addition to mobilising existing data, also generated reams of additional paperwork. Furthermore, the inquiry provides insight into hospital management around 1900 and the practices and logics of hospital accounting in Germany. In the weeks after the initial request, administrators compiled relevant information and calculated the daily rate for the years between 1892 and 1896 and, after further inquiries, expanded upon their calculations. Subsequently, I will highlight three main calculation schemes: about patient figures and income, catering rates, and costing. These schemes, although not necessarily directly related to the initial request in 1897, were indirectly entwined with each other. The first set of tableaus relied on longstanding tabular practices for patient figures and catering days dating back to the early nineteenth century. For example, a large tableau with annual catering days was based on (weekly) patient lists. The calculation of patient fees in the main tableau showed them to be an important source of income (see Figure 4.5).

The tableau broke down by clinical ward the catering days for indigent patients that could be charged to the city of Berlin (including the free contingent of 100,000 catering days) (A) and the days that could be invoiced to patients and health insurance companies (B). At the end of each column, the number of catering days for each rate was summed

4.5 Calculation of catering days for 1902.

up[84] and, in another related table, the overall income from patient fees was calculated per clinical ward.[85] In 1902, altogether 466,166 catering days were calculated.[86] Below the main tableau we find – for each clinic – the number of catering days attributable to patients occupying so-called gratis beds (*Freibetten*). These beds were reserved for patients of medical interest, who were used for research purposes or medical training and treated for free. As a university hospital, the Charité was compensated for teaching and research expenses from a different government source.[87]

The second set of tableaus was similar to the dietary scheme Esse had published forty years earlier. In responding to ministerial inquiries, each item on the dietary schedule of the first and second tables had to be retrospectively (re)calculated for the past five years (see Figure 4.6). To the left of each schedule the diet was listed as it was originally planned on the weekly *Speisezettel* (diet scheme). For instance, on Thursday, 14 January 1897, the schedule for first table lunch included semolina soup, boiled beef, peas and sauerkraut, corned pork, and potatoes; and for dinner roast veal, cheese, butter, and beer. The quantities for each ingredient and their current price were calculated on the right side of the schedule. At the end of the week, averages were calculated for each item in order to arrive at rates per person and day. In addition, another separate sheet of paper listed bread, butter, coffee, and other food consumed at breakfast or during the day. In determining the hospital's overheads, the cost of food served to staff was calculated by multiplying the number of staff in each group by the daily catering rate and the number of days.[88]

In March of 1898 it seemed, to tortured administrators, that every report they submitted simply elicited further inquiries from Prussian officials. After receiving a nine-page report in January, the ministry asked why the catering rates of staff groups were compiled differently and higher than the corresponding one for patients and, crucially, why the expenditures on food for hospital staff amounted to one-third of overall food costs and were higher than the expenditures of other municipal hospitals.[89]

In responding to this query, a third set of tableaus merged existing data into a schedule (*Nachweisung*) designed to verify individual catering rates. For the calendar year 1892, for example, expenditures for food were extracted from overall expenses (630,453 Marks) and adjusted to reflect year-beginning (6,206 Marks) and year-end (13,920 Marks)

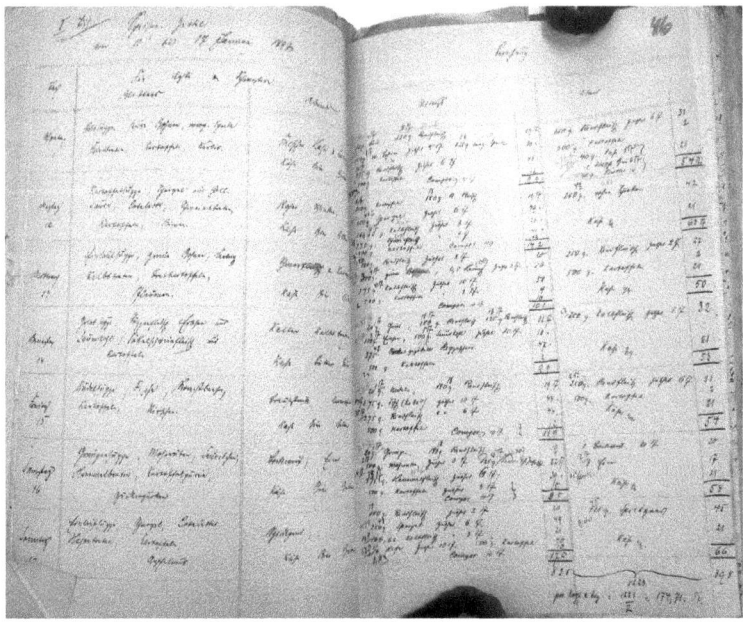

4.6 Recalculation of diet schemes (*Speisezettel*) 1st table, January 1897.

food stocks (technically an accrual and deferral had been made). Any income received from kitchen waste (like bones) was also discounted (3,530 Marks). Finally, expenses for the catering of physicians, apothecaries, clerks, and ward staff were deducted from the adjusted amount (altogether 176,420 Marks) and the remaining expenditures for food (442,789 Marks) divided by the number of patient catering days (576,786). These calculations produced daily rates for food (including wine and extra diets) of 77 *Pfennige* per patient in 1891/92.[90]

And this was only the first calculation! In another tableau, the daily care and catering rate was calculated. Since expenditures for food were dealt with separately, they were deducted from the overall expenses (in 1892: 1,528,577 minus 630,453 resulting in 898,124 Marks). The remaining expenditures were adjusted to account for outstanding balances from other years (resulting in a total deduction of 125,987 Marks). The so-called general expenditures of 772,136 Marks – including linen, maintenance and lodging, water, gas, electricity, but also funeral or ecclesiastical expenses – were divided by the number of catering days (576,786) to produce a daily rate of 1.339 Marks per patient. Furthermore, the overall food expenses for hospital staff and for patients, calculated separately, were also divided by the number of catering days (30.6 *Pfennige* for staff and 77 for patients) and summed to arrive at an overall daily rate of 2.42 Marks per day and patient in 1892.[91]

The Ministry's inquiry illustrates not only the complex cost calculations in German hospitals around 1900, but also helps to explain the motivation and logic behind the calculation schemes and to show that accounting practices were established to control the hospital management and could develop a momentum of their own, as each result elicited further inquiries and calculations. Although the Charité's complex accounting system was somewhat special, it was not unique. At the Düsseldorf Community Hospital in the 1920s, for example, the accounting department likewise calculated each item's proportion of the daily rate.[92] These schemes and accounts were not a uniform system of accounts like that developed and introduced by Henry C. Burdett in the 1890s for voluntary hospitals in Britain.[93] Instead, and not least because in Germany larger hospitals were usually operated by the state, a church, or a municipality, administrators relied on existing, long-established cameralistic accounting practices that generally involved an auditing authority and that were comprehendible and comparable for accountants and civil servants.[94]

The calculation was only the tip of the iceberg: the daily rate was based not only on accounting figures but also on various inventory lists, kept by medical and ward staff, constantly noting the flow of food, linen, and patients. And from the late nineteenth century, newly developed expensive therapies, costly surgical operations, or new diagnostic tools like x-rays were recorded and billed separately. Hospitals began providing detailed information about their dietary schedules and charges for various treatments and therapies, such as x-rays, baths, and surgical operations.[95] Extra billing for the newest and most expensive forms of medical treatment had various consequences: first, it provided an additional source of income for hospitals and an opportunity to showcase their medical prowess. Second, separate billing helped to establish newly developed (expensive) medical therapies because, as their use was not restricted by a lump sum, they were prescribed more often. But third, conversely, extra billing also meant more paperwork for hospital administrators (for instance, before treatment health care insurance funds had to asked for permission in proceed). At the Charité, special charges for medical treatments and diagnostics were noted in patients' files in the decades around 1900 and summarised alongside basic patient data.[96]

The composition of the daily rate changed during the nineteenth century, corresponding to the transformation of the hospital from an infirmary into a medical institution. The proportion of food – both as nourishment and therapy – in the early catering and care-rates decreased and amounted to less than one-third of the overall rate by the 1890s, whereas the number of extra medical services and the proportion of hospital overheads grew.

Although before 1900 disputes about rising medical costs were mainly a preoccupation of health insurance funds and practitioners, this changed after the First World War as hospital expenditures came under greater scrutiny, especially from state authorities, municipalities, and health insurance funds. Rising costs and comparisons between hospitals based on the rate's evolving composition contributed to heated debates about public health and welfare.[97] What ultimately became a major bone of contention between hospitals and health insurance companies in the 1920s had already started around the turn of the century.

Entangled hospital economies

Looking back to the end of the eighteenth and the mid-nineteenth century, we find that calculative practices and accounting at the Charité hospital were remarkably stable. These practices involved counting patients, producing figures, establishing patient groups, and calculating food supplies for staff and patients, tabulating dietary schedules, extrapolating from individual needs to compute overall hospital demand, and balancing budgets to justify past and future expenditures. But aside from these common practices, how did accounting change over more than a century? And how were the hospital economies entangled with accounting? And was the hospital economy of Eller or the 1790s the same as that of 1910?

For all of their stability, accounting practices and their outcome certainly became more formalised. Evolving from the tables used around 1800 that were drawn-up for each purpose by the hospital inspector himself, in the 1850s Esse described numerous standardised forms and tables that were used in everyday hospital practice. The entire process of organising food production, calculating diets, and accounting for food-stocks and expenses became more standardised, not least because it involved far more people gathering information, transferring it onto ledgers, and using it to calculate sums.

Furthermore, administrators came to place greater emphasis on data. Whereas Esse had compiled grams of food and cups of liquid in order to calculate the total intake of food, decades later administrators had become equally, if not more, interested in the *out*flow of financial resources and the *in*come of money from patients fees. The more sophisticated and detailed hospital accounting became in the nineteenth century, the more data and information were needed to operate the hospital and justify its existence.

Beside the figures becoming more standardised (as a precondition for comparisons of income and outcome between different hospitals), the practices themselves became more standardised, professionalised, and institutionalised. As patient care had been professionalised during the nineteenth century,[98] so too had the production of food and cooking. According to Ulrike Thoms, until the 1880s women qualified as housekeepers – often former patients or the wives and widows of wardens – and were employed in (or headed) hospital kitchens. But with rising numbers of hospital patients and enlarged kitchens with more technical equipment, cooking and food supply became rationalised and industrialised.[99] In particular, with the emergence of calorimetry and ecotrophology within nutritional science from 1880s onward, home or household economics in Germany (*Ernährungs- und Haushaltskunde*) also became more scientific.

The relationship between food, diet, and catering-rate manifests itself in the German terms *Kost* (food, diet) and *Kosten* (cost, expenditures). The terms used for feeding patients (*Beköstigung*), the dietary scheme (*Kostplan*), or the institution's food (*Anstaltskost*) can be directly correlated with the verb 'to price' (*kosten*). And just as the word *Kost* for food refers to the noun *Kosten* (expenses), the household economy (as the production site of food) refers to what is now understood as the commercial economy.

More generally, hospital management and accounting, like business management and accounting, became specialised, professionalised, and institutionalised, thus generating a specific medical knowledge: the know-how to run and finance a modern hospital. In the 1780s, hospital inspectors and clerks had no special education and they were often, like Esse, former soldiers. As the number of patients grew and the functional organisation of hospitals became more differentiated, graduates from new commercial colleges and with degrees in public administration (*Staatswissenschaft*) began to influence the civil service, especially in the second half of the nineteenth century. A growing cadre of hospital directors, medical officials, and inspectors composed not just annual hospital reports, but books on hospital management and technology, including hospital accounting and finance.[100] Officials from some of Germany's largest hospitals and leading experts on hospital management joined forces in 1911 to publish *Das Deutsche Krankenhaus* [The German Hospital]. This comprehensive and authoritative tome amassed a wealth of contemporary practical knowledge about hospital organisation, everything from construction (geographic considerations and project planning), equipment and furnishing (for wards, laboratories, operation theatres, kitchens, laundry facilities, etc.), organisation, administration and financing, patient care, and food, as well as legal issues.[101] From the 1920s, an entire genre of publications in this field emerged under the rubric of *Krankenhaus-Betriebslehre*,[102] what in Anglo-American countries was termed hospital management or administration and later hospital economics.

The literature refers to the emerging field of hospital management, expressed in hospital economics as a scientific discipline.[103] The authors and editors of publications on hospital management and accounting were often hospital directors and superintendents. In Germany, this new group of medical officials also organised themselves 1901 in the *Vereinigung der ersten Verwaltungsbeamten der grösseren Krankenhäuser* [Association of Leading Employees of Large Hospitals][104] and founded the *Zeitschrift für Krankenanstalten* [Journal for Hospitals].[105] The creation of such associations and journals helped spawn compendia like *Das Deutsche Krankenhaus* and other handbooks.[106] Finally, knowledge about the hospital and its economy was slowly introduced into higher education, although hospital economics wasn't adopted into the academic curricula until the late 1950s.[107] Since then, both hospital economics (dealing with the management of a single hospital as an organisational entity) and health or medical economics (dealing with health politics and hospitals' role in it),[108] have stressed the financial aspects of capacity planning, rationalisation of work processes, productivity, and efficiency. To the extent that these issues have suffused medical training and practice, as Joris Vandendriessche illustrates in his Chapter 6, physicians have become hospital managers.

Contemporary understanding of a hospital's economy in the 1950s differed from the early nineteenth century. Hospital economy was no longer a set of buildings, nor a household community. Production and consumption were separated from each other, the 'household' and its buildings vanished from hospital grounds, a more pervasive division of labour and rational organisation of resources took hold and drove up demand for trained administrators and accountants. And while accounting in the eighteenth-century hospital economy was already paper-based and complex, it became more detailed and ingrained over time: the more the household *Ökonomie* fell apart, the more accounting came to link production and consumption, care and cure, and the practical challenges of managing a diverse hospital economy with specific knowledge about medical institutions and other health care organisations. The hospital had become a rationalised production unit, an enterprise, an operation, a *Betrieb*. The old *Ökonomie* now existed only on paper, interlinked by and represented in the hospital's accounts.

Acknowledgements

This book chapter is part of a broader project on accounting and bookkeeping in medicine in Germany and Britain between 1750 and 1950. I would like to thank Alexa Geisthövel, Harro Maas, Fritz Dross, and Eric J. Engstrom for their comments and advice on earlier versions of the chapter.

Notes

1 J.T. Eller, *Nützliche und auserlesene medicinische und chirurgische Anmerckungen so wohl von innerlichen als auch äußerlichen Kranckheiten, und bey selbigen zum theil verrichteten Operationen, welche bishero in den von Sr. Königl. Majestät in Preussen gestiffteten grossen Lazareth der Charité zu Berlin, vorgefallen; nebst einer vorangegebenen kurtzen Beschreibung der*

Stiftung, Anwachs, und jetzigen Beschaffenheit dieses Hauses etc. (Berlin: Joh. Andreas Rüdiger, 1730).

2 O. Scheibe, *Zweihundert Jahre des Charité-Krankenhauses zu Berlin. Mitteilungen aus der Geschichte, Entwicklung der Anstalt von ihrer Gründung bis zur Gegenwart* (Berlin: Offprint of Charité Annalen Vol. 34, 1910).

3 I. Richarz, *Oikos, Haus und Haushalt. Ursprung und Geschichte der Haushaltsökonomik* (Göttingen: Vandenhoeck & Ruprecht, 1991).

4 See, for instance, A.H. Murken, *Vom Armenhospital zum Großklinikum. Die Geschichte des Krankenhauses vom 18. Jahrhundert bis zur Gegenwart* (Cologne: Dumont, 1988); G.B. Risse, *Mending Bodies, Saving Souls. A History of Hospitals* (New York: Oxford University Press, 1999); M. Scheutz (ed.), *Europäisches Spitalwesen. Institutionelle Fürsorge in Mittelalter und Früher Neuzeit* (Munich: Oldenbourg, 2008); L. Abreu and S. Sheard (eds), *Hospital Life. Theory and Practice from the Medieval to the Modern* (Bern: Peter Lang, 2013).

5 Eller, *Anmerckungen*, p. 13, figure 1, in which A indicates the lazaret for 'truly sick' (*würcklich Krancke*) and soldiers and B the hospital like an infirmary for the lame, invalid, and old.

6 Eller, *Anmerckungen*, p. 24. More generally D. Gentilcore, *Food and Health in Early Modern Europe. Diet, Medicine and Society, 1450–1800* (London: Bloomsbury, 2016).

7 See, for instance, C.H.E. Moritz, *Treue Erzählung meiner gehabten Schicksale in Berlin, vor, und nach der Aufnahme in die Charité* (Berlin: n.p., 1800); Scheibe, *Zweihundert Jahre*, pp. 57–61 also reports about public grievances.

8 See, for instance, the files about the fraudulent behaviour of the hospital inspector Habermaas in the Archive of the Humboldt University, Charité Direction (henceforth AHU CD), No. 1404.

9 For further literature, see the Introduction.

10 Some exceptions are collected in A. Labisch and R. Spree (eds), *Krankenhaus-Report 19. Jahrhundert. Krankenhausträger, Krankenhausfinanzierung, Krankenhauspatienten* (Frankfurt: Campus, 2001).

11 See, for instance, the contributions in J. Bleker and V. Hess (eds), *Die Charité. Geschichte(n) eines Krankenhauses* (Berlin: Akademie Verlag, 2010).

12 E. Engstrom and V. Hess (eds), *Zwischen Wissens- und Verwaltungsökonomie. Zur Geschichte des Berliner Charité-Krankenhauses im 19. Jahrhundert* (Stuttgart: Franz Steiner, 2000).

13 U. Thoms, *Anstaltskost im Rationalisierungsprozes. Die Ernährung in Krankenhäusern und Gefängnissen im 18. und 19. Jahrhundert* (Stuttgart: Franz Steiner, 2005).

14 Bleker and Hess (eds), *Charité*.
15 Eller, *Anmerckungen*, p. 13.
16 I. Marz, 'Das Charité Lazarett (1710–1790)', in Bleker and Hess (eds), *Charité*, pp. 18–43, esp. p. 32.
17 V. Hess, 'Die Alte Charité, die moderne Irrenabteilung und die Klinik (1790–1820)', in Bleker and Hess (eds), *Charité*, pp. 44–69.
18 Eller, *Anmerckungen*, pp. 20–3. Clemens Hanke notes that it was common for indigent patients to have to work off their hospital stay, see C. Hanke, 'Untersuchungen über die Charité-Patienten von 1743–1752. Eine Studie zur Funktion und Soziologie eines Krankenhauses im 18. Jahrhundert' (Medical Dissertation, Humboldt University Berlin, 1981), p. 255. It seems that this remained common practice until the 1820s, see the file regarding labour of indigent patients in AHU CD, No. 1214.
19 Richarz, *Oikos*; and the article 'Wirtschaft' in *Geschichtliche Grundbegriffe*, vol. 7 (Stuttgart: Klett-Cotta, 1992). Economy in this sense has been idealised by O. Brunner, 'Das "ganze Haus" und die alt-europaische "Ökonomik"', in O. Brunner, *Neue Wege der Sozialgeschichte. Vorträge und Aufsätze* (Göttingen: Vandenhoeck & Ruprecht, 1956), pp. 33–61.
20 See the accounts in AHU CD, No. 1357 (Charité Budgets for 1799 and 1800). The Charité's overall budget at the time was 36,209 Rthlr.
21 See the accounts 'Einnahme und Ausgabe zur Administrations-Geld-Rechnung' 1799/1800 HUA CD, No. 1357.
22 See the files of the inspector Habermaas in HUA CD, No. 1354.
23 See the accounts 'Einnahme und Ausgabe zur Administrations-Geld-Rechnung' and 'Etat der Charité Haus-Casse' 1799/1800 in AHU CD, No. 1357.
24 See, for instance, Scheibe, *Zweihundert Jahre*; Bleker and Hess (eds), *Charité*, especially the site-plan of Charité buildings in 1865 (figure 10.3).
25 See the monthly reports to the Berlin Police, December 1870 and January 1871 in AHU CD No. 1235.
26 See Table 3.1 in Hess, 'Alte Charité', p. 75.
27 See, for instance, the contracts about land sale in Secret Prussian State Archive Berlin, HA I, Rep. 76 VIII D (henceforth cited as GStA), Nr. 240.
28 Scheibe, *Zweihundert Jahre*, p. 72.
29 Hess, 'Alte Charité'.
30 See, for instance, C.H. Esse, *Die Krankenhäuser. Ihre Einrichtung und Verwaltung* (Berlin: T.C.F. Enslin 1857, 2nd edn 1868); or F. Oppert, *Hospitals, Infirmaries and Dispensaries. Their Construction, Interior Arrangement and Management* (London: John Churchill & Sons, 1867, German 1859).
31 E. Hilf, 'Carl Heinrich Esse (1808–1874). Der erste Verwaltungsdirektor der Charité. Ein Beitrag zur Verwaltungsgeschichte des Krankenhauses

im 19. Jahrhundert' (Medical Dissertation Free University, 2003); E. Hilf, 'Zur Geschichte der Charitédirektion im 19. Jahrhundert. Aufbau, Struktur und Personen der Charitéverwaltung zwischen 1820 und 1870', in Engstrom and Hess (eds), *Wissens- und Verwaltungsökonomie*, pp. 49–68.

32 Esse, *Krankenhäuser*. Regarding the role of hospital instructions in early modern Austria, see M. Scheutz and A.S Weis, '"Ordnung im Haus". Das Ordnungsgeflecht in österreichischen Spitälern der Frühen Neuzeit – eine Einleitung in Andeutungen', in M. Scheutz and A.S Weis (eds), *Spital als Lebensform. Österreichische Spitalordnungen und Spitalinstruktionen der Neuzeit* (Vienna: Böhlau, 2015), pp. 31–79.

33 The instructions and regulations about hospital economy and tables on foodstuff calculation comprise one sixth of the publication, see Esse, *Krankenhäuser*, pp. 252–304.

34 Ibid.

35 For examples, see Esse, *Krankenhäuser*, pp. 261–87.

36 Ibid., p. 256.

37 Eller, *Anmerckungen*, pp. 18–21. We can assume that Eller's explications were normative and may have differed from daily reality. On dietary regimes in German institutions, see Thoms, *Anstaltskost*.

38 See the accounts of the 'Consumptions-Etat' calculated from June 1800 to May 1801 in AHU CD, No. 1357.

39 See, for instance, the remuneration budgets for '*Officianten*' and '*Domestiquen*' for 1789 in AHU CD No. 1356.

40 See the weekly reports for the year 1832 in AHU CD, No. 1233, 1348.

41 Ibid. In the early 1830s there were eleven departments: internal diseases, cholera, surgery, ophthalmology, mental illness, venereal diseases, scabies, maternity ward, lying-in ward, paediatric ward, a ward for upper-class patients (*Kranke der höheren Stände*); and in addition a smallpox quarantine station that was generally used for infectious diseases.

42 The table differentiated between patients being newly or readmitted, and those being transferred to other hospital wards. A further column was designated for newborns (as new admissions).

43 The categories included: discharged (cured, improved, not-cured), on leave, escaped, transferred to a different department, and deceased (separately stillbirth, and died within five days of admission).

44 See the weekly reports for the year 1832 in AHU CD, No. 1233, 1348.

45 See, for instance, the monthly reports addressed to the Berlin police between 1871 and 1886 in AHU CD, No. 1235.

46 See, for instance, the deliberations on hospital mortality statistics between the 1830s and the 1850s (AHU CD No. 1230, 1234) and the monthly reports in the 1840s (AHU CD, No. 1241–3).

47 See Litt. A (Enclosure A): Designation of quantities for the meals of the officials and 'Deputanten', calculated for June 1800. See also the accounts 'Consumptions-Etat' calculated from June 1800 to May 1801 in AHU CD, No. 1357, fol. 119.

48 For the Charité House Budget 1800/01, see the accounts 'Consumptions-Etat' calculated from June 1800 to May 1801 in AHU CD, No. 1357, fol. 89–95.

49 By comparison, the salary of officials and *'Deputanten'* was 3,814 Rthlr and of servants and wardens 2,062 Rthlr. Ibid.

50 For the offset of boarding allowances in the Charité's Administrative Budget, the Garden Budget, the Brewery Budget, and the Charité House Budget for 1799/1800, see AHU CD, No. 1357, fol. 50r. As an example of boarding allowances for officials, see ibid., fol. 91–2. The allowances rose and became more detailed over the years. In the 1830s, the annual expenditures for ward staff were 40 Rthlr for real (paid) income, 52 Rthlr for boarding allowances, 7 Rthlr for clothing and linen, 8 Rthlr for heating, 3 Rthlr and 15 *Groschen* for light (candles), 3 Rthlr for soap, and 3 Rthlr and 15 *Groschen* were calculated for wear and tear on inventory. Every group of staff was calculated differently, see GStA, Nr. 240.

51 In the Charité House Budget 1800/1801, item B.1 'Undetermined income [*Unbestimmte Einnahmen*]' corresponded to item IV for current expenditures of the Charité Main Budget; see AHU CD No. 1357, fol. 90 and No. 1355, fol. 24r and 25. From the 1820s there was only one budget for all activities due to the institutional changes in the 1820s (see below) and the declining importance of the hospital's *Ökonomie*.

52 The Prussian Reforms granted municipalities greater autonomy. Until 1819, the Charité hospital was part of Berlin's welfare administration (*Armenverwaltung*) under the auspices of and partly subsidised by the Prussian state. But henceforth, poor relief became the responsibility of the municipal administration, whereas the Charité remained a Prussian state institution. As a result, the city of Berlin now had to pay the costs of care for their indigent patients that the Charité had hitherto treated for free, see A. Förster, *Denkschrift über das zwischen dem Charité-Krankenhause und der Stadt Berlin bestehende Rechtsverhältniß. Im amtlichen Auftrage bearbeitet* (Berlin: Reichsdruckerei, 1892), pp. 22–3. On the Prussian reform movement: R. Koselleck, *Preussen zwischen Reform und Revolution. Allgemeines Landrecht, Verwaltung und soziale Bewegung von 1791–1848*, 3rd edn (Stuttgart: dtv 1981); T. Nipperdey, *Deutsche Geschichte 1800–1866. Bürgerwelt und starker Staat* (Munich: C.H. Beck, 1998); for the welfare and health organisation in Berlin, see R. Münch,

Gesundheitswesen im 18. und 19. Jahrhundert. Das Berliner Beispiel (Berlin: Akademie Verlag, 1995).

53 T.M. Porter, *The Rise of Statistical Thinking 1820–1900* (Princeton: Princeton University Press, 1986).

54 On the history of bookkeeping, see J. Gleeson-White, *Double Entry. How the Merchants of Venice Created Modern Finance* (London: Allen & Unwin, 2013); J. Soll, *The Reckoning. Financial Accountability and the Making and Breaking of Nations* (New York: Penguin, 2014); for Germany, see B. Penndorf, *Geschichte der Buchhaltung in Deutschland* (Leipzig: G.A. Gloeckner, 1913).

55 See, for instance, B. Wunder, *Geschichte der Bürokratie in Deutschland* (Frankfurt: Suhrkamp, 1986); C. Vismann, *Files. Law and Media Technology* (Stanford: Stanford University Press, 2008).

56 Esse, *Krankenhäuser*: instructions for dietary prescriptions for senior house physicians § 13–5 (p. 139), for house physicians §§ 23–6 (pp. 151–2), for *Unterärzte* §§ 12, 15–6 (pp. 164–5).

57 The Charité was primarily a teaching hospital for military surgeons. After their medical training, military surgeons worked as interns or *Unterärzte* in hospitals.

58 See the instructions §§ 15–6, 23 in Esse, *Krankenhäuser*, pp. 165, 168.

59 Esse, *Krankenhäuser*, § 27, p. 169.

60 Ibid., pp. 261–5, Supplement I: Speiseregulativ, A. Beköstigung am dritten Tisch, esp. p. 265.

61 Ibid., pp. 265–6, Supplement I: Speiseregulativ, B. Beköstigung am zweiten Tisch.

62 See the descriptions of the different tables in ibid., pp. 264–70, Supplement I: Speiseregulativ.

63 Ibid., p. 271, Supplement II: Compilation of the ordinary diet (third table).

64 Ibid., pp. 261–5, Supplement I: Diet Schemes, C. First Table, I. Lunch, pp. 267–8.

65 Ibid., pp. 55–9 highlights that the water supply was provided by a separate well and that flooring with inbuilt drains was easy to clean, etc.

66 Thoms, *Anstaltskost*, pp. 209–31.

67 Esse, *Krankenhäuser* 2nd edition 1868. Crucially Thoms, *Anstaltskost*, pp. 241–74.

68 Esse, *Krankenhäuser*, § 15 (*Unterärzte*) on p. 165, and § 64 (ward staff) on p. 204.

69 See T.M. Porter's Chapter 7 in this volume.

70 For the figures, see the Charité budgets in AHU CD No. 1357 and the triennial Charité budget for 1888/1891 in GStA, No. 260.

71 The late 1880s and early 1890s represent something of a turning point. Major renovations and construction work cut the number of patients and increased costs. Also, four new municipal hospitals siphoned off patients, again cutting income, while the costs for new teaching and research facilities grew. In 1913, income from patient fees was 850,000 Marks, from state subsidies 900,000 Marks. See the overview in GStA, No. 269.
72 Scheibe, *Zweihundert Jahre*, p. 129. On daily catering rates, see AHU CD No. 1196.
73 E. Horn, *Oeffentliche Rechenschaft über meine zwölfjährige Dienstführung als zweiter Arzt des Königl. Charité-Krankenhauses zu Berlin nebst Erfahrungen über Krankenhäuser und Irrenanstalten* (Berlin: Realschulbuchhandlung, 1818), p. 54. Horn was the former medical director of the Charité hospital.
74 Ibid., p. 6. See also Hess, 'Alte Charité'. The fees charged by municipal hospitals were partly regulated, see B.J. Wagner, '"Um die Leiden der Menschen zu lindern, bedarf es nicht eitler Pracht": Zur Finanzierung der Krankenhauspflege in Preußen', in Labisch and Spree (eds), *Krankenhaus-Report*, pp. 41–68.
75 Ibid, pp. 48–51.
76 Förster, *Denkschrift*.
77 The lowest rate was 8¾ *Silbergroschen* for adults and 5 *Silbergroschen* for children, see C.H. Esse, 'Ueber die Verwaltung des Charité-Krankenhauses', *Annalen des Charité-Krankenhauses* 1 (1850), 524–70, here 525–7.
78 Daily rates increased slightly after 1900, see AHU CD No. 1200 and 1259; Scheibe, *Zweihundert Jahre*, pp. 129–30; and Wagner, 'Leiden der Menschen'.
79 The Municipal Hospital in Düsseldorf published information about the daily rate in 1910 in a four-page leaflet which, by 1923, had become a twelve-page 'Beköstigungsordnung' and an eight-page pricelist for medical services. See Municipal Archive Düsseldorf, Dept. IV, No. 37800.
80 See, for instance, the audit protocols of the Royal Audit Chamber in AHU CD, No. 1403–5.
81 See, for instance, the requests in the audit protocol for the year 1786/1787 (AHU CD No. 1405) dated 15 December 1788: 'pg. 7. no. 16. The daily rate for Siegesmund Schlitte was charged from 6 April 1787, but according to earlier accounts Schlitte was admitted to the hospital on 6 January 1787, so his hospital fees for three months, 10 Thlr, are missing.' Likewise: 'pg. 117 no. 853–862: Explain the reason why 11,382 purchased sausages are not calculated and accounted for in the foodstuff budget.'

The enquiries illustrate that auditors checked not just single items, but that the different budgets and account books were also cross-checked.
82 R. Freiberg, 'Der Charité-Boykott im Jahre 1893 in Berlin. Eine medizinhistorische Studie über Auswirkungen der Arbeitersozialreformen der 80er und 90er Jahre des 19. Jahrhunderts' (Medical Dissertation Free University Berlin, 1997).
83 See Prussian Ministry of Cultural Affairs to Charité Management, 15 and 30 March 1897 and further requests in the aftermath of previous reports of 10 June and 10 December 1897 AHU CD No. 1259.
84 See the tables for catering days in AHU CD No. 1200, fol. 37, [39].
85 See the tableau for the calculation of actual income for 1902 in AHU CD No. 1200, fol. 44. Besides the calculation of income from patient fees, there was another tableau summing up the number of beds in each clinic, ibid., fol. 43.
86 The total of 466,166 days derived from 456,990 regular hospital catering days and 9,126 days of free board and lodging for research and training purposes, see figure 5 (AHU CD No. 1200, fol. 37).
87 See the calculation regarding the scientific funds for 1904(?) in AHU CD No. 1200, fol. 49; regarding the reimbursement of university hospitals in Prussia, see also Wagner, 'Leiden der Menschen'.
88 See the calculations for first and second table between 1891/92 and 1897/98 in AHU CD No. 1259, fol. 13–52.
89 Prussian Ministry of Cultural Affairs to Charité Management, 17 March 1898, AHU, CD No. 1259, fol. 73.
90 Nachweisung über die Höhe der Verpflegungskosten im Charité Krankenhause, AHU, CD No. 1259, fol. 68.
91 Ibid., fol. 67. See also the draft, fol. 11 and 107–8.
92 The daily rate for 1926/1927 amounted to 9.23 Marks, including for instance 4 *Pfennige* for cleaning material, 42 for heat, light, gas, and water, 25 for linen, 26 (!) for general medicine, 44 for instruments and dressing, [… etc.], 34 (!) for debt service, and 110 for patients' food. Furthermore, salaries amounted to 97 *Pfennige* for physicians (and further rates for various staff groups). See the calculation in the Municipal Archive Düsseldorf, Dept. IV, No. 37800, fol. 72.
93 H.C. Burdett, *The Uniform System of Accounts for Hospitals and Public Institutions, Orphanages, Missionary Societies, Homes, Co-operations, and all Classes of Institutions with Special Forms of Account, Complete Sets of Books, certain suggested Checks upon Expenditure, Forms of Tender, and other Aids to Economy* (London: The Scientific Press 1893); N. Robson, 'A Contextual History of Accounting in UK Hospitals, 1880–1974' (Diss. Phil., Cardiff University 2006).

94 See, for example, K. Eicke, *Buchführung und Bilanz im Rahmen der Organisation einer Kommunalverwaltung. Ein Handbuch für Kommunalbeamte* (Berlin: Deutscher Kommunal-Verlag 1928); idem, *Die Organisation von Krankenanstalten* (Leipzig: Georg Thieme 1930).

95 See the dietary schedule 'Beköstigungsordnung für die allgemeinen Krankenanstalten der Stadt Düsseldorf 1923' and the tariffs 'Aufnahmebedingungen und Kostentarif für die allgemeinen Krankenanstalten der Stadt Düsseldorf für 1923'. The charges were listed in detail: x-rays by the size of the plates, various baths and electrical treatments, dressings for small or large wounds, and numerous surgical operations. The introduction of the dietary schedule and charges had already begun in the 1900s, see Municipal Archive Düsseldorf, Dept. IV, No. 37815, items 20–1.

96 See the discussions about the admission procedure and forms in GStA, No. 269.

97 On discussions about rising expenditures, O. Most, 'Städtische Krankenanstalten im Lichte vergleichender Finanzstatistik', *Zeitschrift für Soziale Medizin, Säuglingsfürsorge und Krankenhauswesen sowie die übrigen Grenzgebiete der Medizin und Volkswirtschaft* 5 (1910), pp. 213–36; O. Krohne, 'Die zunehmende Verteuerung unserer modernen Krankenanstalten und deren Ursachen sowie einige Vorschläge, ihr entgegenzuwirken', *Ergebnisse und Fortschritte des Krankenhauswesens. Jahrbuch für Bau, Einrichtung und Betrieb von Krankenanstalten* 2 (1913), pp. 43–96. Krohne was privy councillor in the Prussian Ministry of Interior. For comparisons of daily catering and cure rates, see the correspondence about cost structures between the city of Breslau and the Düsseldorf Community Hospital in 1926, and in general various tables comparing the daily rates of 45 larger hospitals in the 1920s, Municipal Archive Düsseldorf, Dept. IV, No. 37815. Daily rates had already been published in W. Albrand, *Die Kostordnung an Heil- und Pflege-Anstalten. Zum Gebrauch für Ärzte, Verwaltungsbeamte etc.* (Leipzig: H. Hartung & Sohn, 1903) and for comparisons see 'Kurkosten-Tarife deutscher Grosstädte', *Zeitschrift für Krankenanstalten* 21:2 (1925).

98 A. Faber, *Pflegealltag im stationären Bereich zwischen 1880 und 1930* (Stuttgart: Franz Steiner, 2015).

99 Thoms, *Anstaltskost*.

100 For an early example, see Oppert, *Hospitals*; and later A. Hagemeyer, *Das allgemeine Krankenhaus der Stadt Berlin im Friedrichshain, seine Einrichtung und Verwaltung* (Berlin: August Hirschwald 1879); A. Hagemeyer, *Das neue Krankenhaus der Stadt Berlin am Urban, seine Einrichtung und Verwaltung* (Berlin: August Hirschwald, 1894).

101 J. Grober and E. Dietrich (eds), *Das deutsche Krankenhaus. Handbuch für Bau, Einrichtung und Betrieb der Krankenanstalten* (Jena: Gustav Fischer, 1911).
102 P. Weinstock (ed.), *Krankenhaus-Betriebslehre. Grundsätze und Erfahrungen in wirtschaftlichen und verwaltungstechnischen Krankenanstalts-Betrieben* (Leipzig: F. Leineweber 1924); E. Pütter, *Einrichtung, Verwaltung und Betrieb der Krankenhäuser* (Leipzig: Johann Ambrosius Barth 1926); Eicke, *Organisation*; W. Alter, *Das Krankenhaus* (Stuttgart: W. Kohlhammer, 1936).
103 We can follow this process of knowledge production with reference to L. Fleck, *Genesis and Development of a Scientific Fact* (Chicago: Chicago University Press, 1979, F/E 1935).
104 Many hospital administrators had been members of the Association of Medical Officers, which had published the *Zeitschrift für Medicinal-Beamte* since 1888.
105 Another journal focusing on social medicine and social hygiene was founded in 1905 to deal with hospital issues: *Zeitschrift für soziale Medizin, Säuglingsfürsorge und Krankenhauswesen sowie die übrigen Grenzgebiete der Medizin und Volkswirtschaft*. And with *Modern Hospital* a similar journal was founded in the United States in 1908.
106 See *Handbücherei für das Gesamte Krankenhauswesen*. 7 vols (Berlin: Julius Springer, 1930), edited by A. Gottstein. One volume dealt with the administration of hospitals and another with food supply and dietary schemes.
107 An important contribution to this development was the publication of S. Eichhorn: *Krankenhausbetriebslehre* (Cologne: W. Kohlhammer, 1958), which became a reference work and was later published in numerous volumes and editions as *Krankenhausbetriebslehre. Theorie und Praxis des Krankenhausbetriebes* [Hospital Economics. Theory and Practice of Hospital Business/Management].
108 W.J. McNerney (ed.), *Hospital and Medical Economics. A Study of Population, Services, Costs, Methods of Payment, and Controls*. 2 vols (Chicago, 1962). On the relationship between national health and national economics, see Christopher Sirrs' Chapter 14 in this volume.

5

Contrasting accounting practices in the urban hospitals of England and France, 1890s to 1930s

Barry M. Doyle

Between the mid-eighteenth and mid-nineteenth centuries, most European countries saw the form and purpose of hospitals slowly develop from infirmaries and hospices for invalids, the elderly, the poor, and the incurable to institutions where patients stayed for only a limited period of time with the aim that they would be cured. Admittedly, curing still meant mainly care, through food, shelter, rest, and largely herbal medicines as defined in the *materia medica*. However, the major scientific developments in medicine of the next hundred years, like bacteriology, the x-ray, and the rise of the pharmaceutical industry, saw both diagnosis and therapies change. Moreover, from the 1730s England saw a new type of 'voluntary' hospital appear, while urban expansion in France saw new hospitals supplementing and supplanting the traditional hospice.[1]

This chapter will discuss how these developments influenced accounting practices in hospitals and how accounting practices affected patient treatment. In relation to other chapters in this volume, it will focus mainly on the financial dimension of calculative practices. Yet it is also apparent that published accounts and reports of voluntary hospitals raise questions about the moral economy of accountability, as donors and other external bodies put pressure on the hospitals to make their accounts more transparent and comparable. Moreover, as Neil Robson has demonstrated, the early twentieth-century establishment of Henry Burdett's uniform accounting system for English hospitals shows how a certain financial and administrative knowledge, the know-how to manage and finance hospitals, was generated and disseminated.[2]

The history of finance in hospitals has been a vibrant area of study in Britain for the past twenty years, yet there are only a few studies on the practices of accounting and their relation to medical knowledge. Research has focused on the income and expenditures of medical institutions and, in particular, on whether the charitably funded hospitals were in financial trouble in the run up to the Second World War[3] – with most accepting that the transformation in voluntary hospital fortunes was driven by the introduction of workers contributory schemes.[4] However, there has been less discussion of the finances of the hospitals of the local state,[5] while Florian Gebreiter and William J. Jackson note in their overview on hospital accounting that the literature is particularly UK-centric. Indeed, for France there are only a few studies of the history of hospital finance and accounting, mainly focusing on Lyon,[6] while increasing attention is being paid to the role played by the *prix de journée* in French hospital accounting.[7]

The following chapter will explore these topics, analysing and comparing hospital finance and accounting practices in France and England. Drawing, in particular, on evidence from the hospitals of the northern English cities of Leeds, Sheffield, and Middlesbrough, and the northern French cities of Lille, Rouen, and Le Havre,[8] it will examine how hospitals were financed; who paid for hospital care and cure? Which groups of patients had access to hospitals? And how (by what means) were hospitals managed and by whom? For hospital accounting was linked to medical knowledge and patient care, as the knowledge about (sources of) income and (future) expenditures shaped the nature of the services delivered. Focusing on the period between the 1890s and 1930s, this chapter discusses both the transformation of hospitals from civic charitable institutions to semi-charitable bodies and the economic factors that underpinned the shift from care to cure. It will compare the differences in hospital accounting and accounting practices in England and France. In particular, it will consider how goods and services were provided, free or through charitable income, including the work of doctors; how the cost of treatment, especially between different types of patients, was calculated; and finally what effects this had on who could be treated and how.

The main sources utilised for the English case are the published annual reports of voluntary hospitals along with some unpublished records including minute books.[9] The sources for the French cities are more diverse. Some hospitals had a so-called *compte moral*, though often only for a few years. Similar to an English annual report, they list income and expenditure under particular headings and provide considerable detail on spending at various levels.[10] In addition, there are manuscript *compte administrative* showing the working out of the annual budget[11] as well as good general committee minutes and reports that include financial data and discussions of disputes, like that concerning the level of the *prix de journée* for the Lille hospitals.[12] The following section will describe patient types and their access to hospitals, along with the finance, management, and accounting practices in French and English hospitals around 1900. It will then discuss subsequent changes in the structure of patients, medicine, and finance and the effects of these changes on hospital accounting and accounting practices in France and Britain until the 1930s.

Finance, accounting, and calculative practices in French and English hospitals around 1900

At the turn of the century, there were three types of hospitals in England. Charitable hospitals that developed from the 1730s as new voluntary institutions were based on a subscriber system, with individuals and groups providing regular payments towards the operating costs of the institution in return for various privileges.[13] Although some ancient hospitals had substantial endowments and investments, most modern (post-1750) hospitals relied on donors to meet operational costs. Certainly, many English hospitals did increase legacy income after 1900, but investments were usually used for capital projects rather than operating costs.[14] Running alongside the voluntary hospitals – that undertook most of the general and specialist surgical and medical treatment – was a system delivered by the local authorities split between two providers: municipal hospitals responsible for infectious diseases, tuberculosis, and some maternity services; and poor law institutions treating a substantial number of the poorest patients, especially the elderly, infirm, and chronically ill.[15] Third, there was a small private sector for the middle and upper classes. This chapter will focus on voluntary hospitals and not deal with the private sector or with England's separate state provision.[16]

In France, a unified system developed based on a network of medieval charitable hospitals and hospices.[17] The early nineteenth century saw the financial and managerial merger of all institutions in a locality under the control of one main provider – *le commission administrative de hospice*. The hospital commissions were responsible for the hospitals dealing with acute diseases and the hospices that managed the care of both sick and healthy social groups.[18] Modern specialist institutions were poorly distributed across the country leaving many non-urban areas dependent on hospice services similar to England's poor law infirmaries – although religious and mutual institutions and a private sector were also present.[19]

Until the 1890s, French hospitals drew on traditional charitable sources of income based on long-term endowments, donations, and legacies, some accrued over hundreds of years.[20] As with subscriptions in England, this was the main source of operational income in the nineteenth century. These funds were used to acquire investments of two types to provide a regular, stable income: rural (farm) and urban (residential rental) property; and stocks and shares (*rentes sur l'état*), especially government bonds.[21] Some hospitals had military wings for treating soldiers for a fee, while many towns received a municipal subvention. This varied from small sums in cities like Lille to a substantial proportion of operating costs as in Le Havre, where the subvention was an established element of commission income provided annually as a fixed lump-sum to meet the cost of the city's sick poor.[22] Moreover, from the 1880s there was a growing number of paying and paid for patients, including those from other communities, those covered by their employers, and those paid for under state schemes like *Assistance Médicale Gratuite* (AMG) for the poor, *Assistance Obligatoire* (AO) for the elderly and infirm, and coverage for industrial injuries.[23]

But access to hospital treatment was rarely based solely on medical need. In most cases the income level of the patient determined admission. In English voluntary hospitals care and medical treatment was free, but only for those defined as 'sick poor'; while in France, patients eligible for institutional care had to be 'indigent'. But defining these groups proved difficult and was as much a social convention as an economic or medical definition.[24] Thus, in most English hospitals until the turn of the century, patients had to secure a letter of recommendation from a subscriber, thus demonstrating their socio-economic status as fit for treatment. Policing this category, especially among outpatients, proved highly controversial as seen in London in the 1880s; but with the rise of contributory schemes, increasing numbers of hospitals abandoned the subscriber letter, Gosling seeing this as a decisive shift towards the medicalisation of the hospital.[25] In France, admission was similarly strictly limited by income and residence, with patients required to supply a certificate of their indigence and residency, as well as providing a medical recommendation from a local doctor.[26]

In addition to social or financial categories, the English voluntary institutions explicitly excluded a range of patient types. For example, at Leeds General Infirmary women close to giving birth, those with mental health problems, suspected of having smallpox or other infectious diseases, venereal disease, tuberculosis, or those 'who are adjudged incurable' were to be denied admission.[27] These groups were excluded for a variety of reasons – financial, reputational, or preventative. Thus, those who could not be cured were likely to incur considerable cost with both financial and reputational damage to the institutions. Pregnant women and their babies stood an above average chance of dying, while those suffering from infectious diseases and the insane were a threat to the other patients and staff and to the efficient working of the institution. There was also a time limit on treatment with a maximum of two months being the norm before discharge and, as a result, hospital managers and doctors preferred surgical cases. Although surgery was more expensive in the short term, patients could be discharged more quickly and an efficient and timely cure was conceivable. In general, the restrictions on admission sought to limit the number of days of maintenance a patient could run up rather than the medical cost of treatment or cure.

But this limitation on patients had consequences for the research undertaken by Medical Schools.[28] Although moderate and curable cases might be easy to handle and, as routine cases, useful for teaching, the severe or interesting cases that formed the basis for medical research were missing. Moreover, during the heyday of microbiology and bacteriology there were few patients with infectious diseases in English general hospitals – though medical schools, like those in Leeds, did form partnerships with municipal infectious diseases institutions.[29] In France, there were fewer medical restrictions, with the main hospitals of Lille treating venereal and infectious diseases, as well as taking in maternity cases and mental health patients for observation. Only children under eighteen months were explicitly excluded.[30]

A range of freely provided services underpinned the voluntary character of English hospitals. The most significant of these was the expertise of the honorary medical staff that treated all patients admitted without receiving payment from either the hospital or the patient. The medical staff did this in part from an obligation to the sick poor, but also to improve their skills and in many cases to advance medical knowledge and build a speciality. They saw the reputational benefits of voluntary hospital work, which might attract paying patients to their private practice, as worth more than a small salary. Moreover, such honorary positions provided power with little responsibility as well as access to the facilities and support of the institution.[31] In France, medical services were provided by trainee doctors (*internes*) and by specialists on a fee basis with local indigent patients treated free of charge.

In both countries there was a dual system of responsibility and operational delivery. English voluntary hospitals were run by a voluntary management committee elected by the subscribers. The board appointed honorary officers, including a chairman, secretary, and treasurer. This voluntary executive committee was legally responsible for the finances of the institution, although daily control was in the hands of paid officials. At Leeds General Infirmary, for instance, a general manager and an assistant, along with an accountant, a cashier, and a collector, oversaw the administration.[32] However, hospital administrators were also more or less responsible to their funders. In the English case this included the subscribers – who had to approve an audit of the accounts – but also the external funders who provided income, such as the increasingly powerful contributory schemes, and other interests like the medical profession.[33]

In France, the local hospital commission comprised seven members: the mayor, two citizens nominated by the council, and four by the prefect. The mayor was chairman while a secretary (*ordonnateur*) and treasurer were appointed. Their responsibilities were similar to those in England though more closely circumscribed by law. The secretary was responsible for preparing the budgets and accounts and paying the bills. The secretary was supported by the *receveur de hospices* who managed the commission's finances and in particular the income and investments and the housekeeper (*économe*) who collected, stored, conserved, and distributed the commodities needed by the hospitals.[34] In France, hospitals were overseen but not run by the municipality, although they could challenge the setting of the daily rate and the allocation of costs in their budgets, while the prefect had to approve the accounts and future budgets.[35]

English hospitals had increasingly transparent accounting procedures based on the publication of detailed income and expenditure figures made available to subscribers, stakeholders, and the general public through an annual report. From the mid-eighteenth century the report – and the Annual General Meeting to which it was presented – demonstrated the transparency and propriety of the institution and its actions. The opportunity for scrutiny ensured that the democratic body of subscribers could hold the committee to account and be sure that their money freely given was being used for the purposes intended.[36] The main system of accounting was 'retrospective' – the accounts reported on the income raised and how it was spent in the previous year. The procedures for presenting the accounts had considerable local variation, but by 1900 the larger voluntary hospitals were influenced by Burdett's Uniform Accounting System, the key innovations of which were the separation of ordinary and extraordinary income and the use of a balance sheet.[37]

In France, transparency came through the external oversight provided by the prefect and city. As with much of Europe, French institutions presented 'prospective' budgets anticipating future income and expenditure. Based on the previous year's activities and the expected income, a budget for the current year was sent to the city council and the prefect of the department for approval. The budget included a proportion of income allocated for extraordinary expenditure (usually 10 per cent) and could be enhanced with supplementary credits. At the end of the year the accounts were signed off and any deficit either met by the municipality or carried forward.[38] The categories utilised were notionally universal but considerable diversity existed even in the three cities examined here.

Shifts in hospital treatment and changes in accounting practices between 1900 and the 1930s

Aiming to treat the majority of the sick poor or indigent for free was not a significant problem as long as demand, supply, and income levels were broadly in alignment.[39] But after the turn of the century, several factors in this equation changed.

From the late nineteenth century, the charitable class of patients began to shrink as working-class incomes rose. At the same time, an increasing number of patients were seeking admission who could meet their own cost or were eligible to have their costs met for them. In both countries these included patients from other local authority areas, those covered by state schemes like industrial injuries, people insured by friendly societies, private companies, the state, or mutual contributory schemes.[40] In Leeds the General Infirmary (LGI) allowed admission to paying patients, while in Lille a wide range of non-indigent could be admitted, including various workers as well as paying patients on the *surety* of a local citizen.[41] Furthermore, communities without general or specialist facilities could send patients at an appropriate *prix de journée*. Residents of other communities taken ill or injured in the city would be treated, but attempts might be made to recover the costs.[42]

In addition to these paying patients, new groups expected access during and after the First World War. In France, inflation and economic crisis had the consequence that many lower middle-class families, unable to meet the full cost of their treatment, were seeking access to the hospitals.[43] In Le Havre in 1926 the administrative commission noted that:

> It is remarkable how many people there were who in the past, when they fell ill, could have supported the cost of the doctor and medication but, due to the increased cost of living, find it impossible to pay their doctor and pharmacist. This category of people – small landlords, modest employers, are today more and more numerous in the hospital admissions and […] they have to be treated at the cost of the community.[44]

Similar trends were noted in England by 1930 as an increasing number of lower middle-class patients sought free treatment through membership in contributory schemes.[45] Although there was a trend to admit patients on medical grounds and then to seek payment, universal admission was still opposed, especially by the medical profession, that saw the potential for loss of income, and hospital administrators, who feared free-riders accessing services underpinned by charity.[46]

The increase of non-charitable cases admitted to hospitals presaged the shift from care to cure, as both the number of patients and their profile changed. Patients requiring care were more likely to be indigent, economically inactive, and to stay in the institution for prolonged periods.[47] Those seeking a cure were likely to be relatively prosperous, economically active, and looking to return to work quickly. The former were invariably dependent on charity or state support while the latter were acquiring access through contributory schemes and ultimately French state insurance. Moreover, the shift from care to cure had positive effects on the length of the patients' hospital stay, with evidence of substantial reductions in the length of stay in English hospitals in the 1920s, although a similar trend was not seen in France before the 1930s.[48]

The shift from care to cure also had consequences for hospital costs, as a range of essential improvements in medical diagnostics and treatment were deployed in clinical practice. In predominantly caring regimes, food and housekeeping were central to the budgets of hospitals with routine treatment usually administered by nursing staff, whereas salaries, pharmaceuticals, and medical technologies were of limited importance. But after the turn of the century, scientific and technological tools became more important as laboratory facilities, x-ray units, and electrical departments began to appear.[49] Much of the cost associated with these new treatments was bound up in capital costs – operating theatres, x-ray departments, light treatment, radium treatment, and laboratories – although further expenses could result from new medicines like serum therapy or Salvarsan.[50]

By the early decades of the twentieth century, English hospitals were employing a small number of paid trainee doctors and salaried specialists, although both hospitals and doctors resisted the pressure to provide payment for senior medical staff who continued to give their services for free.[53] By the 1930s, there was a complex debate around how to recognise the contribution of the honorary medical staff without undermining the charitable work the hospitals did for the poor. In some cases, the hospitals allocated a proportion of the income raised from contributory schemes to a staff fund for research, travel, or other non-remunerative activities. In some small general practitioner hospitals, medical staff received a direct payment and in other schemes direct payment was being considered by 1938. But in general, the medical profession preferred to rely on income thresholds for contributory scheme membership to ensure that doctors were not losing lower middle-class patients to the free hospital system.[54]

The rising number and changing types of patients and the increasing cost of their treatment, along with economic crises, inflation, and reduced legacies and donations, required new solutions for hospital finance in both countries. The late nineteenth-century agricultural depression saw a decline in farming incomes while urban property was also increasingly problematic due to low yield, long leases, poor returns, and high maintenance costs that had to be met from operational income. As a result, stocks and shares became more significant in France, where managers in Lille, for example, were keen to extricate themselves from urban property in the early 1920s as very long leases came up for renewal.[55] But this policy faltered when investment returns collapsed as inflation and a weak currency ate into the value of stocks and bonds.

Thus, extended access for patients and rising costs made it necessary to restructure hospital income, and in the years after 1914, new schemes for patient payment transformed hospital finances – which in turn raised questions about the charitable status of the institutions. The continuing presence of charitable resources for both English and French institutions had an effect on how hospitals chose to account for the growing number of paying and paid for patients on their wards. Questions emerged about how to measure the cost of these patients when the hospitals were now only partially charitable institutions. Did they expect someone to pay and if so by what method? To meet this challenge new charging models were developed – lump sum allocations in England versus individual daily fees for treatment in France (Figures 5.1 and 5.2).[56]

In England, the National Health Insurance Act, introduced in 1911, only covered payments to the doctor and for medicine, but not for hospital treatment.[57] As a result, the early twentieth century saw the

	1910 %	1920 %	1928 %
Staff	24	25	30
Domestic	19	21	19
Food	30	23	19
Medical	19	18	17
General	8	13	15

5.1 Expenditure, General Voluntary Hospitals Leeds and Sheffield, 1913–28.[51]

	1910 %	1920 %	1928 %
Staff	9	13	13
Domestic	14	33	23
Food	70	46	49
Medical	5	5	10
General	2	3	5

5.2 Expenditure, Lille Hospital Commission, 1910–28.[52]

growth of worker-led mutual contributory schemes that provided free treatment in exchange for a small weekly payment. Somewhat later in France, the introduction of state insurance opened up the hospitals to around a quarter of the population. Both of these initiatives raised the issue of upper and lower salary limits for membership, especially in England where schemes had limited regulation and no uniform rules.[58] Moreover, for French institutions new accounting issues were raised, in particular what costs should and should not be included in the day rates charged to insurers?[59]

In England, no attempt was made to link the patients treated to the financial support provided by external funders. Instead, many of the larger contributory schemes took 'the easier path in dealing with hospitals by giving block grants allocated usually in ratio to the mass of work done, not by making payment of accounts in respect of individual members of schemes actually treated. Doubtless much clerical and accountancy work is thereby avoided.'[60]

To meet these challenges, English hospitals came to rely on a combination of lump sum and standardised weekly charges while the daily rate was rarely used. In some cities, weekly charges were published from the early 1920s and information on the average cost of all patients was collected,[61] although this was rather meaningless as an accounting or charging tool. Indeed, the published weekly charges rarely covered the full cost of treatment. Thus, the 1921 Sheffield tariff stated 'in-patients other than contributors to the Joint Hospitals' Scheme, their dependents and the necessitous poor should be asked to pay a standard rate of £1 15s 0d per week towards the cost of their maintenance'. This was not the actual cost of treatment and most patients paid significantly less than the figure – somewhere nearer to one pound.[62] Moreover, unlike France, there was no attempt to calculate the medical cost of different classes of patients with charges levied only for maintenance costs.

The reason English hospitals were reluctant to opt for precise charging was the central importance of both charitable/voluntary ideals and charitable/voluntary resources to the system. As in France up until the 1940s, receipts were comprised of voluntary subscriptions and donations along with direct and indirect patient payments – a mix of charitable and commercial income. However, the mutual contribution schemes challenged the fundamental basis of the voluntary hospital system. In these schemes, workers paid small weekly contributions to a fund that entitled members to free treatment if admitted to a hospital that was part of the scheme. As was noted in 1930, larger schemes collected contributions and then redistributed to member hospitals based on the average number of patients treated. This allocation did not meet the cost of the patients; it merely reflected the relative workload. Administrative simplicity aside, the schemes recognised that it was essential to distance the hospitals from a straightforward commercial transaction, foregrounding instead the ongoing charitable function of these institutions.[63]

Thus, the key feature of the English system was the absence of a link between the patient and the direct cost of the treatment. There were a number of reasons for this, some of which were derived from accounting practices, but at root it was because many of the costs were met from voluntary sources. As S. Clayton-Fryers, Secretary of LGI, noted in 1938: 'Even if contributory schemes met the full cost of maintenance their members would still be the recipients of charity in so far as they were using buildings and equipment provided at great cost by the philanthropic public.'[64]

This contrasted markedly with the situation in France where increasingly complex clerical and accountancy work was undertaken to establish an appropriate fee to charge both paying and paid-for patients.[65] From the late nineteenth century, the key accounting model was the *prix de journée*, a form that shaped and was shaped by the practices of health care in the hospital. It was emblematic of the transfer from charitable to social medicine as it reflected a growth in the number of patients for whom the cost of treatment was recovered and therefore needed to be known. *Prix de journée* initially emerged in the 1890s to charge other communities for extra-mural patients: since hospitals were for local people, the cost of non-resident patients had to be recovered.[66] Daily rates were then devised for AMG in 1893 and these were extended as other patients whose costs were met by state schemes emerged, such as industrial injury cases (1899) and AO in 1905.[67] The *prix de journée* was also used for military patients treated in communal hospitals, although the rate was set by the Ministry of War without considering the local cost of treatment. This proved problematic during the First World War when a sharp increase in military patients placed considerable strain on the financial and physical resources of hospitals in *Seine Inférieure*.[68]

In 1918, a law permitted separate *prix de journée* for medicine and surgery, with the latter calculated as a 1.33 multiple of the former. The basic resource unit emphasised maintenance and was to be calculated by summing all institutional expenses minus medical personnel, purchase of medicine, dressings, clinical instruments, and laboratory equipment divided by the total number of patient treatment days. These costs were further differentiated for hospice cases, with the elderly, incurable, medical, and surgical patients charged at progressively higher rates. These rates were revised upwards in 1926 when the hospital day-rate was set at twice the hospice cost. Moreover, costs could vary enormously with the rate for surgical cases in 1926 priced at 7.5 French francs (FF) in Bayonne but 24.27 FF in Paris. These rates were based on highly differentiated real costs for patients: evidence from Lille in 1922 showed that spending on patients in the Hospice Generale was less than half that in the Charité hospital – a difference accounted for by lower food and drink rations and large numbers of unpaid religious nurses.[69]

The *prix de journée* was supposed to capture the real cost of treatment. But significant problems emerged, as seen in the hospitals of Lille and Le Havre.[70] The tariff was retrospective. Initially, the law decreed it should be based on the average cost of treatment over the preceding five years, although this was gradually reduced to three years. This proved problematic in periods of inflation like 1914–28, yet pricing based on previous years remained the practice until 1943.[71] In Le Havre, this accountancy practice hampered the activities of the hospitals as it limited their ability to increase their income and therefore their expenditure. There was also uncertainty about what costs could be included when calculating the daily rate. The law favoured direct operational costs only, but hospitals wanted to include capital outlay, renovations, administration, new equipment, etc. This caused considerable problems, for example in Lille in 1926, when the commission argued for the inclusion of capital costs in the daily rate for non-indigent patients on the grounds that the income that had built and maintained the hospitals had been given to the poor of the city and should not subsidise the treatment of the relatively better off.[72]

The fall in other sources of income, especially after 1914, meant the *prix de journée* became central to meeting rising costs and increased demand. Hospitals began to utilise it in negotiations with all patient providers. It was applied to flat rate payments such as those made by the military and lump sum municipal subventions for indigent patients, usually to show that these were inadequate. In Le Havre in 1926, for example, the hospital commission insisted the council pay its subvention in line with the charges the town imposed on the 'charitable establishments' in a way that represented the money they spent for 'the treatment of the sick poor of the town'.[73] The following year it proved necessary to utilise a department subsidy to allow the hospital to set 'actual figures' for the *prix de journée* while an agreement was finally made with the municipality for a substantial increase in the subvention from 600,000 FF to 1.4 million FF in 1928 and 2 million FF in 1929. The move pleased the commission which commented, enigmatically, that this meant they could 'present honest budgets'.[74] The fraught negotiations in Le Havre showed that the *prix de journée* made hospitals more aware of their costs but also limited their actions.

In response to the ongoing financial crises of many hospital commissions in northern France, the first elements of the French social insurance programme were instituted between 1928 and 1932. This met the cost of treatment for around 25 per cent of the population in the social groups just above the indigent, the elderly, and the infirm and provided both increased access and substantial additional income.[75] Thus, the key difference that developed between the two nations in the 1920s was between the lump sum/flat rate payment system in England and French schemes that aimed to meet the full cost of individual patients. The decision not to seek full cost payments either from patients or the contributory schemes displayed a tension in the development of English hospitals. For while patients may have demanded access to the hospital and have seen their payment of 3 pence a week to the contributory scheme as entitling them to treatment, the hospitals, doctors, and scheme managers all retained an interest in maintaining the fiction of charity. Certainly, the published and private accounts of English hospitals became more sophisticated and detailed. Average costs were calculated per patient and per bed while weekly charges were set. There was even a trend toward calculating actual costs (reckoned to be about £3 per week by 1930) but these were not applied to patients on the general wards. Moreover, the mixture of charitable and patient payment made accounting potentially difficult and accurate charging even more so – as the French found in the 1920s.

Accounting for health and the shift from care to cure between 1900 and the 1930s

To some extent, the accounts do reflect a movement from care to cure in the activities of interwar hospitals. In general, charitable care included hospice care. The costs were relatively low and the purpose was to keep the patient – for whom little could be done medically – safe and comfortable. In institutions delivering this kind of service, much was not accounted for, including much of the nursing and the time provided by doctors. In both England and France, religious orders and able-bodied inmates provided care in ways that rarely appeared in the account books,[76] with French nursing and domestic staff accounted for in the same way as patients, namely by days of maintenance.[77] Finally, these institutions rarely revealed their management costs, other than a small heading for administration. In both nations, most management was undertaken by voluntary or political appointees and not by paid managers.[78]

Medicalisation heralded important shifts in the accounting process. The key changes included the diminishing importance of food in the accounts (see Figures 5.1 and 5.2). From prior to the First World War into the 1920s, the detailed recording of foodstuffs and other household items took up a significant part of the published accounts with year on year comparisons of costs and spending.[79] This could include listings of important household items like candles, coal, and wood for lighting and heating. But these products slowly disappeared from the published accounts in English hospitals as food and household took up less of the annual cost of the institutions and the introduction of electricity, gas, and central heating moved the cost from commodities to utility bills. On the other hand, salaries became increasingly prominent. From the turn of the century, hospitals employed more and more people. There were more junior doctors and nursing was largely professionalised in England, though less so in France. Domestic staff were employed and increasingly lived outside the institution, while the administration grew as more complex department structures and the need to track and account for patients required the employment of more clerks and managers. Ironically, it was only the pharmacy and the medical technology costs that remained stable (proportionately), although the amount spent under these headings did increase in cash terms. For example, at the Leeds General, expenditure on the pathology laboratory had reached £1,500 by 1938. Furthermore, the city's specialist Maternity Hospital and Hospital for Women joined together to establish a laboratory paid for by donations and income from private patients. Similarly, although much of the scientific research in Sheffield was carried out in the university labs, thanks to the donation of a large house on the outskirts of town an isolation centre for mothers was established that cut cases of puerperal sepsis and provided research facilities. In all these cases, the capital for expansion came from donors rather than from operational income.[80]

The shift from care to cure was most evident in capital expenditure – and ironically it was the charitable nature of the English institutions that allowed them to modernise more rapidly than their French counterparts. Investment in new technologies like x-ray, pathology, radium treatment, and improved operating theatres was met entirely by individual donation or public subscription – from Lord Manton's gift of an x-ray unit to LGI in 1922 to Alderman Graves' £100,000 donation to found a Sheffield Radium Centre in 1940.[81] In some cases, the focus of facilities was determined by outside agencies, such as the Yorkshire Miners' Welfare donating £25,000 for a new wing in Sheffield that included an orthopaedic unit.[82] Until the 1930s it is clear that the French hospitals outside of Paris, with their limited sources of income, were severely restricted in their opportunities to expand. Le Havre could not afford to paint its wards for eight years, let alone develop new specialities, while in Lille conflict raged over the appropriate use of the 10 per cent allocation for extraordinary expenditure.[83] The situation improved in the later 1920s when more generous allocations from the municipality allowed Le Havre to open a laboratory suite and Rouen instigated plans for a maternity block and a new surgery wing.[84]

During the period under investigation, hospital wards opened to wider social groups while the costs of treatment passed from elite philanthropists and local tax payers to direct payment, indirect mutual insurance, and, in some cases, state-backed social insurance.[85] The key observable differences between England and France were that: England adopted a mutual model while France eventually instituted state insurance; England funded most hospital treatment through lump sum allocations while France funded most hospital treatment via reimbursement for the daily cost of the patient (*prix de journée*). Moreover, where the lump sum had been used, for example in well-established municipal subventions like that in Le Havre, by the late 1920s this was increasingly accounted for and remunerated on a *prix de journée* basis.

Thus, it would seem that the development of the *prix de journée* was central to the transformation from charitable to social medicine in France. It aimed to allow institutions to recover much of the cost of the treatment they provided and to develop a more modern, medicalised service that rejected the restrictions of traditional and municipal charity.[86] Yet, it would appear that the English voluntary hospital accounting method of lump sum allocation did not accept the shift from charitable to social medicine. This was partly a conscious decision to retain the free services of consulting staff and partly a desire to keep administrative and transaction costs to a minimum. Yet it was a discourse as much as it was an accounting practice – a way of working that continued to prioritise medical need over ability to pay. It facilitated a substantial expansion of hospital provision and treatment in interwar England, while at the same time managing entitlement and ultimately keeping costs down. Indeed, many of the practices learned in this period were transferred into the NHS allowing it to deliver universal health care free at the point of delivery while managing costs and expectations.[87]

It is apparent that the economic crises faced by the two nations after 1914 and the expansion of hospital access to a wider range of social groups shifted the main function of accounts from providing information on efficiency for use by funders to establishing a framework for fair and effective pricing in the context of a mixed economy of provision. In the process it raised significant issues around how to account for the hospitals' charitable resources and obligations. Thus, the changes in hospital finance and the calculation of lump sum, weekly and daily charges influenced accounting practices. For France, proper accounting in the hospitals as the basis for the calculation of the *prix de journée* had wide-ranging implications for the value of charges for hospital treatment. This was even more true for English hospitals where the meaning of accounting practices changed more than in France, corresponding to the shift from care to cure.

Notes

1 B. Abel-Smith, *The Hospitals, 1800–1948: A Study in Social Administration in England and Wales* (London: Heineman, 1964); J. Imbert, *Les Hôpitaux en France* (Paris: Presses Universitaires de France, 5th edn, 1988).
2 N. Robson, 'A contextual history of accounting in UK hospitals, 1880–1974' (PhD Dissertation, Cardiff University, 2006).
3 S. Cherry, *Medical Services and the Hospitals in Britain, 1860–1939* (Cambridge: Cambridge University Press, 1996); M. Gorsky, J. Mohan, and

M. Powell, 'The financial health of voluntary hospitals in interwar Britain', *Economic History Review* 55 (2002), 533–57; N. Hayes and B.M. Doyle, 'Eggs, rags and whist drives: Popular munificence and the development of provincial medical voluntarism between the wars', *Historical Research* 86 (2013), 712–40. For hospital accounting, see the overview of F. Gebreiter and W.J. Jackson, 'Fertile ground: The history of accounting in hospitals', *Accounting History Review* 25 (2015), 177–82.

4   M. Gorsky, J. Mohan with T. Willis, *Mutualism and Health Care: British Hospital Contributory Schemes in the Twentieth Century* (Manchester: Manchester University Press, 2006).

5   A. Levene, M. Powell, J. Stewart, and B. Taylor, *Cradle to Grave: Municipal Medicine in Interwar England and Wales* (Bern: Peter Lang, 2011).

6   M. Garden, *Histoire Economique d'une Grande Enterprise de Santé: Le Budget des Hospices Civils de Lyon, 1800–1976* (Lyon: Presses Universitaires de Lyon, 1980); and J-P. Domin, *Une Histoire Economique de l'Hôpital, XIXe-XXe Siècles: Une Analyse Rétrospective du Développement Hospitalier*, 2 vols (Paris: La Documentation Française, 2008); T.B. Smith, *Creating the Welfare State in France, 1880–1940* (Montreal and Kingston: McGill-Queen's University Press, 2003); T.B. Smith, 'The social transformation of hospitals and the rise of medical insurance in France, 1914–1943', *Historical Journal* 41 (1998), 1055–87.

7   J-P. Domin, 'L'expérimentation du prix de journée dans les hôpitaux publics. Naissance d'une organisation de soins socialisés (1893–1945)', Unpublished paper presented to XXe Journées d'Histoire du Management et des Organisations: La Santé, Lille, 2015.

8   B.M. Doyle, 'Healthcare before welfare states: Hospitals in early twentieth century England and France', *Canadian Bulletin of Medical History* 33 (2016) 174–204.

9   For example, Leeds General Infirmary, *Annual Reports* (Leeds: LGI, annually); Sheffield Royal Hospital, *Annual Report* (Sheffield: Sheffield Royal Hospital, annually).

10 Le Havre has a good set of *compte moral* running from 1908–34. Lille only has one *compte moral* – for 1912 and Rouen five from 1928–32. Hospice de Lille, *Compte Moral Administratif de L'Exercice 1912*, Archives Départementale du Nord (ADN) 96J/3rd supplement 10; Vice President de la Commission Administrative, *Rapport Annuel sur La Gestion des Hopitaux de Rouen* (Rouen, annually 1928–32); Hospices du Havre, *Compte Moral du Exercise* (Rouen: annually) Archives Municipales Le Havre (AMLH), Mhop 121–125.

11 These exist from 1906 to 1936 for Lille and intermittently for Rouen, Commission Administrative des Hospice de la Ville de Lille, *Hospices – Comptes*

Administratifs, 1905–35, ADN 96J/2303; Registres de délibérations de l'Hospice General et de l'Hotel Dieu, Rouen, Archives Départementale du Seine Maritime [ADSM], H-Depot 3, L162.
12 Hospices de Lille, 'Situation Financière Rapports, 1924–30', ADN 96J/2396.
13 See B.M. Doyle, *The Politics of Hospital Provision in Early Twentieth-Century Britain* (London: Pickering & Chatto, 2014), pp. 35–40.
14 Gorsky, Mohan, and Powell, 'Financial health'.
15 A. Levene, J. Stewart, and B. Taylor, *Cradle to Grave. Municipal Medicine in Interwar England and Wales* (Oxford: Peter Lang, 2011); J. Reinarz and L. Schwarz (eds), *Medicine and the Workhouse* (Rochester: University of Rochester Press, 2013).
16 B.M. Doyle, 'Les soins hospitaliers en Grande-Bretagne pendant l'entre-deux-guerres: un marché de la santé?', in B. Valat (ed.), *Marches de la Sante en Europe au XXe Siecle* (Toulouse: Presses Universitaires du Midi, 2020).
17 Imbert, *Les Hôpitaux en France*.
18 Doyle, 'Healthcare before welfare states'.
19 C. Chevandier, *L'Hôpital dans la France du XXe Siècle* (Paris: Perrin, 2009).
20 In Lille they amounted to around 45 million francs worth of assets by the 1920s – although in newer urban areas like Le Havre they were small. Hospices de Lille, 'Situation Financière Rapports, 1924–30' ADN 96J/2396, Hospices du Havre, *Compte Moral 1924*, AMLH, Mhop 123.
21 A. Lemay, *Etude Historique et Pratique de L'Assistance Publique en France: Les Hôpitaux et Hospices Civils de Lille* (Lille: Dubar, 1912); Domin, *Histoire Economique*. Lyon favoured urban rentals, Garden, *Histoire Economique*.
22 Lemay, *Etude Historique*; Hospices du Havre, *Compte Moral 1912*, AMLH, Mhop 121.
23 Lemay, *Etude Historique*, pp. 72–102 and 302–6; Smith, 'Social transformation', 1082–5.
24 G.C. Gosling, *Payment and Philanthropy in British Healthcare, 1918–48* (Manchester: Manchester University Press, 2017); Lemay, *Etude Historique*.
25 K. Waddington, *Charity and the London Hospitals, 1850–1898* (Woodbridge: Boydell and Brewer, 2000); Gosling, *Payment and Philanthropy*.
26 LeMay, *Etude Historique*, pp. 331–5, 343, 359.
27 'Extracts from the Rules and Bye-Laws', LGI, *Annual Report 1920*, p. 140.
28 S. Sturdy, 'The political economy of scientific medicine: Science, education and the transformation of medical practice in Sheffield, 1890–1922', *Medical History* 36:2 (1992), 125–59.
29 Doyle, *Politics*, p. 30.
30 Lemay, *Etude Historique*.
31 G. Weisz, *Divide and Conquer: A Comparative History of Medical Specialization* (Oxford: Oxford University Press, 2006); A. Digby, *The Evolution*

    of British General Practice, 1850–1948 (Oxford: Oxford University Press, 1999).
32 LGI, *Annual Report*, 1932, p. 10; Doyle, *Politics*, pp. 142–3.
33 Gorsky et al., *Mutualism*.
34 LeMay, *Etude Historique*.
35 Mairie de Rouen, *Rapport documentaire et critique sur la politique hospitalière de la ville de Rouen* (Rouen: Presse Autographique, 1925), p. 19; Hospices de Lille, 'Situation Financière Rapports, 1924–30', ADN 96J/2396.
36 A. Holden, W. Funnell, and D. Oldroyd, 'Accounting and the moral economy of illness in Victorian England: the Newcastle Infirmary', *Accounting, Auditing and Accountability Journal* 24 (2009), 525–52.
37 Robson, 'Contextual history'.
38 LeMay, *Etude Historique*; Hospices du Havre, *Compte Moral 1924* AMLH, Mhop 123 and subsequent years.
39 Domin, *Histoire Economique*; Cherry, *Medical Services*.
40 Gosling, *Payment and Philanthropy*; Domin, *Histoire Economique*.
41 'Rules', LGI, *Annual Report*, 1920, p. 140; Hospice de Lille, *Compte Moral 1912*.
42 Domin, *Histoire Economique*.
43 Smith, 'Social transformation'.
44 Hospices du Havre, *Compte Moral 1926*, AMLH, Mhop 123, p. XVIII.
45 *Hospitals Yearbook 1931* (London: British Hospital Association, 1932), pp. 56–68.
46 Doyle, 'Les soins hospitaliers'.
47 G. Weisz, *Chronic Disease in the Twentieth Century: A History* (Baltimore: Johns Hopkins University Press, 2014).
48 R. Pinker, *English Hospital Statistics, 1861–1938* (London: Heinemann, 1966), p. 11; Hospice de Lille, *Compte Moral Administratif de L'Exercice 1912*, p. 137; 'Rapport établis par les bureau d'hygiène de différentes ville du department', ADN, Séries X 220–87349.
49 R. Wall, *Bacteria in Britain, 1880–1939* (London: Pickering & Chatto, 2013).
50 For developments in Leeds and Sheffield, see Doyle, *Politics*, pp. 49–52.
51 Sheffield Royal Hospital, Sheffield Royal Infirmary, Leeds General Infirmary, Leeds Public Dispensary, *Annual Reports*, 1918–47.
52 Commission Administrative des Hospice de la Ville de Lille, *Hospices – Comptes Administratifs*, 1905–35, ADN 96J/2303.
53 *Hospitals Yearbook 1931*, pp. 56–68.
54 Doyle, 'Les soins hospitaliers'; *Sheffield Independent*, 7 and 8 September 1938.
55 A.J. Vancostenobel, *Le Bien des Pauvres de Lille: cent ans de la vie des arrentements des hospices* (Lille, 1929); Garden, *Histoire Economique*.

56 Domin, 'Prix de journée'.
57 G. Finlayson, *Citizen, State, and Social Welfare in Britain 1830–1990* (Oxford: Clarendon, 1994).
58 Smith, 'Social transformation'; Doyle, 'Les soins hospitaliers'.
59 Hospices de Lille, 'Situation Financière Rapports', 1924–30' ADN 96J/2396.
60 *Hospitals Yearbook 1931*, p. 59.
61 Gosling, *Payment and Philanthropy*; LGI, *Annual Report 1919*, p. 11.
62 SRH, *Annual Report, 1921*, p. 6; SRI, *Annual Report, 1922*, p. 9.
63 For example, Leeds Workpeople's Hospital Fund, *Annual Report, 1937* (Leeds, 1938), pp. 18–20.
64 *Manchester Guardian*, 26 November 1938.
65 Domin, 'Prix de journée'.
66 Domin, *Histoire Economique*.
67 Smith, 'Social transformation' for the schemes; Domin, *Histoire Economique* for the development of *prix de journée*.
68 'Registres de délibérations de l'Hospice General et de l'Hotel Dieu, Rouen' 1 Decembre 1926, ADSM, H-Depot 3, L162; Hospices du Havre, *Compte Moral 1918* AMLH, Mhop 122.
69 'Rapport sur le prix de journée des pensionnaires à leur charge' ADN 96J/1763.
70 Domin, 'Prix de journée'.
71 Domin, *Histoire Economique*; 'Rapport sur le prix de journée' ADN 96J/1763.
72 Garden, *Histoire Economique*; Domin, *Histoire Economique*; 'Rapport sur le prix de journée' ADN 96J/1763, pp. 6–7.
73 Hospices du Havre, *Compte Moral 1926*, AMLH, Mhop 123 p. XIX.
74 Hospices du Havre, *Compte Moral 1928*, AMLH, Mhop 123 p. XX.
75 Smith, *Welfare State*, pp. 132–5.
76 K. Schultheiss, *Bodies and Souls: Politics and the Professionalization of Nursing in France, 1880–1922* (Cambridge, MA: Harvard University Press, 2001); B.M. Doyle, *A History of Hospitals in Middlesbrough* (Middlesbrough: South Tees Hospitals NHS Trust, 2002).
77 Vice President de la Commission Administrative, *Rapport Annuel sur La Gestion des Hopitaux de Rouen, 1928* (Rouen, 1929), pp. 46–7.
78 For case studies of hospital management, see Waddington, *Charity and the London Hospitals*; Doyle, *Politics*, chapter 6.
79 LGI, *Annual Report, 1919*, pp. 40–7; SRI, *Annual Report, 1920*, p. 9; *Rapport Annuel sur La Gestion des Hopitaux de Rouen, 1928*, p. 40.
80 Doyle, *Politics*, chapter 2.
81 Doyle, *Politics*, pp. 127–30.

82 SRH, *Annual Report, 1937*.
83 Hospices de Lille, 'Situation Financière Rapports', 1924–30" ADN 96J/2396, Hospices du Havre, *Compte Moral 1924*, AMLH, Mhop 123.
84 'Les diverses améliorations des hospices civil de Rouen ont été inaugurées hier', *La Dépêche de Rouen*, 24 April 1932.
85 Gosling, *Payment and Philanthropy*; Smith, *Welfare State*.
86 Domin, *Histoire Economique*.
87 M. Gosky, 'The British National Health Service 1948–2008: A review of the historiography', *Social History of Medicine* 21 (2008), 437–60.

6

Reforming on paper: Accounting practices in the Leuven Academic Hospitals, 1920–60

Joris Vandendriessche

During the Second World War in Leuven, governing the teaching hospitals of Belgium's largest university was an uphill battle. German troops had occupied St. Pieters Hospital and part of St. Raphael Hospital and converted them into a military hospital. The evacuation of these buildings required the redistribution of medical services, patients, and physicians across the remaining space. Fear of German demands for additional hospital resources remained a preoccupation throughout the war.[1] Inflation jeopardised the financial health of the hospitals, as prices for coal and food rose rapidly, while the income from patients and local authorities remained stable or even declined. Under these circumstances, Gerard Van der Schueren began his tenure as the first director of St. Raphael Hospital. While he acted primarily as a 'crisis manager', he also envisioned opportunities for a permanent, far-reaching reorganisation. In his view, the war offered 'a unique opportunity for our generation to carry out reforms'.[2] But in response to Van der Schueren's reform plans, most professors of the medical faculty simply retorted: 'After the war!'[3]

Ultimately, however, although he had hoped for more speedy reforms, Van der Schueren was successful. His wartime plans were implemented in the late 1940s and 1950s. The Second World War thus proved a turning point in the administrative history of Leuven's academic hospitals.[4] Van der Schueren's elaborate correspondence with the university's rector, Honoré Van Waeyenbergh, offers a glimpse into a professionalising administration that included, as a crucial component, a centralised 'accountancy department'. This professionalisation took place parallel to – and this was no mere coincidence – the development of the Belgian welfare state. As elsewhere in Western Europe, access to health care was expanded through public investments. Such access became a 'right' for all citizens. And this, in turn, fortified a process that had begun in the late nineteenth century: the transformation of the hospital from a site designed to care for the poor into one designed to deliver specialised medical treatment to all social classes.[5] The archival holdings for the Leuven academic hospitals in this period include the products (budgets, balances, and reports) of a massive paper machine. These documents allow us to ask new questions about the functioning of administrators like Van der Schueren and of the bookkeepers in his accountancy department. How was 'accountability' organised and who was accountable to whom? And more importantly: to what extent did bookkeepers and administrators – through their accounting practices – steer the expansion of academic health care?

To answer these questions, I will examine an extended period of time, including the interwar period. I will consider the hospital reforms in Leuven as part of a broader trend toward 'rationalisation' in the mid-twentieth century – a trend that comprised new forms of management and budgetary control. These techniques were introduced well before the establishment of a centralised hospital administration. To uncover them, I will investigate the early history of St. Raphael Hospital, which was comprised of financially autonomous institutes led by 'professor-directors'. By exploring their prewar managerial roles, we can better assess the impact of Van der Schueren's postwar reforms. These reforms, it should be clear, considerably diminished professors' power to make decisions autonomously. But there is more to this story. I will argue that accounting practices became more performative in the postwar period, in the sense that by creating new administrative realities (on paper) bookkeepers also influenced – to a far greater extent than in the interwar years – the actual organisation of medical care in the hospital. Put differently, accounting became central to the redistribution of responsibilities in a hospital that was increasingly structured around an expanding range of medical specialties. It proved an essential tool of the integrated postwar hospital model of the academic health centre or *centre hospitalier universitaire*. The restructuring of the Leuven academic hospitals offers a telling example of this.

Class-based bookkeeping

In the years after the First World War, St. Pieters Hospital was still governed according to nineteenth-century customs. It was owned and financed by the Social Service Agency of the city of Leuven, which had reached an agreement with the congregation of Augustinian Hospital Sisters. The latter were in charge of nursing and daily housekeeping. Medical services were provided by the medical faculty of the Catholic University of Leuven, for which St. Pieters served as a teaching hospital. Faculty members received a fixed annual fee from the Social Service Agency and a salary from the university for teaching and organising practical training for medical students.[6] The patients belonged to the lowest social classes, the so-called indigent population. They were hospitalised on the wards and received free treatment. In a sense, they 'paid' with their bodies by being subjected to the examinations of medical students. Other costs such as meals, drugs, and accommodation were covered by the Social Service Agency. This type of hospital governance, which relied on a collaboration between local authorities, religious congregations, and universities, existed in most major Belgian cities. It was modelled on the French health care system, which had been introduced during the French Revolution in the Southern Netherlands, the region that would become Belgium in 1830. This model also included a *Commission d'Assistance Publique* that was comprised of local politicians and members of the urban elite and that acted as a hospital board.[7] The major difference with France, however, was that besides these public hospitals, religious congregations were much more active in setting up their own socio-medical institutions (e.g. hospitals, hospices, asylums), resulting in a firm grip of the Catholic Church over the provision of care.[8]

It is therefore telling that most bookkeeping in St. Raphael Hospital before the Second World War was done by the Sisters of Love (whereas after 1945 a central university hospital administration would be established). The contract of 1929 between the university and the congregation not only entrusted the daily care for all patients to the religious sisters, but also stipulated that they would be in charge of collecting fees. To this end, they set up an administrative bureau on the ground floor of the Clinic of Internal Medicine. The fee was set at 25 Belgian francs per day of hospitalisation and per patient, following the principle of the *prix de journée*, an accounting unit created in the late nineteenth century.[9] It was agreed that the religious sisters were entitled to two-thirds of this sum (to cover their expenses: meals, furniture, drugs, etc.); the remaining third was to be passed on to the university, which spent it on small wages for interns training to become specialists, medical equipment, and building maintenance. One employee of the university – Jules Robberechts – was charged with administering the university's share in these revenues. By the middle of the 1930s, it was clear that the university's share was insufficient to cover its expenses and so the contract with the religious sisters was re-negotiated: the *prix de journée* was raised by 5 francs that would go entirely to the university, while the sisters were now allowed to charge patients for drugs separately (instead of them being included within an aggregate price). To the dissatisfaction of the university, the sisters described this arrangement to patients as '5 franks of tax for the university'.[10]

If the price for hospitalisation was independent of one's social class, fees for treatment and laboratory analyses that required specific medical technologies were not. For having x-ray photos taken, undergoing radiotherapy for cancer, doing fitness training with special equipment after surgery, or having a Wassermann test for syphilis, patients were charged one of three possible tariffs based on their social status.[11] The resulting income was deposited in separate accounts for each of these treatments and managed by different professors. For example, Richard Bruynoghe, director of the Institute of Bacteriology, controlled the fees for the blood tests of patients who had been admitted to academic hospitals and who were sent to his institute for the tests. Bruynoghe used the funds to cover expenses for materials and laboratory workers.[12] This meant that even though private patients could not be used for clinical demonstrations, they were an important source of income for the university and helped to cover the costs of medical equipment. For the professors, however, private patients were much more important because they could be charged fees for private consultations and thus considerably supplement academic salaries. This resulted in tensions between the interests of the university (attracting sufficient indigent patients) and the economic interests of the members of the medical faculty (attracting sufficient private clientele). The university proposed class-based prices for the medical services offered by the university, whereas the medical faculty preferred to keep the costs incurred by (private) patients for using the university's equipment as low as possible. All agreed, however, that patients belonging to the 'superior' classes needed to be well isolated from the other patients, otherwise it was feared they would shun the hospital.[13] This involved not only private rooms (some with separate bathrooms) instead of wards, but also different waiting rooms, and even a different office to collect their fees.

These diverging interests can be illustrated in several discussions about patient fees between the rector Van Waeyenbergh and Gerard Van der Schueren, on the one hand, and Joseph Maisin, a radiotherapist and director of the Institute of Cancer, on the other. Since the late 1920s, the smallest kind of x-ray photograph was priced at 25 francs for indigent patients and 60 francs for private patients. For indigent outpatients, a supplement of 30 francs was requested 'to prevent them from insisting too strongly on being examined without hospitalization [and thus] to escape being put under observation.'[14] In this case, a difference in price was intended to make a hospital stay more attractive and thus recruit more patients for the purpose of clinical instruction. A proposal by Maisin to increase the cost for all radiographies by 10 francs in 1944 was greeted cautiously by Van Waeyenbergh: 'We should make sure that the price of the radiographies does not turn away the indigent clientele that is most necessary for education.'[15] Van der Schueren was equally critical of such a flat rate increase. He pleaded for a proportional increase in terms of percentages of the existing rates in order to avoid disturbing the balance between the fees charged for different social classes. In Maisin's proposal, he added, 'the modest people pay the difference.'[16] For Maisin, however, the greater complexity that different tariffs implied for his institute's bookkeeping was in itself a reason to prefer flat rates. In 1937, he had introduced a standard price of 45 francs per patient-day at the Institute 'because the bookkeeping became too difficult'. This sum covered the costs of both hospitalisation and treatment, regardless of the nature of that treatment (e.g. radiotherapy with radium or x-ray therapy).[17] This higher patient fee turned the Institute of Cancer into an anomaly within St. Raphael Hospital as all other institutes separated hospitalisation costs from class-related treatment fees. The measure revealed that for Maisin the institute, as an administrative entity, was more important than the over-arching structure of St

Raphael Hospital. Turning this around was one of Van der Schueren's ambitions that proved most difficult to realise.

Professors-turned-managers

What is striking about the financial apparatus of the academic hospitals in the interwar years is the relative absence of the university's central administrative services. Certainly, if one keeps in mind the mechanisms of control installed after the Second World War, it seems surprising that so much financial autonomy was left to medical faculty. They collected fees from private patients and spent the budgets generated by the income from specific medical services, such as x-ray photography. Most of them hired secretaries and medical assistants to run their consultations and paid their salaries without interference from the university. In fact, they operated their own private clinics within St Rafael Hospital. We are able to reconstruct this modus operandi through the lens of later complaints once the university sought greater control over the hospitals' finances and professors' prerogatives came to be regarded as symptoms of outdated 'patriarchy'. Yet such a reading also ignores the trust that was placed in academics' managerial abilities in the early twentieth century – a trust that resulted from the way in which the university had been able to realise and finance its remarkable expansion since the late nineteenth century.

The organisational model of the institute was central to this success. By the 1920s, institutes had become an integral part of the university structure (alongside the traditional division into faculties). They had been a means of facilitating laboratory-based scientific research that required more manpower and teamwork than older individual forms of scholarly research. A strict staff hierarchy led by 'professor-directors' was typical of their operation. In the medical field, several institutes had been established before the First World War, such as the Institute of Bacteriology in 1894 and the Institute of Pathology in 1906. When new hospitals had to be set up in the 1920s, the model of the institute was employed to organise disease- or patient-specific institutions, such as the Institute of Cancer or the Institute of Pediatrics. In the late 1920s and 1930s, St Rafael Hospital was in fact nothing more than a series of loosely connected institutes, each run by its own director. This meant that a strong managerial role, which also involved particular financial practices, was already part of the range of duties of early twentieth-century medical academics.

Fundraising comprised a part of these practices. Contrary to the relative absence of the university's leadership in the daily financial governance of the academic hospitals, rector Paulin Ladeuze, Van Waeyenbergh's predecessor, had coordinated efforts to obtain sufficient funding for the construction of St Rafael Hospital. In the 1920s, a nation-wide subscription campaign was launched among the Catholic community for the first of these new hospital buildings, the Institute of Cancer. The medical faculty had acted as the executive committee of this campaign, holding lectures across the country on the hopeful, but also expensive new techniques used to fight cancer (e.g. radiotherapy) and coordinating local committees (often composed of alumni) in many local parishes.[18] Subscriptions were an old technique. They were regularly employed to fund British voluntary hospitals in the nineteenth century or French scientific institutions such as the *Institut Pasteur* in Paris. But the use of mass media and the wide recruitment strategy – for just 5 francs parishioners of modest means could 'buy a brick' for the Institute of Cancer – gave the Leuven campaign a modern hue.[19] Catholic nobility, longtime supporters of the university, nevertheless remained the most important group of donors (Figure 6.1). Their financial help involved specific forms of accountability, which meant demonstrating that their money was being well used and simultaneously recognising their generosity. Joseph Maisin, for example, made calls to the countess Jean de Mérode and showed her around the construction site of the Institute of Cancer.[20] And one of the treatment rooms in the Institute – the *Salle Comtesse de Mérode* – was named after her.[21]

New forms of government funding complemented these traditional means. Since 1922, the state had allocated annual subsidies to the two private and ideologically opposed universities in Belgium: the Catholic University of Leuven and the Free University of Brussels. During the same period, a new set of national scientific and socio-medical agencies, such as the National Work for Child Welfare (1919), the University Foundation (1920), the National League Against Cancer (1924), and the National Science Foundation (1927), distributed government funds for specific purposes.[22] They formed a crucial element of interwar social politics: the improvement of workers' health became a tool designed to prevent social chaos (which to some meant stopping the

BULLETIN DE SOUSCRIPTION

Je soussigné désire participer à l'érection de l'Institut du Cancer de l'Université de Louvain, en qualité de (1) :

Membre fondateur (50,000 francs au moins) ; *Membre donateur* (5,000 francs au moins) ;
Membre protecteur (25,000 francs au moins) ; *Membre adhérent* (pour la somme de fr. _____).
Membre bienfaiteur (10,000 francs au moins) ;

Je verserai le montant de ma souscription au Compte-chèques postaux n° 126.433 *(Université de Louvain, Cancer)*.

Je désire que le montant de ma souscription soit touché par la poste.

Je ferai parvenir le montant de ma souscription au Recteur de l'Université de Louvain, (100, rue de Namur, Louvain), ou bien au Trésorier du Comité de _____
par _____

(Nom et prénoms) (2) _____
(Adresse complète) _____
(Lieu et date) _____

(1) Biffer s. v. p. les mots inutiles.
(2) Ecrire très lisiblement le nom et l'adresse.

Louvain. — Impr. Van Linthout.

6.1 Forms such as this 'Subscription Ticket' were used during the fundraising campaign for the Institute of Cancer in Leuven during the 1920s.

rise of socialism). A competition between Catholics and socialists arose over workers' bodies in so far as providing access to health services (e.g. through the intermediary of mutual societies) was regarded as a road to the socio-political affiliation of the working class.[23] Leuven professors learned to move within these new structures which shaped nascent Belgian science and health policies, ridden as they were by ideological conflict. These policies, moreover, developed their own paper technologies. For unlike philanthropic gifts, subsidies needed to be negotiated and accounted for much more concretely in the form of budgets and reports.

Administrative reform

The postwar changes to the mechanisms of governance and accountability at the Leuven hospitals were triggered by external factors. Without going into too much detail about Belgian social history, debates over several health insurance reform proposals raged between workers and employers during the war years and resulted in a Social Pact that was endorsed by the Belgian government on 28 December 1944. It was the 'birth' of the Belgian Social Security Administration. The new law made health insurance mandatory for all employees, but did not challenge the prewar system of private ideologically-based mutual societies, the most important of which were the Christian and Socialist Health Funds. The state did, however, create a new agency that centralised the collection of employee contributions. Employers would deduct a portion of employees' wages and pass it on to the state, which then distributed it to the private mutual societies.[24] This latter system was grounded in an ideal of *administrative rationalisation* in that it avoided the immense bureaucratic machinery that mutual societies themselves would otherwise have had to set up in order to collect the fees. Nevertheless, opposition to such centralisation soon arose. Catholics believed it neutralised the moralising effects of personal contributions to mutual societies. The medical profession opposed it because it entailed far-reaching state control over health expenditures. The fees paid by the mutual societies for specific treatments now became legally fixed, eroding the ability of physicians to set prices themselves.[25] The 'Leburton Law' of 1963 (named after the Secretary of Social Precaution, Edmond Leburton), which further expanded the system of mandatory health insurance, therefore resulted in a nation-wide physicians' strike.[26]

The impact of these shifts in Belgian social policy on the Leuven academic hospitals can hardly be overestimated. They entailed a further democratisation of health care, granting many more patients access to the hospital. Socially insured employees also challenged the traditional divisions between 'indigent' and 'private' patients: the treatment of many of the former was now paid for by the mutual societies resulting in demands for higher quality care than traditional forms of 'free' treatment.[27] In the long run, the prewar hospital wards no longer sufficed and were gradually abolished. For the purposes of this chapter, however, I want to highlight another type of influence exerted by these postwar social reforms: they helped comprise the context in which *administrative rationalisation* came to be regarded as a tool for progress. What transpired at a macro-political scale, in particular the debates over the benefits of centralised fee collection and the opposition of 'liberal' physicians concerned about their loss of autonomy, also occurred at a micro-institutional scale in the Leuven hospitals. There, too, a clash between 'socialised' and 'liberal' medicine took place. The cause of this clash relates directly to the fact that the university's leaders seized upon the new income from the Belgian Social Security Administration as an occasion to professionalise and centralise their hospital administration. Their efforts included a new way of bookkeeping that inevitably decreased the financial autonomy of the medical faculty and inaugurated a radical shift in the governance of the academic hospitals.

This reform potential of bookkeeping practices was essential to the plans of Gerard Van der Schueren, the first director of St Rafael Hospital in 1940. The creation of this position by rector Honoré Van Waeyenbergh, who succeeded Paulin Ladeuze in the same year, is in itself indicative of the ambitions that drove more centralised governance. Van der Schueren shared with Van Waeyenbergh a new style of leadership, a vision of a 'healthy' and rational administration – a phrase that both continuously repeated in their correspondence – in which sound bookkeeping comprised an important component. Both had won their spurs as administrators during the Second World War, organising the hospitals and the university as a whole in an era of rising inflation and German troops occupying many of the academic buildings.[28] During these years and inspired by earlier visits to American hospitals, Van der Schueren drafted several plans to reform St Rafael Hospital.[29] His vision of 'integrated' hospitals, fully organised on the basis of the medical needs of patients and realising cost reduction by employing a form of scientific management, did indeed come from across the Atlantic. Van der Schueren was convinced that such modernisation required a centralised administration that could quantify care by drawing up effective occupancy rates, comparing these and the income they generated between services, and thereby informing decisions about future investments. It was the only way to assure that empty beds in one institute would be immediately filled with surplus patients from another, that young specialists could develop their (sub)disciplines by setting up a small service (since sitting professors rarely handed over beds voluntarily), and that *all* patients would somehow be mobilised for the purposes of medical education, even though private patients required more discretion.[30] He was well aware that these reforms would evoke considerable opposition among the professors.[31]

The collection and management of the new social security fees, a considerable source of income, became a major issue of debate. For Van der Schueren and Van Waeyenbergh, it called for centralised bookkeeping in the hospital, whereas a committee of professors preferred to leave it to the different services themselves.[32] In Van der Schueren's view, the committee's proposal was simply 'the continuation of liberal medicine in the hospital'.[33] Nevertheless, a consensus on how to spend these revenues was easily reached. All agreed that they should not be included in the general budget of the university, but instead employed for the benefit of the academic hospitals. Particularly 'physician-assistants', i.e. those doctors seeking specialisation through internships – whose numbers were rising – should be among the beneficiaries. In addition, the new positions of 'clinic head' (*kliniekhoofd*) and 'assistant clinic head' (*adjunct-kliniekhoofd*) were created for those physicians who, although working within the academic hospitals, had no formal teaching obligations. In other words, those doctors who had worked in the formerly 'private clinics' of individual professors were now integrated into university staff.[34]

The question was thus not so much what the social security fees would be used for, but rather how they would be divided among the different services and to what degree professors would have a say in the expenditures. To what extent could the university, on the one hand, leverage those financial resources to push its own agenda (e.g. to make sure students would be exposed to all sorts of specialised medical treatments)? And to what extent would professors, on the other hand, have the autonomy to build and expand their own clinical services and research activities? The position of the university was strengthened, somewhat ironically, by the sentiments expressed by senior, high-status faculty members. Collecting fees for the treatment of 'indigent patients' who now benefitted from health insurance, they claimed, devalued the 'moral prestige' of their professorships.[35] Related to this was the fear that if these patients paid for their treatment, they would also require more attention, resulting in less time for research and teaching. Already in the interwar years, patients on the 'margins of the indigent clientele' and those privately insured by mutual societies had challenged the practices of the Leuven teaching hospitals.[36] 'Should we not foresee some rooms at a low price, where the head of the department [the professor] would accept a low fee and interns would have no access?'[37] The eventual outcome was different: the disappearance of the class of indigent patients meant that private patients would gradually be used for the purposes of medical education.

In 1946, the university's leadership and the medical faculty reached a compromise.[38] Social security fees would henceforth be collected by a new, central accounting service. Five per cent of all fees would be used for a central library, while 10 per cent would cover administration costs and unforeseen deficits. The remaining amount would be divided across the different medical services and could be spent by the professors to cover the salaries of physician-assistants or to buy new medical equipment. But these expenses were to be made 'in consultation with' the university's leadership. Such consultation – and this is essential – was organised through accounting practices. It was agreed that the new centralised service would draw up full and separate annual budgets for each medical service, carefully mapping the expenditures and profits of each specialism. These financial overviews were sent to each professor and informed further negotiations. Professors, in turn, were obliged to submit a budget proposal for the next year by 15 September.[39]

Bookkeepers and accountants

Van der Schueren's reforms were soon reflected in the spatial organisation of the hospital. Henceforth, patients were registered in a new hospital building, of which the ground floor would function as a general entrance. The central hospital administration was housed on that floor as well, including the 'accountancy department' (*service de comptabilité*). The blueprints for this new building illustrate the way this department was designed to function. The staff would include an accountant-in-chief, two assistant-accountants, and one cashier.[40] Its location was chosen in such a way that patients needed to pass by the window of the cashier to pay their fees. For 'ward patients', Van der Schueren added, the accountancy department acted as a means of surveillance, because patients required a voucher from the cashier in order to retrieve their personal clothing after payment. Private patients would pay their bills in the office of the accountant-in-chief.[41] 'The reception of the patients by the Accountancy Department,' Van der Schueren explained in another letter, 'is of the utmost importance for the impression the sick would retain of the hospital.'[42] The function of the hospital accountant, as it was described in the 1950s, was thus one of a remarkably 'visible' person that represented the hospital as a whole. In another plan, a door from the accountants' offices to the adjacent monastery was added to ensure collaboration with the bookkeeping service of the religious sisters.[43] However, the university soon took over this function entirely.

Who were these accountants? And how were they received by medical professors? The archival record contains only a few traces of these employees. Jules Robberechts, who had controlled the finances of the university's share of hospitalisation revenues in the interwar years, became part of the new accountancy department.[44] A Mr Crab, director of the university's central administration, regularly contacted medical professors to elicit financial data for the annual budgets. His complaints to Van der Schueren reveal that this cooperation did not always run smoothly. Joseph Maisin, the personification of the autonomous 'professor-director', seemed to have rejected the growing presence of bookkeepers in the hospital. Van der Schueren concluded that his collaboration with Mr Crab was no success: 'contact with the secretariat [the central administration] to draw up the budget is systematically avoided.'[45] Maisin pleaded instead for a decentralised administration: 'I strongly believe, based on past experience, that the accounts cannot be established correctly if not by the Services themselves. It seems impossible that an employee, who does not have the slightest idea of what is happening in the different services, will end up with correct accounts.'[46] For the university's leadership, however, the presence of these employees was essential to help better integrate the different medical institutes. New appointments of staff became opportunities for negotiation. When Maisin requested an additional nurse for the Institute of Cancer in 1946, Van der Schueren appointed Frans Polfliet instead. Polfliet was a member of the university's administrative service who 'knows well the workings of the [Institute of Cancer] service'. By taking over the administrative duties of the nurses, his appointment would generate more time for actual medical care.[47] It was both a means to gain more control over the financing of the institute and a money-saving measure, given that the salary of administrative personnel was lower than that of certified nurses.

The accounts of the hospital were also reviewed by outsider auditors who checked the annual balances. Their professional gaze upon these documents made previous bookkeeping attempts seem 'amateurish'. In 1951, Nicholas Falkovsky, an accountant and former employee at the Belgian Ministry of Finance, reviewed the books of the different institutes. In his first report, he stated boldly that in fact 'there exists no [real] bookkeeping' at the hospital.[48] His report revealed that by 1951, double-entry bookkeeping had still not fully replaced older customs. The introduction of this new system proved difficult because it necessitated a full inventory of assets, debts, loans, accounts, etc. Much of this information was difficult to acquire from the university's central services, or remained on their budget rather than on the hospital's balance sheet. Information was also needed from the religious sisters who were in charge of all nursing and who owned much of the furniture and medical equipment. Disentangling this jumble of accounts and possessions proved frustrating and tiresome. Both Van der Schueren and Falkovsky, for example, regretted that the large government subsidies for the Institute of Cancer remained on the balance sheet of the university, thus creating an artificial deficit for the hospital.[49]

Budgets and 'strength reports'

What little archival information about the accountants themselves remains contrasts with the well-preserved documents that their paper machine produced which grant us better insight into the function of budgets and reports. Their format, in particular, illustrates the way in which they represented the 'academic hospitals' as a single entity. Much like the accountant of the 1950s represented the clinics to the patient (Van der Schueren stressed this exemplary role), these reports conveyed to professors an integrated vision of all institutes belonging to a larger entity. As agreed in the 1946 compromise, the central administration drew up standardised annual budgets for each service, employing the same categories to arrange receipts and expenditures. The pre-printed forms, to which only the name of the service and the figures were added, were likely to have left professors wondering about the finances of other services, thereby perhaps unwittingly stimulating greater competition between them. The structure and length of the forms changed several times over the course of the 1950s and 1960s (Figure 6.2). Moreover, new types of documents were introduced that represented the hospital in its totality. Among these were Van der Schueren's notorious 'strength reports', which (although effectively drawn up by mostly anonymous accountants) became associated with his style of governance. These daily reports documented the number of

6.2 A standardised form, filled out for the service of Pediatrics, 1952.

patients per room or ward, the number of new and discharged patients, and the number of the deceased patients so as to calculate the 'occupancy rate' of the academic hospitals. These reports also allowed the effective costs per patient per day to be calculated.[50]

It is difficult to pinpoint the effect of these accounting practices on the traditional managerial roles of medical academics. Their interaction with professional bookkeepers was clearly new. But the influence of these practices was more far-reaching in the sense that they changed the ways in which the recruitment of new assistants and the acquisition of new medical equipment was negotiated. The postwar expansion of the service of radiotherapy in the Institute of Cancer offers a telling example. Here, financial reports assisted in resolving an old conflict within the

Institute: that between Dutch-speaking and French-speaking physicians. Since the 1930s, the former had pushed for more autonomy and more opportunities within the still unilingual French-speaking university, resulting in the splitting up of several medical services, e.g. Surgery A (French-speaking) and Surgery B (Dutch-speaking).[51] The prestigious service of Radiotherapy, however, had remained undivided, one of the arguments being that it would be too expensive to set up two services given the high costs of radiation equipment. A second-rate service for the Dutch-speaking physicians didn't seem to be an option. Van der Schueren, himself a Dutch-speaking physician and radiotherapist, opposed this view. He deemed it possible to provide such a service on one of the wards of St. Pieters Hospital. 'Its necessary financial organization forms no objection, as I can prove', he added to Van Waeyenbergh.[52] In 1952, the service of 'Radiotherapy B' opened its doors. It was indicative of the role that administrative arguments, grounded in practices of accounting, were increasingly playing in settling linguistic conflicts at the university.

The creation of Anaesthesiology as an independent medical service further illustrates the impact of bookkeeping on hospital organisation. Beginning on 1 April 1951, the Belgian Social Security Administration started reimbursing the costs of anesthesia separately from those of the surgical intervention itself, de facto recognising it as a unique specialism. In response, the hospital board decided to administratively split Anaesthesiology from the service of Surgery 'to avoid difficulties' when tallying these new receipts.[53] Paying anaesthesiologists and the costs of their equipment using revenues from surgical operations had previously led to contentious debates. Part of these new revenues would be used to create a hyperbaric room, to improve the intensive care units, and to organise an emergency service – measures in which the Leuven anaesthesiologists took the lead. The case of anaesthesiology shows how the interwar model of the 'institute' as an accounting unit no longer sufficed to organise postwar health care.[54] The major institutes – surgery, cancer, and internal medicine – were now subdivided into different medical services and each drew up its own budget. As a corollary to this development, 'professor-directors' lost much of their prestige. In the 1960s, 'department heads' would replace these directors, bringing a degree of unity to different sets of specialisms, but without the same financial control as their predecessors had been able to exercise.

Budgets and balances thus oiled the administrative machinery that dismantled the bastions of medical academics in the 1950s. They shifted strategic decision-making about specialisation and medical expansion to a higher level of governance: that of the university's leadership and the board of directors of the Academic Hospitals. Here the deficits of 'weak' services were counterbalanced by the profits of 'strong' ones in the name of the overall mission of offering the best possible care and medical education. Non-medical experts were integrated into this inner circle. Under the leadership of Jan Blanpain, Van der Schueren's successor as director of St Rafael Hospital, this reliance on specialists to help guide hospital reform was continued. Blanpain would also further professionalise the hospitals' administration in the 1960s by introducing a strict separation between 'bookkeeping', 'registration', and 'reception'. The hospital accountant, as a result, became even more of a specialist, but also moved increasingly into the background, out of view of patients.[55]

Conclusions

Writing the history of hospital reform in Leuven, it is tempting to sympathise with Gerard Van der Schueren and his attempts to introduce new forms of rational administration, including 'healthy bookkeeping'. The available archival sources clearly reinforce his point of view. His letters to Honoré Van Waeyenbergh reveal his frustrations over the resistance of medical faculty, led by the radiotherapist Joseph Maisin, who protected their professorial prerogatives regarding the running of 'their' hospital services. But such a reading has its own risks. We may underestimate their experience of losing autonomy and of seeing their established professorial status being eroded by the introduction of a new class of non-medical experts: the accountants and auditors, the lawyers and economists. This counter narrative of possible resistance has remained underexplored in this chapter.[56] We lack the personal correspondence of professors to assess whether or not ideals of 'caring' for patients clashed with the quantitative logic of accountants and administrators. This was certainly the case during periods of cost-saving in the late twentieth century.[57] Was there also a sentiment among professors in the middle of the century that care could not be reduced to a set of numbers?

Conversely, looking too closely through Van der Schueren's lens as a reformer, we may overestimate the novelty that accountants brought to the way the hospital was organised and managed in the postwar era. I have tried to compensate for this by also analysing the managerial roles of medical academics in the interwar years. Accounting practices, which could take different forms, were clearly part of their duties as directors and heads of service. Those practices served – both before and after the Second World War – as tools for use in negotiating the interests of different stakeholders: the university, the professors, religious congregations, socio-medical agencies, mutual societies, etc. This meant that professors were well acquainted with how to draft budgets or use reports to account for subsidies before professional accountants arrived at the hospital. The state's interwar health care initiatives (e.g. subsidies for cancer treatment) had already established new mechanisms of control and accountability that had been absent in the philanthropic economy of the nineteenth-century hospital. To partake in these mechanisms of state funding, professors developed specific administrative and financial skills.

What was it, then, that professional accountants and administrators brought to hospital governance in the postwar era? An important observation on the debates about hospital reform in the 1940s and 1950s is that the modalities of accounting became *themselves* the subject of debate. Discussions were not only about each stakeholder's share in the revenues; they were also about who would collect the fees and control the finances. These debates about the benefits of centralisation versus decentralisation reveal an awareness of the impact of administrative decisions – such as the drawing up of individual balances per medical service – on the (future) organisation of the hospital. Aggregate budgets and strength reports did more than just help visualise the academic hospitals as a single entity; in fact, they created a new unity that had not existed before the Second World War. While they withdrew financial autonomy from established professor-directors, they also redistributed it to specialised services that gained greater independence by virtue of them now having their own administrations, allowing them to make choices about how to use their allocated budgets. In other words, accounting practices functioned as the wheels of medical expansion. Through the paperwork of accountants, the health policies of the government and the educational ambitions of the university transformed academic hospital care.

Notes

1 University Archive Leuven (UAL), Archive of Honoré Van Waeyenbergh (AVW), 3760, Plan van inrichting van een klinische afdeling in de voorwaarden van [de Duitse dienst] luchtafweer [Outline of the organisation of a Clinical Service following the conditions of the (German service of) Anti-Aircraft Defence, undated (c. 1941–44)].
2 UAL, AVW, 3760, Universitair Gasthuis [Academic Hospital], undated (c. 1941).
3 UAL, AVW, 3757, G. van der Schueren to H. van Waeyenbergh, 21 December 1941.
4 On the twentieth-century history of the Leuven academic hospitals, see J. Vandendriessche, *Zorg en wetenschap. Een geschiedenis van de Leuvense academische ziekenhuizen in de twintigste eeuw* (Leuven: Leuven University Press, 2019).
5 The modalities of these expanding health systems differed considerably from one country to the next. For an introduction, see C. Webster, 'Medicine and the welfare state, 1930–1970', in R. Cooter and J. Pickstone (eds), *Companion to Medicine in the Twentieth Century* (London: Routledge, 2003), pp. 125–40.
6 In a letter to Van Waeyenbergh, Van der Schueren looked back on the evolution of the wages of the professors working at St. Pieters Hospital after the First World War. UAL, AVDS, 304, G. van der Schueren to H. van Waeyenbergh, 22 March 1950.
7 For a discussion of this French model of hospital financing, see B.M. Doyle, 'Healthcare before welfare states: Hospitals in early twentieth century England and France', *Canadian Bulletin of the History of Medicine* 33:1 (2016), 174–204, 179–80.
8 For an overview of Catholic health care in Belgium, see J. de Maeyer, L. Dhaene, G. Hertecant, and K. Velle (eds), *Er is leven voor de dood: tweehonderd jaar gezondheidszorg in Vlaanderen* [There is Life before Death: Two Hundred Years of Health Care in Flanders] (Kapellen: Pelckmans, 1998).
9 UAL, Archive of Gerard van der Schueren (AVDS), 304, Personeel, 304, Ligdagprijs [Price of Patient Day]. On the introduction of the *prix de journée* in nineteenth-century France, see J.-P. Domin, *Une Histoire*

économique de l'hôpital (XIXe–XXe siècles). Une analyse rétrospective du développement hospitalier (Paris: Comité d'histoire de la Sécurité sociale, 2008).

10 UAL, AVW, 3757, Report of 13 March 1946 of the Study Group. This latter body was a commission that was to debate the postwar organisation and expansion of the academic hospitals.

11 UAL, AVW, 3760, Untitled note, undated (1940–45), containing the different tariffs for different laboratory tests and therapies (e.g. radiation).

12 On this Institute of Bacteriology, see G. Vanpaemel and J. Snaet, *Medisch laboratorium of universitair bedrijf? Het Instituut voor Bacteriologie te Leuven* [Medical Laboratory or Academic Company? The Institute of Bacteriology in Leuven] (Leuven: Lipsius, 2016).

13 UAL, AVW, 3757, Plan van organisatie der universiteitsklinieken Sint-Raphaël [Outline of the organisation of St. Raphael Academic Hospital], 1941.

14 UAL, AVW, N, 3607, Tarif du service de Radiographie de l'Institut du Cancer [Tariffs of the Service of Radiography in the Institute of Cancer].

15 UAL, AVW, N. 3611, H. van Waeyenbergh to J. Maisin, 12 March 1944.

16 UAL, AVW, N. 3611, Note of 3 March 1944 titled Radiografie [Radiography] by G. van der Schueren for H. van Waeyenbergh.

17 UAL, AVW, 3607, Prix de la journée d'hospitalisation dans les salles et des malades traités à l'Institut du Cancer [Price of the Patient Day in the wards and for the patients treated in the Institute of Cancer], undated.

18 In a letter to the Countess Jean de Mérode, rector Paulin Ladeuze explained how the fundraising campaign worked and the role of the medical faculty. UAL, ACA, 1048, Copy of a letter of 11 June 1924 of P. Ladeuze to J. de Mérode.

19 UAL, ACA, 1049, List of deposits by local committees.

20 UAL, ACA, 1048, J. de Mérode to P. Ladeuze, 2 January 1926.

21 UAL, ACA, 1050, Plaques du Cancer. (The document contains a list of the commemorative nameplates in the Institute of Cancer.)

22 On Belgium's science policy in the interwar years, see R. Halleux, *Tant qu'il y aura des chercheurs. Science et Politique en Belgique* (Brussels: Luc Pire, 2015), pp. 60–74; K. Bertrams, *Universités et entreprises: milieux académiques et industriels en Belgique, 1880–1970* (Bruxelles: Le Cri, 2006).

23 G. Vanthemsche, *De beginjaren van de sociale zekerheid in België, 1944–1963* [The Early Years of Social Security in Belgium, 1944–63] (Brussels: VUB Press 1994), pp. 13–44.

24 For an overview, see K.P. Companje, R.H.M. Hendriks, K.F.E. Veraghtert, and B.E.M. Widdershoven (eds), *Two Centuries of Solidarity. German,*

Belgian and Dutch Social Health Care Insurance, 1770–2008 (Amsterdam: Aksant, 2009); D. Rigter, 'Belgian mutual health insurance and the nation state', in B. Harris (ed.), *Welfare and Old Age in Europe and North America* (London: Pickering & Chatto, 2012), pp. 189–206.

25 On this opposition in the late 1940s and 1950s, see Vanthemsche, *De beginjaren*, pp. 123–64.

26 G. Marchildon and K. Schrijvers, 'Physician resistance and the forging of public healthcare: A comparative analysis of the doctors' strikes in Canada and Belgium in the 1960s', *Medical History* 55 (2011), 203–22.

27 At the end of the Second World War, several members had already suggested creating 'small rooms at low cost' where 'the clientele at the margins of the indigent clientele' could be treated. UAL, AVW, Conseil de directions des cliniques universitaires. Suggestion de programma pour la seconde réunion [Meeting of the Board of the Academic Hospitals, Proposal for the Agenda of the Second Meeting], undated (1944).

28 *De Universiteit te Leuven, 1425–1985* [The University in Leuven, 1425–85] (Leuven 1986).

29 Van der Schueren had been a Rockefeller Fellow in New York in 1933–34, see K. Geboes, 'Schueren, Gerard Leon Joseph van der', *Nationaal Biografisch Woordenboek* 20 (2011), 885–97.

30 American hospitals were an example, for Van der Schueren, of how to avoid empty beds. He also admired them for their organisation of a 'Social Service', which welcomed patients and guided them throughout the hospital. UAL, AVDS, 304, Untitled document, 6 February 1953; UAL, AVW, 3760, Verzorgend Gasthuis [Nursing Hospital], undated (1940).

31 In a letter to Van Waeyenbergh, he pleaded for a gentle implementation of his reforms to avoid 'a revolution' in the hospital. UAL, AVDS, 304, G. van der Schueren to H. van Waeyenbergh, 9 January 1952. For a detailed overview of his plans in the early 1950s, see UAL, AVDS, 304, Regeling van de sociale veiligheid in haar 2de phase [Agreements on Social Security in its 2nd Stage], undated (c. 1950–52).

32 UAL, AVW, 3758, Comité d'Études des Cliniques Universitaires. Rapport de la réunion du mardi 15 mai 1945 [Study Group of the Academic Hospitals. Report of the Meeting of 15 March 1945].

33 UAL, AVDS, 304, Inning van de honoraria van de sociale veiligheid [Collection of Fees for Social Security], undated.

34 Ibid.

35 UAL, AVDS, 304, Note sur l'application de la loi sur les assurances sociales [Note on the Enforcement of the Law on Social Security], 1946.

36 UAL, AVW, 3757, Conseil de directions des cliniques universitaires. Suggestion de programma pour la seconde réunion [Meeting of the Board of

the Academic Hospitals, Proposal for the Agenda of the Second Meeting], undated (1944).
37 Ibid.
38 UAL, AVDS, Note sur l'application de la loi sur les assurances sociales [Note on the Enforcement of the Law on Social Security], 1946.
39 UAL, AVDS, 304, H. van Waeyenbergh to G. van der Schueren, 6 February 1954.
40 UAL, AVW, 3757, Plan van organisatie der universiteitsklinieken Sint-Raphaël [Outline of the organisation of the Academic Hospital St. Raphael], 1941.
41 Ibid. See esp. 'Addendum I'.
42 UAL, AVW, 3757, G. van der Schueren to H. van Waeyenbergh, 21 December 1941.
43 UAL, AVW, 3760, Note 'Het administratief ziekenhuis' [The Administrative Hospital], undated (c. 1940).
44 UAL, AVDS, 304, Inning van de honoraria van de sociale veiligheid [Collection of Fees stemming from Social Security], undated (1945).
45 UAL, AVW, 3612, Institut du Cancer. Compte du second semestre de 1944 [Institute of Cancer. Accounts of the Second Semester of 1944], 1944.
46 UAL, AVW, 3612, J. Maisin to G. van der Schueren, 21 September 1944.
47 UAL, AVW, 3612, G. van der Schueren to H. van Waeyenbergh, 20 April 1946.
48 UAL, AVDS, 274, N. Falkovsky, Système comptable en vigueur et ses inconvénients [Current System of Bookkeeping and its Drawbacks], 20 May 1951.
49 UAL, AVDS, 274, N. Falkovsky, Cliniques Universitaires St. Raphaël [St. Raphael Academic Hospital], 13 December 1956.
50 UAL, AVW, 3757, Plan van organisatie der universiteitsklinieken Sint-Raphaël [Outline of the organisation of St. Raphael Academic Hospital], 1941.
51 On these linguistic conflicts in Leuven academic medicine, see J. Vandendriessche and L. Nys, 'Expansion through separation. The linguistic conflicts at the University of Leuven in the 1960s from a medical history perspective', *BMGN – The Low Countries Historical Review* 132:1 (2017), 38–61.
52 UAL, AVW, 3760, Untitled document by G. Van der Schueren, undated (c. 1945).
53 UAL, AVDS, 287, G. van der Schueren to H. van Waeyenbergh, 1 April 1951.

54 Special thanks to Barry Doyle for suggesting the idea of the Institute as an 'accounting unit'.
55 UAL, AVDS, 286, J. Blanpain, Nota's omtrent de oprichting van de opnamedienst en van de aankoopdienst [Notes on the Creation of an Admission and Acquisition Service], 1959.
56 Special thanks to Christopher Sirrs for suggesting the idea of such a 'demedicalisation' that paralleled the well-known medicalisation of the hospital.
57 Vandendriessche, *Zorg en wetenschap*, pp. 173–206.

7

Asylum accounts in health and in money

Theodore M. Porter

The insane asylums that began to spring up in the early nineteenth century in Europe and North America were mostly state institutions. Even if not, they were likely to be supported as charitable organisations or to take in patients whose expenses were covered by public funds for the indigent. Hence, recordkeeping at these institutions drew as much from the expectations of state administrative reporting as from specifically medical traditions. Even the medical numbers were adapted to budgetary purposes. Basic elements of patient identity – such as place of birth and of residence, immigrant status, onset of illness, marital state, and religious confession – all had a role in determining who was entitled to admission, where they would be lodged, and who should bear the costs. Beyond that, the value of the work of these institutions was judged in part according to their ostensible effectiveness in restoring the reason of these suffering souls. A second goal, never forgotten by state authorities, was to control the public nuisance caused by madness and to protect the families of the mad from descent into pauperism. Without cures, however, there was little justification for taking on the high costs of asylum treatment. The nineteenth-century asylum movement was launched by reformers who argued that insanity was a disease like other diseases and no less curable. Records of outcomes were thus an indispensable form of asylum data, the basis for the most crucial calculations.[1]

The massive expansion of these institutions from the early nineteenth century was attended by a no less remarkable intensification of recordkeeping. Hospitals in these years confronted ever higher standards of accountability. A notable moment in this history of evolving mores of data was the descent into madness of King George III of England in 1788–89, posing an acute political question: whether it was necessary to appoint a regent to govern in his place. The Reverend Dr Francis Willis, brought in from the provinces to treat the king, claimed in his private practice to have cured nine in ten of those patients whose treatment was begun in a timely fashion. He had, however, no records to support his claim, and with so much at stake, parliamentary authorities were certainly not going to put blind faith in the bald assertions of an outsider physician. The search for more authoritative data led naturally to the gates of Bedlam. William Black, a leading public-health physician, found that Bethlem, the royal asylum in London, held no official records of patient outcomes, but that, unofficially, the apothecary there had kept data on the diverse characteristics of each patient. Black seized the opportunity to analyse these records, which he soon presented in a new edition of his just-published book on causes of death, including tables of cures for Bethlem patients in relation to diverse variables such as age and assigned cause.[2]

The push for public asylum statistics was soon felt in the United States and Continental Europe as well as Britain. The Anglophone countries, especially, began including basic statistics in printed annual reports, which circulated as public documents. This was partly a gesture of public accountability, but was also allied to campaigns for public support of these burgeoning institutions. The statistics indicated that many patients were cured, and further that prompt admission to an asylum led to greatly improved outcomes. In France and Germany, the annual report remained somewhat exceptional, but Continental asylum doctors, too, were soon required to keep routine statistics for submission to regional or central governments and to state ministries. Everywhere, they wanted the public to be informed of the benefits of asylum care, and so they passed along their experience in multi-year reports for local or professional journals. Alienists (doctors for the insane) also competed with other institutions near and far to show the best outcome statistics.[3]

Inscription

The conditions for entering patient data in books were usually left implicit, without reference to the circumstances of an interview or even the person supplying the information. It seems, however, to have been generally recognised that such records derived from a medical examination, to be carried out by a doctor as in effect a case history. Until the late 1860s, many asylums had just one physician. In the simplest case, the patient was brought in by a 'friend', meaning the legally-responsible person, who was most often a close relative. The doctor kept a big admissions book, with categories of data arrayed in columns from left to right, and with lines for about ten or fifteen up to as many as fifty patients running from top to bottom. Books lined by hand with a pencil and straight-edge gradually gave way to printed volumes from a medical supply house. A typical layout begins with the patient admission number and name and follows with sex, place of residence, marital state, occupation, religious confession, and so on, all the way across facing pages, verso and recto. As a rule, we do not get the impression of a probing inquiry, but rather of routine data entry. At first, the doctors almost never thought of imposing uniform categories – for example, of occupation – but entered a category or description based on what they were told. Even the medically significant information, such as the first signs of mental breakdown, appear often to have been filled out in a routine way, though sometimes there are hints of scepticism on the part of the doctor. On the basis of such reports, sometimes including a written medical report from home as well as direct observation, the newly admitted patient would typically receive a diagnosis. No one but a physician could be allowed to specify the disease form, not even for statistical purposes. One of the earliest censuses of insanity, carried out in Norway and beginning in 1825, was held up for three years owing to the difficulty of lining up enough physicians to make proper medical determinations. The doctors would have liked to rely on personal observation to fix the causes of insanity and the duration of illness prior to admission. But since they would almost never have been present to witness early signs of mental disturbance, they had to rely on the assessment of someone in the household. As for designated causes, they signalled their scepticism in the statistics as well as the admission books by referring to the causes as 'presumed', 'assigned', 'alleged', or, in German, *'mutmaßlich'*. Almost every table of causes in every language was qualified in this way. Physicians also often complained of the unreliability of causal attributions arising from the experience of untrained lay observers.[4]

The outcome, of course, could not be assigned until the patient departed from the institution. This, the most important datum of all, was fixed by the asylum physician, who relied on experience and discernment rather than on any formalised standard. The admission books included on the right side of the right-hand page a set of columns for ticking off the outcome of treatment, which usually included cured, improved, not cured, and dead. Other outcomes, such as 'removed by family' or 'eloped' (escaped), as well as entries in the right-most column for 'observations', might also bear on statistical indicators of successful treatment, since they were sometimes invoked to exclude certain patients from the statistics. This could include patients whose prospects for cure were ruined, they supposed, by too long a delay prior to admission and others who left while a promising treatment was still underway. Asylum directors were acutely aware of the effect of patient transfers, sometimes between different kinds of institutions. If a prison or poorhouse managed to move someone with a deadly infection into an asylum, their responsibility for the death, and with it a failure to cure, would be transferred as well. Asylum officers considered this inappropriate, and whenever possible they excluded such persons from the statistics.

There were other complications to the system of registration. Patients transferred from other institutions, especially non-medical ones, might arrive with a constable or other attendant who knew nothing of the patient's background or medical history. Sometimes, however, welfare officials or prison wardens had detailed records of a prospective patient, which the asylum doctors sought to extract as information. The proliferation of asylums led to increasingly stringent rules for admission, including one and then two medical certificates. These doctors seem often to have relied mainly on families for data on patient history and causes, but the referring doctors might sometimes also function as a source of information. Some institutions sent out a questionnaire to the families of prospective patients, which might run to dozens of questions, many of them pertaining to patient history. Especially in Germany, the public health officer (*Physicus*) had a role in authorising admission, and would examine the prospective patient and provide information as part of the process.

Physicians, in the guise of healers, preferred to think of this accumulation of data as a guide to medical treatment. In practice, the information was likely to be more relevant to keeping order in the asylum than to curing individual patients. Admission forms increasingly incorporated this aspect of asylum management, specifying which newly admitted patients were noisy, dirty, or violent. The prolonged, twisting development of a case, often tightly interwoven with childhood experiences, education, work relations, and family affairs, provided possible material for a rich narrative. Not for nothing did madness become a favourite theme for plays, novels, and operas. Doctors developed the genre of the insane history, ferreting out in their spare time – for the instruction of their colleagues and of the public – evidence of mental disturbance in kings, artists, and religious leaders from the past. Narrative histories of their own patients, however, were the rare exception throughout the nineteenth century. There are occasional exceptions to this characteristic brevity, such as the stories put together by a London asylum director at Hanwell in the 1840s.[5] The requirements for record-keeping became more strenuous in the later part of the nineteenth century. In England, the admissions procedure increasingly dictated the structure of patient casebooks. In this new configuration, details of insane behaviour were recorded on medical certificates within an unwieldy folio casebook, which formed the legal basis for admission of the new patient. The familiar patient data – including age, residence, occupation, religious confession, and disease form – having been entered into labelled boxes at the top of the left-hand page, were then rearranged into paragraph form as the principal elements of a case history.[6]

In Britain and America, casebooks remained the principal repositories for patient information right into the twentieth century. German asylums, by contrast, had long since gone over to files in which to keep patient data. These offered the obvious advantage that the records for any particular case would be found in a single folder, so that all this information – whatever its medical value – could more readily be taken into account. The first casebooks in Worcester, Massachusetts began by setting aside eight or ten pages per patient, which rapidly contracted to two pages. Long-term patients, even the most uneventful cases, would fill these pages, then continue in the spaces left behind during the early phase of profligacy, and continue after that in the pages of new casebooks. The casenotes of a single patient could easily be divided into five or more sections. Even with indexing of the volumes and cross-referencing, it must have been extremely unusual for a doctor to inspect the complete file of a long-term patient. In the early years, it may not have mattered too much, since most asylums were small enough for the physician to know something of all his patients. As institutions grew immoderately large, from the 250 patients once idealised into the thousands, the improvement of case record storage emerged as a great desideratum.[7]

It is far from clear that this effort had much effect on medical treatment. The real purpose of data recording had as much to do with administration and reporting as with medicine. Production of tables seems to have been paramount. Almost every category of inscription, corresponding to a column in the admission book, provided the basis for a table in the annual report. In the early years, until about 1860, most of these tables provided totals for some variable, for example of patients by township or county of residence, religious confession, disease form, or imputed cause. Most of the rest created a little distribution – for example the number of patients in five-year age intervals, or the delay from outbreak of illness to admission into an asylum – at less regular intervals. Almost everywhere, but especially in America, asylum superintendents emphasised the essential role of data and statistics in the operation of their institutions. There is little evidence in these documents of medical numbers being used to sort out patients for different sorts of treatments. The destiny of the data gathered on every new patient was to be merged into institutional statistics. Their purpose was partly to demonstrate the effectiveness of the institution and partly to suggest ways to improve mental health in the population at large. Asylum numbers were understood to show the decisive role of certain causes of insanity, notably vicious or unwise behaviour in the form of alcohol consumption, masturbation, and heredity.

Statistics and accounts

Asylum reports distinguished between medical and administrative numbers. The former were denominated in numbers of persons, the latter most often in money terms. The alienists endeavoured to maintain a distinction between these forms of accounting, but they inevitably ran together in some respects. Alienists understood well enough that the high cost of treatment demanded results. Doctors consistently rejected direct comparisons of their institutions with the various forms of poor relief on the basis of cost, but to those who paid the bill for indigent patients, the value of maintaining a patient under treatment was similar to that of residence in a prison or even a poorhouse.

From early in the nineteenth century, advocates of subsidised asylum care emphasised the injustice of treating the mad as criminals. They also insisted on the advantage to everyone of providing treatment for a disease that had been proven curable. This could be shown by calculation. American institutions may seem to have pioneered this sort of calculation. The Ohio Lunatic Asylum, which published a German version of its earliest reports, was modelled in many ways on the asylum in Massachusetts, sharing, in particular, its intense optimism about cures. The opening ceremony, on 25 May 1838, was graced by a sermon delivered by Charles Fitch, identified as an instructor in the Ohio State Prison. He preached that the best hope for curing lunacy

> 'is to be met, not by miraculous agency, – God having confined that agency to special times for special purposes, when the great ends for which it was employed were not to be accomplished by any means to the men of those generations, – but by human agency in the application of means, developed in the progress of science, and forming a treatment peculiar, appropriate, and decisive.'

He was particularly proud of the scrupulous care with which the institution managed its expenses. The state had relied on the labour of convicts from the penitentiary to put up its impressive building. 'And thus has she made the crimes of one portion of the population to contribute largely to the benefit of another; converting the poison, drawn by the one from the body politic for their destruction, into a rich nutriment and healing balsam for the support of the health of the other.'[8]

The Ohio Asylum had, during its first years, a few paying patients, who contributed about a fifth of its budget. Mainly it provided care at little or no cost to indigent residents – and madness could reduce most families to indigence. On these terms, unfortunately, this asylum, like most, rapidly filled with patients, so that it soon was impossible to admit all those in need. William M. Awl, the founding superintendent, expressed deep regret on this point, since he – like almost every other alienist – insisted on the need to admit patients early, before the disease lodged itself so deeply in the brain as to make the patient incurable.

Still worse, they were often compelled to admit old and unpromising patients while younger and more recent ones were being turned away. 'Without professing to be always minutely and perfectly correct in our data, upon a subject so mysterious and obscure, as that of mental derangement, we, nevertheless, attach great importance to our statistical researches', and these, Awl claimed, provided management a firm basis for defence of the institution. Some comparative tables in the annual report for 1843, borrowed from a 'sister institution' (Worcester), showed that results of treatment in Ohio were better than average. How regrettable that so many young persons must be deprived of its benefits![9]

In 1850, the newly appointed asylum superintendent in Ohio went beyond such lamentations and calculated the consequences. He was Samuel Hanbury Smith, who had studied in England with John Conolly, famous for liberating the patients in the giant asylum at Hanwell from mechanical restraints. Smith had been teaching at the Starling Medical College in Columbus Ohio and editing a medical journal there when he was chosen to succeed Awl at the asylum. He served for two years and prepared two annual reports there before succumbing to the spoils system; and the second of these, in particular, deserves recognition as a classic of the genre. It includes a passionate defence of the publicly funded state asylum, partly on the grounds that support for needed treatment would dry up if the rich broke off into their own institutions. Nor would the affluent gain anything from separate asylums, since the beneficial effects of asylum care evaporated for patients who did not labour. Smith also went beyond the familiar lament over lost opportunities to restore disturbed young persons to productive good health and provided worked-out numerical proofs of the monetary advantages to the state of ample provision of asylum care.[10]

He began with the recent US census, which showed 1,351 lunatics and 1,399 idiots in Ohio. The figure for lunatics, at least, was probably low, he surmised, for Massachusetts already had 1,512 insane in its asylums – a ratio of about 1 patient to 750 inhabitants. Ohio would require space for more than 2,000 patients even to lower its ratio to 1 to 1,000. Consider, then, the monstrous financial losses that accrued in Ohio in consequence of delayed treatment. The cure of a patient brought early to the asylum cost less than $100, including costs for the journey and admission proceedings. Owing to a lack of adequate space, he had been forced to turn away more than 200 patients in the last year. 'Now, supposing, of all these but 25 were curable, *and we have in one year an expense of $50,000 entailed on the community*', screamed his italic letters. He estimated that 500 more insane persons in Ohio had been made incurable by admission delays, implying a still more horrifying cost of '*one million of dollars!* A sum monstrous enough to build five such vast establishments as this.' Beyond these costs, there was the 'loss to society in human minds and powers and influences', not reducible to dollars and cents.[11]

Despite these promises of long-term savings, local governments seem generally to have done whatever they could to avoid paying the added cost of asylum care, resorting instead to what he regarded as the spurious cheapness of prisons and poor relief. No doubt they were reluctant to face increased poor rates now for the sake of the savings promised for later. Probably they were not quite convinced by the promises of medical reformers bearing the gifts of supposed savings. They had other ideas for lowering their costs. Poor relief in most places was a local responsibility. Although American states took on the expense of constructing the new asylums, they did not pay the costs of running the institutions or feeding the patients. Families with means were expected to pay these charges, and costs for the insane poor were billed to local jurisdictions. But what if the new patient was already insane before arriving in this part of the state? The arrival of undesired immigrants, such as the Irish in the 1840s, created tempting opportunities to push these costs onto the state. A Worcester director told of Irish immigrants, already ill due to alcohol when they left the old country, and argued that the burden should be shifted from local rate-payers to the state. Interestingly, the data kept routinely by asylums, especially the determination of cause and the assignment of a longer duration of illness, was relevant to this question.[12]

The states were not very happy to find that their initial investments in asylum care began almost immediately to create new obligations. They grew increasingly sceptical of the promise of the asylum. Was the expense of doctors and therapies even necessary? The 'moral treatment', as Andrew Scull has insisted, did not seem to depend on medical expertise, but was rather a matter of a quiet, orderly life in the country and of regular physical labour, supplemented by behavioural management based on teaching the insane to respond to incentives for good behaviour. Although the doctors succeeded in warding off the notion that curative asylums might have no need for doctors, there remained the problem that more and more patients showed little hope of being cured.[13]

In practice, madhouses and asylums were never just medical, but also partly about relieving a public nuisance. In the 1830s, the Prussian Rhine Province refused for a time to accept Maximilian Jacobi's insistence that the Siegburg Asylum, which he directed, was strictly a curative institution. They threatened to turn over much of the work to members of a religious order rather than relying on doctors, and they argued that protecting the population from disorderly lunatics was an important task of asylums even if there was no hope of curing them. In the end, the doctors could not maintain their image of the asylum as a strictly medical institution. As cure rates declined and asylum populations skyrocketed, the budget-watchers pushed to separate off the insane who showed little prospect of a recovery and to put them in custodial institutions. Physicians argued that they might just as well inscribe Dante's famous slogan on the gates of the asylum: 'Abandon hope all ye who enter here.' Even asylums that held on to their curative goals were beginning to look like scenes of hopeless despair by the 1860s.[14]

Balance sheets

While Smith drew back from equating the value of health and life with monetary sums, his numbers declared that asylum care could yield a net surplus, even in budgetary terms. The ordinary asylum tables giving costs in the administrative part and treatment outcomes in the medical report cannot quite be equated with a balance sheet, but it was clear that patient outcomes were the most significant factor to be weighed against the costs of building and running an asylum. In America, especially, asylum advocates like Dorothea Dix promised wondrous results for madhouses. Insanity was a disease like any other, they emphasised, and more easily cured than many. The argument, made often enough in words, appeared in an implicitly numerical form in every table of outcome numbers. It was summed up still more simply in a number that, by 1830, was beginning to provide a universal basis for assessing the effectiveness of asylums: the cure rate. Nothing, it seemed, could be simpler than using such a number to compare the success of different institutions. Americans loved to print up tables comparing their results with the most famous Old-World institutions in Paris, London, and York. The Connecticut Retreat in Hartford showed cure rates in the 1830s of more than 90 per cent, matching and then surpassing the previous champion, a private asylum in London. A decade later, the Massachusetts asylum matched it, and Awl even achieved a perfect 100 per cent in 1843, earning the nickname cure-Awl.[15]

But what is a cure rate? Insanity was a special kind of disease, one that, as asylum tables showed, might clear up within weeks or linger for decades. It was hard to know whether recovery should be attributed to medical treatment, and difficult to specify when a case had become hopeless. Everyone agreed, however, that the prospects of cure were much more favourable in new cases than in old ones. The impressively high cure rates achieved by some American asylums were not calculated for every admitted patient, but only for patients who offered a reasonable prospect of being cured. In the early years, this usually meant 'new patients': those who had come to the asylum within a few months up to perhaps a year of the initial outbreak of insanity. This made the recorded figure for duration of illness before admission a consequential one. Yet it was a figure in which alienists put little faith, since the observation almost always depended on members of the household rather than qualified doctors. American asylums typically calculated a separate cure rate for new cases. The cure rate for old cases was always much worse.

The formula used to calculate those nearly perfect figures for new patients were little discussed in these best of times, when it looked as if the only serious impediment to curing the insane would disappear once the public was properly informed. Alas, cure rates soon came down as the institutions filled up with hopeless patients, requiring new or expanded institutions to make room for new patients. It eventually came out that the brilliant success of alienists in that era of the giants depended on specific practices for admitting, discharging, and classifying patients. For a chronic condition like insanity, the experienced doctor should not give up easily, and serious doctors like these were rewarded with excellent numbers. Such doctors hesitated a very long time before pronouncing their ministrations a failure. As long as the patient lived, there remained a chance of success. Even a death could be treated as an unfortunate consequence of infection or disease rather than a failure of treatment. In the year when John Galt of the Eastern Virginia Asylum in Williamsburg achieved a 100 per cent cure rate, he excluded one patient who died as well as many still under treatment. A sufficiently unscrupulous asylum superintendent would almost never be obligated to accept even a single failure. These men, however, were not being simply dishonest, just stubbornly hopeful. When families insisted on removing a patient who was getting worse, the superintendents regretted as much the loss of hope for this poor soul as they did this blemish, possibly avoidable, on their record of treatment. Death remained, like taxes, inescapable, but it might still be removed from the accounts. And the doctors need not necessarily be blamed. Prisons and poorhouses, solicitous to maintain good health statistics, would sometimes exploit the breakdown of an inmate's last days to transfer their ward to a mental hospital, where death might ensue within days or even hours. Should such a failure to cure, and such a death, be put on their account? Superintendents argued that it should not. But they did not, in fact, exploit every possible loophole for the sake of their statistics.

Reclassification of data was one way to sharpen the statistics. Another was to choose a favourable formula. The basis for calculation of cure rates was almost never made public, though a comparison with the statistics might enable a clever arithmetician to reverse engineer it. Especially for a chronic condition like insanity, there was no fully satisfactory measure. The doctors definitely did not want to divide the number of cures by the total of all patients, which would in almost all cases produce unsatisfactorily low numbers. A more acceptable alternative was to divide the cures either by the number of patients admitted each year, or perhaps by the total number of discharged patients. The (nominally) international French effort to standardise asylum statistics in the late 1860s chose to divide cures by the customary intake of new patients.[16] This solution, like most of its predecessors, tended to prevent patients who remained in the institution from weighing down the cure rate, without authorising the superintendent to exclude patients who appeared hopelessly deranged from the calculation. Deaths, of course, were at best only partly within the control of the physician. Although the doctor in most cases had the authority to pronounce a cure, the admission and discharge of patients depended on a legal determination and could be influenced by the views of family members. The physician's sovereign power to shape the statistics was thus real but incomplete.

Still, the patient accounts were clearly the physician's responsibility. These were in most cases submitted annually to a legislature or government ministry. Asylum medicine was mainly a field of public health rather than of individualised patient treatment, and the physician dealt with numbers all the time. He could scarcely avoid developing at least rudimentary quantitative skills, and some asylum doctors even learned, for example, to calculate statistical error coefficients using Poisson's formula. Faced with cure rates that were already declining by 1850, and that got much worse after that, they wanted to understand what was happening. The catastrophically low cure rates that seemed to prevail in so many institutions by the 1870s were in fact different numbers than their cure-all predecessors. Increasingly, asylums calculated the number of patients discharged as cured divided by the total population of patients. A hopeless long-term patient could weigh against the cure rate for decades, and the tendency over the decades was for institutions to be filled to overflowing with cases of this kind.

Public asylums in Britain never engaged in the kind of manipulations that worked so well for a time in the United States. John Thurnam, appointed as medical superintendent of the York Retreat, took a dim view of very high cure rates, arguing that rates of about 40 per cent for permanent cures were probably the best that could be hoped for. He quickly gained an international reputation as an expert on asylum statistics. He showed, for example, how differently measured cure rates would not only give different results, but also manifest a different trajectory of development, so that one measure could decline while another rose. Hence, an apparent improvement or deterioration of cure rates could be meaningless, reflecting, perhaps, nothing more than changes in the number of long-term, incurable patients.[17] The level of statistical criticism was higher than we are accustomed to expect for mid-nineteenth-century doctors. It reflected the character of mental medicine as an important area of public health, and also, perhaps, Thurnam's relative independence from pressures to demonstrate high rates of cure. Others, however, such as the well-known American alienist Pliny Earle, were led to recognise some of the problems of asylum data or calculations by their embarrassment at the catastrophic decline of measured cure rates from the 1830s to the 1870s. He emphasised the initial lack of attention to relapses, which had allowed some patients to be entered in the statistics as cured scores of times.[18] In any case, these were numbers that mattered. Support of asylums as curative institutions seemed to hinge on statistical evidence that such expenditures were buying cures, and thus, in the long term, would lower the financial cost of insanity even to the state.

Numerical incentives

William Farr had only recently assumed his position in the new General Register Office when he discussed in a pamphlet the problems of asylum statistics. He was by then the leading medical statistician in England and known throughout Europe and North America. He absolutely refused to put implicit faith in numbers, at least not until they were made more uniform and reliable. At the time, asylum figures were feeble and often misleading, since medical superintendents could always find excuses for bad numbers. The original London asylums at Bethlem and St Luke's, he complained, admitted patients as 'incurable' and thus excluded them from the calculations if they had been sick for just one year. At the nearby Middlesex county asylum at Hanwell, where John Conolly was then introducing his system of non-restraint, the cure rate was only 18.8 per cent. This could be compared, unfavourably, with the English average of 40.34 per cent. The alienist William Ellis explained it away as a consequence of admitting so many incurable patients.[19]

Farr did not claim that such explanations were necessarily false. The demand for measures of 'permanent' cures seemed to him quite meaningless, since it could never be known at the time of dismissal whether a cure would last. The per cent of 'cured' patients readmitted, an inverse measure, would at least provide some insight on this matter. In an essay on measures of death rates, which he published in 1841 in the *Journal of the Statistical Society of London,* Farr tried out an analogy of insanity statistics with mortality rates. While an effective treatment for death could of course never be permanent, social medicine could certainly hope to reduce the annual death rate. Incorporating a temporal dimension into these measures, he used the percentage cured per year as his index of the quality of asylum treatment. He also worked with numbers of final outcome: the percentage of asylum patients who in the end died sane or insane.[20]

Farr contended that statistics meant nothing until they were clearly defined, and that they required close policing. The psychological and medical condition of each asylum patient, he declared, should be registered upon admission and discharge by an impartial officer. He insisted particularly on the need for inspection of lunatic asylums, which, after all, had witnessed some extraordinary scandals. Asylum personnel, he complained, keeping their own statistics under the indulgent supervision of idle gentlemen whose visits were announced well in advance, could not be trusted to keep good statistics. The walled-off asylum, cutting the patients off from their families, created a system that invited abuse. He even defended the old Bethlem model of easy public access, greatly maligned by the champions of 'moral treatment' for allowing visitors to enter for a few pennies and gawk at the mad. Accurate statistics and decent treatment, he thought, depended on openness to inspection.[21]

Properly regulated statistics, however, were precious. They could very nearly replace the commissions and commissioners charged to regulate asylums. Farr aspired, in what we might describe as a neoliberal way, to create better health systems by turning measures into incentives, a system of results-based payment. For example, let a pauper asylum receive £20 per admitted patient plus £100 for a recovery, and let it be charged £50 for each death. 'At this rate the finances of Hanwell would rapidly decline', he declared while other (unnamed) asylums would flourish. Since there would also be large fluctuations, it might require a life insurance office to even out the peaks and troughs. The greatest obstacle, he conceded, lay in determining 'the reality of the recovery'. With expert commissioners charged now to assure the quality of statistics rather than to impose their decisions, the future was bright. Under such a system, 'what ardour would they not give to the search after remedies for a most deplorable class of diseases that attack man in his very essence – darken his understanding – pervert and desolate his affection.'[22]

Dollars and sense

Alienists of the early nineteenth century thought they could relieve the burden of this most terrible of diseases. That charitable vision attracted unprecedented state support. Concern for the suffering of the mad had an important role in the success of campaigns for asylum treatment, even if more mundane concerns to preserve public health were also involved. As legislation requiring state provision of asylum care – first enacted in France in 1838 – spread over Europe and North America, idealistic motives increasingly gave way to mundane, practical ones. The institutions could not achieve their mission but instead filled up with unappealing pauper patients who were almost impossible to manage, never mind cure. Instead of containing or even reversing the terrible increase of insanity, the creation of so many asylums seemed only to accelerate its growth, almost without limit. The promise of cures under a system of firm but kindly paternalistic treatment gave way to an ideal of maintenance. The old patient accounts, which had shown sufficient cures to give a rationale for large expenditures, could no longer provide a basis for optimism. Yet it was impossible to reverse the initiatives that had begun with so much optimism, to send tens and hundreds of thousands of unruly and unreasonable people back to their distressed spouses, parents, and offspring, or to abandon them in alleys, gutters, and barns. They could not even close the gates to the newly mad who somehow kept appearing there.

The division of patients into curable and incurable, as we have seen, originated as the statistical basis for an argument that the vast majority of patients could be cured if only their institutions were well run and sufficiently numerous. The ambition then was to preserve curability by checking disease before it could penetrate more deeply into the brain. The new desideratum was to avoid wasting funds on patients whose treatment must be futile. The implicit accounting that tallied up cures to justify such expenditures was losing its credibility, or at least was applied more narrowly now to incoming patients with a favourable prognosis. And the bold quantitative scheme to demonstrate that asylum care could pay for itself ended in failure. In the less hopeful atmosphere of the late nineteenth century, the promise of cures was downgraded in the accounts. The noted psychiatrist and eugenicist Ernst Rüdin spoke in 1911 of an 'avalanche' of medical expenditures and of the duty of psychiatry to contain it, 'to preserve the state'.[23] To be sure, he worried also about the quality of the population, but again, for the sake of the state. Nineteenth-century states had for a time taken a remarkable interest in mental illness, but medical outcomes could not readily be monetised. Ministries and legislatures had always balanced monetary expenditures against other expenditures. In an era that was losing faith in the worth of suffering individuals with poor prospects of becoming productive, the bottom line was bound to privilege monetary values over human ones.

Notes

1. On the functioning of these institutions, see T.M. Porter, *Genetics in the Madhouse: The Unknown History of Human Heredity* (Princeton: Princeton University Press, 2018); also A. Scull, *'The Most Solitary of Afflictions': Madness and Society in Britain, 1700–1900* (New Haven: Yale University Press, 1993).
2. Committee appointed to Examine the Physicians who have attended His Majesty During His Illness, Touching the present State of His Majesty's Health, *Report*, Ordered to be printed 13 January 1789; W. Black, *An Arithmetical and Medical Analysis of the Diseases and Mortality of the Human Species* (London: C. Dilly, 2nd edn, 1789); I. Macalpine and R. Hunter, *George III and the Mad Business* (New York: Pantheon Books, 1969), esp. pp. 297–9.
3. Porter, *Genetics in the Madhouse*.
4. Porter, *Genetics in the Madhouse*, chapters 2, 4.
5. By late in the nineteenth century, psychological/psychiatric biographies of political, religious, and literary figures were becoming rather common in alienist journals such as the *Allgemeine Zeitschrift für Psychiatrie*. See London Metropolitan Archives H11/HLL-B20/1 Case Book Males 1845–50 for a rare collection of case history biographies.
6. *London Metropolitan Archives*, H11/HLL/B19/24 Female Case Book 1873–74 and H11/HLL/B21/13 Male Case Books 1873–74 showcase writing of this kind; see Porter, *Genetics in the Madhouse*, p. 201.
7. Harvard Countway Library, Center for History of Medicine, Records of the Worcester State Hospital, Patient Case Books, 1833–37.
8. *First Annual Report of the Directors and Superintendent of the Ohio Lunatic Asylum … for the Year 1838*, p. 9.
9. *Sixth Ohio Asylum Report for 1843 Report*, pp. 14–15, 37.
10. D.M. Schullian, 'Dr. Samuel Hanbury Smith of Cincinnati, Columbus and Hamilton, Ohio', *Bulletin of the Medical Library Association* 39 (1951), 146–54.
11. *Thirteenth Ohio Asylum Report for 1851*, pp. 14–19; Porter, *Genetics in the Madhouse*, p. 44.
12. Porter, *Genetics in the Madhouse*, p. 93; see the 20th and 22nd annual reports for the Worcester State Hospital for 1850 and 1852.
13. Scull, *Most Solitary of Afflictions*, pp. 188–202.

14 See the report on Jacobi's institution, *Bericht über die Verwaltung der Irren-Heil-Anstalt zu Siegburg während der Jahre 1833, 1835, und 1836* (Koblenz, 1837), p. 13.
15 On cure rates and asylum statistics, see T.R. Beck, 'Statistical notices of some of the lunatic asylums of the United States', *Transactions of the Alban Institute* 1 (1830), 60–83; C.M. McGovern, *Masters of Madness: Social Origins of the American Psychiatric Profession* (Hanover: University Press of New England, 1985), p. 76.
16 L. Lunier (in the name of a commission of doctors) 'Projet de Statistique applicable à l'étude des maladies mentales arrêté par le Congrès Aliéniste International de 1867. Rapport et exposé des motifs', *Annales médico-psychologiques*, series 5 volume 1 (1869), 32–59.
17 Porter, *Genetics in the Madhouse*, p. 73; J. Thurnam, *Observations and Essays on Statistics of Insanity and on Establishments for the Insane* (London: Simpkin, Marshall, 1845), pp. iii–xii; Dr Bernhardi, 'Irrenstatistische Bemerkungen zu dem Vorschlage eines Normalschemas für tabellarische Uebersichten', *Allgemeine Zeitschrift für Psychiatrie* 2 (1845), 264–95, 277–8.
18 P. Earle, *The Curability of Insanity* (Philadelphia: J. B. Lippincott, 1887), first study (1876), pp. 7–63.
19 W. Farr, *On the Statistics of English Lunatic Asylums and the Reform of their Public Management* (London: Sherwood, Gilbert, and Piper, undated [date given in worldcat 1840]). See also J. Eyler, *Victorian Social Medicine: The Ideas and Methods of William Farr* (Baltimore: Johns Hopkins University Press, 1979).
20 Farr, *On the Statistics*; W. Farr, 'Report upon the mortality of lunatics', *Journal of the Statistical Society of London* 4 (1841), 17–33.
21 Farr, *On the Statistics*; Farr, 'Report upon the mortality of lunatics'.
22 Farr, *On the Statistics*, esp. pp. 38–41.
23 E. Rüdin, 'Einige Wege und Ziele der Familienforschung mit Rücksicht auf die Psychiatrie', *Zeitschrift für die gesamte Neurologie und Psychiatrie* 7 (1911), 487–585, 571–2.

Part III
Production

8

Charitable accounting: The Royal Jennerian Society and vaccine production

Andrea Rusnock

On a December afternoon in 1802, at the City Coffee House on Cheapside in London, a group of prominent physicians pledged to advance the new practice of smallpox vaccination by creating a society that would provide free vaccinations to the poor and supply vaccine at no charge to practitioners around the world. Named in recognition of Edward Jenner and his pioneering work in vaccination, the Royal Jennerian Society for the Extermination of Small Pox (RJS) would accomplish these lofty goals by collecting charitable subscriptions and recruiting a network of surgeons who would volunteer their time to vaccinate the poor. Its financial model shared many similarities with other British medical charities, such as voluntary hospitals and outpatient dispensaries. All of them depended on careful and transparent accounts – both financial and medical – to assure their benefactors that monies were well spent and health care goals were met. For the RJS, accountability thus embraced both the fiduciary duty to subscribers and duty of care to their patients.

This chapter highlights the mutually reinforcing nature of financial accounting and medical accounting in medical charities. In doing so, it draws together several strands of research on eighteenth- and early nineteenth-century medicine: the rise of hospital medicine and the birth of the clinic, the medicalisation of society and the increased government involvement in public health and welfare, and the growth of more experimental and numerical approaches to medical knowledge.[1] Financial aspects of these trends have generally been neglected by historians, or treated entirely separately as a branch of accounting history. Much is to be gained by considering financial and medical accounts together.[2]

Competition among medical charities in eighteenth-century Britain was fierce. According to historian Bronwyn Croxson: 'Demonstrating that funds were used properly was vitally important to successful fundraising.'[3] Charities adopted a variety of accounting practices to document and publicise the appropriate and successful use of donations. Financial and medical information were merged into a single document presented first to the governing body of the charity and then to the public in order to solicit subscriptions to maintain the charity. In the case of the RJS, its secretary prepared quarterly reports for the Board of Directors of the revenue from subscriptions along with an account of expenses combined with a record of the number of vaccinated individuals and vaccine packets distributed. In 1803, the RJS made public the full list of subscribers and the amount of each donation in its *An Address of the Royal Jennerian Society*.[4]

The RJS provides a particularly fruitful example to examine the role of accounting in medical charities because its mission was controversial in Britain. Opposition to vaccination centred around two issues: the concerns that cowpox came from an animal; and that it did not produce lifelong immunity. Jenner was convinced that vaccination protected individuals from smallpox throughout their lives, but as the practice spread, cases of vaccinated individuals getting smallpox surfaced and the need for revaccination was increasingly recognised. Smallpox inoculation, on the other hand, did produce lifelong immunity; however, it also triggered dangerous epidemics, a realisation that eventually led to the 1840 act that made it illegal.[5] Nonetheless, scepticism toward vaccination remained in Britain long after the practice had been strongly embraced in other countries. This contested feature of vaccination placed even greater emphasis on accurate accounting, and the creation of a special type of account – the vaccination register.

This third type of account – the vaccination register – functioned epistemologically as a paper tool for the members of the Royal Jennerian Society to investigate and assess the quality, safety, and efficacy of the vaccine.[6] The leaders of the RJS created specially designed registers to be used only by members of the RJS, not the public, to track the

The Royal Jennerian Society and vaccine production

number of individuals who had been vaccinated as well as the different strains of the vaccine. RJS vaccinators recorded the source of the vaccine for each individual they vaccinated. If the vaccinated patient subsequently became ill or had an unusual reaction, the information recorded in the register provided a method of identifying and evaluating the safety and efficacy of the vaccinating matter. This latter function proved essential to investigating reports that attempted to discredit vaccination.

This chapter begins by reviewing the establishment, organisation, and accounting practices of medical charities in eighteenth- and early nineteenth-century Britain. It then discusses the creation of the RJS, highlighting the structural and financial similarities to other medical charities, including the types of accounting practices it adopted to attract and maintain subscriptions to finance its goals. The third section examines the operations of the RJS, reconstructed from the minutes of the Board of Directors and the Medical Committee, focusing on the financial and social functions of its accounts that detailed the costs and extent of vaccinations performed by the RJS. The last section analyses the vaccination register, which served the epistemological functions of establishing the safety and efficacy of vaccination. In short, an analysis of specific examples of RJS accounts underscores the intertwined nature of their financial, social, and epistemological functions.

Medical charities in eighteenth- and early nineteenth-century Britain

In eighteenth-century Britain, new types of medical philanthropy supported the development of hospitals and dispensaries in towns and cities. These new hospitals – called voluntary hospitals because they were supported by voluntary subscriptions from benefactors – shaped hospital and outpatient care.[7] Unlike older hospitals, many of which dated back to the medieval period, that served as almshouses for the poor, voluntary hospitals sought to limit the provisioning of care to deserving poor patients who could be cured. The first voluntary hospital, the Westminster in London, opened its doors in 1720; by 1800, London had five general voluntary hospitals, and outside the metropolis, twenty-eight provincial towns had established voluntary hospitals.[8] In addition, specialised charitable institutions for lying-in, fevers, smallpox, and other conditions opened their doors. Funded by subscriptions and other forms of charitable giving, voluntary hospitals provided free care to the poor by physicians and surgeons who donated their services.[9] Similar arrangements supported the development of dispensaries throughout Britain, which provided outpatient care.[10] As a benefit, subscribers were entitled to refer a certain number of patients to the charity for medical care. Donors who gave significant sums served as governors to these institutions, meeting at least quarterly to oversee their operations.[11] These organisations relied upon financial and patient records to encourage subscriptions and guide decisions about the operations of the charity.

The accounting practices of charities in the eighteenth century evolved from custom, borrowed from those used by early businesses. According to Frances Miley and Andrew Read, 'extant evidence suggests commercial accounting practices permeated society during the eighteenth century and were adopted by other types of organisations',[12] such as medical charities. Most eighteenth-century charities issued annual reports with detailed information about the finances of the charity, the services provided, and a list of subscribers (benefactors).[13] These annual reports publicised the charity's financial soundness in order to attract new donors. Good accounts signalled good governance, and eighteenth-century charities created rules to guide accounting practices.[14] For example, the Governors of the London Foundling Hospital, founded by Thomas Coram in 1739 to provide care for abandoned children, issued rules in 1757 to formalise its accounts; according to Miley and Read, these rules 'describe the entire recordkeeping system, referring to the hospital's financial and non-financial records collectively as the hospital's accounting system.'[15]

Non-financial records listed the names of patients, frequently their age and sex, their ailment, and most importantly, the outcome of their treatment. These records were valuable not only to benefactors, but also significantly to medical practitioners.[16] Physicians often shaped the types of accounts that were kept in the new medical charities. John Lettsom, a prominent Quaker physician who founded the first dispensary in London at Aldersgate in 1770, maintained registers with information about the types of diseases patients suffered from and whether they survived or died. Using these accounts, Lettsom calculated the mortality of each type of disease by month and sought to evaluate the impact of new therapies like cinchona and ventilation.[17] The motivations for accounting – financial stability, charitable subscriptions, patient care – blended together into medical charities' accounting systems.

Edward Jenner, smallpox vaccination, and the establishment of the RJS

The Royal Jennerian Society was created in 1803, a little less than five years after the publication of Edward Jenner's *An Inquiry into the Causes and Effects of Variolae Vaccinae, or Cow-Pox* (1798), which detailed the use of cowpox to prevent smallpox. Vaccination provided an alternative to the earlier procedure of inoculation, where smallpox lymph or scabs were inserted into a scratch on a patient's arm to induce a mild case of smallpox. Securing lymph for inoculation was fairly easy because of the widespread incidence of smallpox. By contrast, acquiring cowpox lymph proved more difficult. The disease appeared sporadically in dairy herds in the western counties of England, making it hard to collect lymph directly from infected cows. Thus, one of the first obstacles proponents of the vaccination faced was maintaining a supply of cowpox lymph.

Doctors and surgeons developed a variety of methods to produce and distribute cowpox. The method deemed most successful had been pioneered by Jenner himself: arm-to-arm transmission in humans. Vaccinators harvested lymph from the vaccination site roughly eight days following the initial incision. In some cases, the lymph would be immediately used to vaccinate other individuals (literally arm-to-arm). Otherwise, the harvested cowpox lymph was dried on threads and ivory lancets, or kept fluid in sealed quills or between glass plates.[18] The success of these methods was often more miss than hit: frequently, the gathered lymph failed to produce an active case of cowpox.

Proponents of vaccination thus realised the need for human repositories to keep the cowpox active. George Pearson, a doctor and chemist who became one of the first advocates of vaccination, established the London Vaccine-Pock Institution in June 1799, but it collapsed within a year because Pearson snubbed Jenner, who refused to support it.[19] The idea, however, proved lasting: surgeons in large cities would vaccinate individuals (often children) and harvest cowpox from their arms in order to maintain a supply of cowpox lymph that could be supplied to correspondents who requested it at home and abroad.

The need for a more centralised and organised system of distribution became clear as demand for cowpox lymph grew. A meeting chaired by the Lord Mayor of London on 19 January 1803 formalised the initial proposal for the RJS with the support of the Duke of Clarence (the future King William IV), four peers, at least one financier (John Julius Angerstein), several aldermen and clergymen, London businessmen and printers, and an impressive list of prominent physicians and surgeons. At the end of January, the society named itself the Royal Jennerian Society, after securing the patronage of King George III.[20] According to its charter: '[t]he unspeakable benefits which may be expected to arise from an extensive diffusion of this salutary practice will be much accelerated by the establishment of an Institution in a central part of the Metropolis'.[21]

The society pursued this goal in several ways: it set up twelve vaccinating stations throughout London that provided free vaccinations and kept records of all vaccinations performed,[22] it published a comparative view of inoculation and vaccination to demonstrate the advantages of the latter,[23] it petitioned clergy of all faiths to promote vaccination among their parishioners,[24] it served as the centre for correspondence and personal visits from foreign doctors,[25] and finally it sent cowpox lymph to anyone who requested it. The RJS never charged for the vaccine it distributed and this largesse was regarded as central to the spread of vaccination. 'This gratuitous diffusion of Vaccine Virus,' claimed a newspaper article in 1805, 'has been a principal means of spreading the Vaccine Inoculation throughout the British Empire and the World.'[26]

To do all of these things required money, and the society's organisers successfully solicited high-status patrons, patronesses, and clergy, whose annual subscriptions provided key support. These contributions, along with larger donations from the Corporation of London (the governing body of the city of London) (£500) and the East India Company (£100), supplied the funds to run the society.[27] By 15 June 1803 – six months after it had been established – the RJS had raised £3,226 through subscriptions (which included the donation from the Corporation of London).[28] Additional support from the British government came in the form of franking privileges, which covered the society's postage costs to send vaccine and communications around the world.[29]

The original charter for the RJS set up a Board of Directors and a Medical Committee. The Board of Directors oversaw the charity's finances, while the Medical Committee supervised the vaccination stations and attended to the quality and safety of the vaccine. The Board of Directors comprised three bankers (Robert Barclay, Robert Ladbroke, and Felix Ladbroke), two printers (John Nichols and William Phillips), and the Reverend Rowland Hill. The printers were especially important for overseeing publicity during the first months of the society. Reverend Hill, an early proponent of vaccination, served as minister to two churches, one in London and one in Gloucestershire, and at the end of his sermons, he vaccinated parishioners for free.[30] Reverend Hill, along with other RJS board members, encouraged religious leaders of all faiths – 'Church of England, Kirk of Scotland, Protestant Dissenters, Society of Friends, Hebrew nation and the Ministers of all other religious bodies' – to promote vaccination in their sermons.[31]

Doctors and surgeons made up the Medical Committee, with Jenner appointed as president.[32] Members of the Board of Directors and the Medical Committee were considered governors and as governors were expected to pay 1 guinea a year to the RJS.[33] For the first few months, both the Board of Directors and the Medical Committee met weekly, with reports shuttling between the two bodies. Four times a year, a general court convened representatives from the Board of Directors and the Medical Committee. Charles Murray, a lawyer, was appointed secretary to the RJS and his quarterly reports summarised its work. The minutes from both the Board of Directors and the Medical Committee of the Royal Jennerian Society record the details about expenses and debates over the necessity of particular expenditures that underscored the different aims of the two bodies: the Board of Governors focused on finances – keeping the society solvent; and the Medical Committee concentrated on ensuring the safety and quality of the vaccine.

The operations of the Royal Jennerian Society

The RJS headquarters – called the Central House – were located in Salisbury Square, off Fleet Street, where the Resident Inoculator and the Secretary for the society rented rooms. The key figure for the RJS, the Resident Inoculator, was expected to carry out vaccinations daily between the hours of 10:00 am and 3:00 pm,[34] collect lymph from satellite stations in London, maintain a supply at the Central House, and, finally, send vaccine to those who requested it. For these services, he received £200 per year and free lodging. Dr John Walker became the first Resident Inoculator in 1803, overseeing twelve stations located throughout London from Mile End in the east to Westminster, and from Southwark (south of the Thames), to Clerkenwell (in the north).[35] Prior to his appointment, Walker had served as an assistant vaccinator to Dr J.R. Marshall for the British navy in the Mediterranean. Upon his return to London, Walker joined the medical group that created the RJS.

One of the first actions of the RJS was to create and publish a comparative view of inoculation and vaccination that highlighted the advantages of vaccination. John Nichols, one of the printers on the Board of Directors, published the resulting table (see Figure 8.1), which had been condensed into a single page. The Board of Directors supported this effort to publicise the virtues of vaccination, but it kept an eye on printing costs. At the meeting on 17 March 1803 at St Paul's Coffee House, the Board resolved 'to print a very large impression of the comparative view' but wanted it 'in such a form' that it would 'impose the least possible burthen upon the funds of this Society'.[36] One week later it reviewed the revised comparative view and commended 'its economical format that allowed for 'some useful additions to be printed upon one side of the same paper whereby a considerable expence to the Society will be saved'.[37] The 'useful additions' on the reverse side of the comparative view were details about the locations of the vaccination stations, when they were open, and the names of surgeons who performed the vaccinations. On 31 March, the printing committee of the RJS was 'instructed to procure twenty thousand copies of the small Edition and 5,000 of the larger to be printed'.[38] These were distributed to subscribers, and to each of the vaccination stations.[39]

The Board of Directors engaged in other types of promotion for the RJS, including printing 5,000 copies of a flyer with a list of RJS subscribers and a set of vaccination instructions to be distributed to each subscriber, to members of both Houses of Parliament, and to the London aldermen.[40] The Board also ordered a large painted and framed

The Royal Jennerian Society and vaccine production 217

8.1 A Comparative View of the Natural Small-Pox, Inoculated Small-Pox, and Inoculated Cow-Pox, by John Addington, by Order of the Medical Council of the Royal Jennerian Society for the Extermination of the Small-Pox.

sign to be hung at the Royal Exchange as well as similar signs for other London neighbourhoods to complete the publicity effort.[41]

Both the Board of Directors and the Medical Committee recognised the importance of careful accounting to the successful operation of the RJS. The initial job description for the Resident Inoculator placed heavy emphasis on clerical duties. According to the Medical Committee, 'a large share of his (the Resident Inoculator's) Employment will be in the Capacity of Medical Secretary and Register; he be fully competent to conduct with credit and reputation the Important business of Registering the Medical transactions of the Society, and of carrying on the extensive correspondence which he shall be required to undertake'.[42] More specifically: 'He shall keep a register of the Inoculating practice at the Central House, and lay a monthly abstract of all the

Stations before the Council. He shall also register the names and residence of all persons to whom the matter of Inoculation shall have been distributed on behalf of the Society.'[43]

To fulfil these duties, the Medical Committee ordered several large register books to record vaccinations, distribution of vaccine matter, and anomalous cases. The Board of Directors, however, questioned the necessity of this expense. John Addington, the surgeon who had ordered the books, conceded that 'the Blank Book designed for keeping an account of Anomalous Cases, which for the sake of uniformity had been ordered the same size as the other books of the set was very much larger than would be at all necessary'. Addington proposed substituting a smaller, less expensive book in its place.[44] Presumably, there were to be few, if any, anomalous cases. Again, like the table comparing the advantages of vaccination and inoculation, financial constraints and optimistic expectations for vaccination shaped accounting practices.

The registers documented the number of vaccinations and justified expenses to the society's patrons. Each vaccination station was furnished with 'one desk with Lock and two keys for keeping the Books and paper furnished with Pens, Ink and paper'.[45] Addington created 'certain forms for the registers of Inoculations, distribution of Matter and Consultations respecting Vaccination', and the Medical Committee asked Addington to 'superintend the preparing the same for the various stations'.[46] The surgeons at each station were charged to 'register the whole of the Inoculating practice' in the account books supplied by the society.[47] The form Addington created was quite detailed (see Figure 8.2), and listed information about the name, residence, and age of the patient, the method of the vaccination and the source and state of the vaccine matter, observations about the vaccination sites for both right and left arms for the 4th, 8th, 12th, and 16th days following the vaccination, general observations about the patient's constitution, and if vaccine matter was harvested from the patient on the 8th day. Separate tables recorded information about additional consultations with patients to manage unusual symptoms and to record the distribution of vaccine matter.[48]

The Board of Directors mandated that the surgeon at each vaccination station send an account to the Resident Inoculator on the twentieth of each month detailing the number of vaccinations performed since the last account.[49] The Board also specified that the Resident

The Royal Jennerian Society and vaccine production 219

8.2 Register of Inoculations, *Address of the Royal Jennerian Society, for the Extermination of the Small-Pox. With the Plan, Regulations, and Instructions for Vaccine Inoculation. To Which is Added, a List of the Subscribers.*

Inoculator present a summary of the total number of vaccinations and include 'how many plates charged with [vaccine] matter have been distributed.'[50]

The vaccination registers: tables of trials to tables of practice

In addition to the financial and social roles of accounting, the RJS registers played a pivotal role in establishing vaccination and drew on prior efforts to document and evaluate the quality, safety, and efficacy of the cowpox vaccine. Edward Jenner, in his initial pamphlet, had published a series of case histories of vaccinations that he had performed. Each case history included personal information about the patient (name, age, residence), the source of the vaccine, primary symptoms, and the outcome. While Jenner's pamphlet was organised as a narrative, subsequent publications by other physicians frequently relied on tables or registers with similar information to guide, evaluate, and legitimise the practice of vaccination.[51]

One of the first and most influential advocates, Dr William Woodville, physician to the London Smallpox and Inoculation hospitals, began vaccinating with cowpox just two months after Jenner announced his discovery. Woodville vaccinated roughly 600 individuals and summarised his work in brief case histories of each patient. Then, Woodville took the further step of constructing tables of the case histories. The columns of the tables listed the source of the vaccine, the name of the vaccinated individual, and the number of pustules the patient exhibited. (The number of pustules served as a visual gauge for how serious the illness was.) Woodville stated his goal for the table: 'In order that the progressive descent of the Cow-pox infection from patient to patient, as well as the magnitude of the disease which was excited by the inoculation, may be comprehended at one view, I have subjoined the following tabular statement.'[52]

'At one view' was optimistic: Woodville's table was over 20 pages in length, but patterns were visible. For example, on the first page of the table, the individual Collingridge had 170 pustules following vaccination; George, who was vaccinated with lymph from Collingridge, had 530 pustules. By contrast, most others had 10 pustules or fewer. What could account for these differences? Did smallpox matter somehow get mixed with cowpox? Did smallpox effluvia infect patients who had been vaccinated? Questions such as these directed Woodville's and Jenner's research into the behaviour of cowpox vaccination and the tables contributed both to raising and answering these type of enquiries.

Woodville's table also functioned as an instrument or paper tool, permitting readers to trace a strain of cowpox through many vaccinations, but the process was cumbersome. As cowpox production (mainly through arm-to-arm transmission) and distribution became more widespread, doctors revised Woodville's table to record the source and to ensure the 'goodness' of the vaccinating lymph. The register designed by Addington for the RJS (see Figure 8.2) was an ambitious effort to collect and record vaccination details, but it proved to be too unwieldy for practitioners, as shown below.

The investigation of anomalous cases of failed vaccinations – patients contracting smallpox after the vaccination or patients contracting smallpox from the vaccine – and the resulting news or rumours thereof were critical to the success and spread of vaccination, and Jenner took a particular interest in policing the reputation of vaccination. The Board of Directors recognised the vital importance of refuting adverse reports and resolved that it 'will defray all expences attendant upon the same'.[53] The RJS pursued many avenues to maintain the reputation of vaccination. For example, the RJS carefully monitored the London Bills of Mortality. In 1803, two deaths were attributed to cowpox in the Bills, and the Board of Directors immediately asked the Medical Committee to investigate.[54] A special committee interviewed one of the searchers, a woman appointed by the parish to examine the bodies of the deceased to determine cause of death, and filed a report with the RJS alleging that the searcher had listed cowpox as the cause of death solely based on her opposition to the practice and not on the physical signs present on the corpse. The special committee noted that 'It may be proper to add, that the Searchers did not look at the arm of the deceased', which would have revealed whether the dead woman had in fact been vaccinated.[55] Two months later, a deputation of the RJS met with the Company of Parish Clerks, who agreed that it had been an error to list cowpox as a cause of death and they would correct the mistake.[56] The doctors of the RJS prevailed in this instance.

In March 1804, the Medical Council appointed another special committee to investigate the case of Mrs Minton and her child who had been vaccinated two years previously. It is not clear how this case came to the attention of the RJS, but it responded quickly. The child had an eruption that looked like smallpox and the special committee was instructed 'to endeavour to trace the progress of the matter taken from the child for the purpose of propagating the infection'.[57] The special committee presented the results of their investigation three months later: the child did indeed have smallpox (evidence came from two children who were inoculated with matter taken from his pustules). This investigation revealed that lymph had been harvested from the child and used to inoculate other patients before doctors realised that it was smallpox, not cowpox. According to the report, the committee then became concerned about the original vaccination: 'the only doubt which can be now entertained respects the efficacy of his vaccination'.[58]

The case of Mrs Minton and her child led to a change in the way the RJS recorded vaccinations. In the summer of 1804, it created a new

Number	Source of Matter	Name	Residence	Age	Days of Attendance	Event	Remarks
2549	251	Maria James	9 Elliott Court	2Y 7M	4.8.12		

8.3 Excerpt from RJS vaccination register, September 1804

register and mandated its use at each of the London vaccinating stations beginning in September 1804 (Figure 8.3). The form would 'occupy two pages instead of one'[59] and was much simpler than the one created by Addington in 1803. Many of the details were removed, leaving a chart that required only short, well-defined entries in each of the columns.

The following spring (1805), the Medical Committee issued detailed instructions on how to fill in this form, indicating that the vaccinators were not complying with the Committee's initial requests. Each column was to be filled: the first column kept a running tally of the number of patients vaccinated at the particular station. The second column specified the source of the vaccine matter by using the number listed for the patient from whom the cowpox had been harvested; this reference facilitated the process of tracing the lineage of a particular vaccine. The third, fourth, and fifth columns provided identification of the patient, and the sixth column detailed information about the days the vaccinator had seen the patient following the initial vaccination. The last column, titled event, asked the vaccinator to enter one of the following letters: P for perfect vaccination; D for doubtful vaccination; and F for failed vaccination. The designation of P, D, or F was based on the visual inspection of the vaccination site at several specific times following the vaccination.[60]

The register kept a running account of the number of individuals who had been vaccinated, and it provided a method to evaluate the success of the vaccination by the appearance of the vaccination site (Perfect, Doubtful, or Failed) and to trace the source of the vaccine if something should go awry – a type of quality control. Like the alphabetical index, the enumeration of patients made this table easy to use. It became a working, dynamic instrument that effectively documented the spread of cowpox by linking bits of information in an ongoing chain and using enumeration as an index.

The limitations of charitable institutions

In May 1803, just five months after its establishment, the RJS reported 'upwards of 300 charges of Matter which were distributed to Medical gentlemen residing in and near London and in various parts of England and Ireland, to the East and West Indies, to Holland, Germany, Italy and America'.[61] After eighteen months, the RJS had vaccinated 12,288 individuals in London and '19,352 charges of Vaccine virus were supplied from the central-house to most parts of the British empire, and to foreign countries'.[62] The London Bills of Mortality recorded the dramatic impact of the free vaccinations offered by the RJS on smallpox mortality in London: in 1800, 2,409 individuals died of smallpox; in 1804, 622 died (roughly a quarter of the number for 1800).[63] By all measures, the RJS's promotion of vaccination was a success.

Throughout its short existence, however, the Royal Jennerian Society struggled financially. Initially sustained by subscriptions, the society's funding became increasingly precarious as the novelty of vaccination waned and philanthropic donations decreased. At a general meeting held on 2 March 1807, the RJS voted to reorganise, merging the Board of Directors and the Medical Committee into a single entity composed of 36 members, 12 of whom were physicians. This vote tacitly acknowledged the failure of the original governing structure. At the same meeting, the terrible finances of the Society were reviewed: £450 annual income, £800 annual expenses. By 1808, when urged to come to London immediately because of the imminent collapse of the RJS, Jenner reflected 'What can occasion our Soc[iet]y to fall into ruins? Nothing I conceive but the want of that grand Pap Money.'[64]

The RJS continued to operate in deficit for another year until Parliament intervened. A series of hearings were held during which Jenner confessed that the 'Royal Jennerian Society was now so impoverished from want of subscriptions'.[65] Parliament readily acknowledged the importance and value of the work of the RJS and authorised the establishment of 'a central institution in London, for the purpose of rendering Vaccine Inoculation generally beneficial to his Majesty's subjects, to be superintended by a certain number of the Royal College of Physicians and of the Royal College of Surgeons in London.'[66] The annual cost was estimated to be £2,500 to £3,000 – far more than the expenditures of the RJS. One of its mandates was to supply vaccine to the British army and navy, which it did until 1861.[67] Indeed, by the second decade of the nineteenth century, in the midst of the Napoleonic wars, the British, French, and American governments had stepped in to finance and oversee the production of vaccine. The National Vaccine Establishment officially opened in December 1808, and by August 1809 the RJS dissolved.[68]

The dissolution of the RJS points to the limitations of financial and social accounting to the survival of medical charities. Despite the best efforts of the RJS to document and publicise its success through financial accounts (how much money was raised and how much was spent) and social accounts (the number of individuals vaccinated and the number of vaccine packets sent to correspondents), the RJS failed to raise the funds necessary to carry on its work. Transparent accounting was important to charities, but it may not always have been sufficient.

While the finances of the Royal Jennerian Society failed, the medical goal of the charity to supply safe vaccine without charge succeeded. This success in part depended on the accurate accounts maintained by the RJS, which allowed special committees to investigate instances of vaccination failure. The RJS pioneered a new type of accounting practice, the vaccination register, which created a continuous log of individuals who were vaccinated and the source of the vaccine. The vaccination register marked an important shift in the presentation and use of case histories (a key form of medical knowledge) from a narrative format to enumerated tables – in short, an epistemological accounting function. The accuracy of this log was key to investigating accusations that vaccination had done harm. The registers – a type of paper tool – provided a method to reconstruct the pedigree of the vaccine. The willingness of the British government to take over and pay for the administration of a national vaccine institution endorsed this success.

Acknowledgements

Research for this chapter was supported by NLM Grant 5 G13 LM 011206–02 from the National Library of Medicine. I would like to thank the contributors of this volume for their insightful comments and suggestions. And I am indebted to Paul Lucier for his business acumen.

Notes

1. G. Risse, 'Medicine in the age of enlightenment', in A. Wear (ed.), *Medicine in Society – Historical Essays* (Cambridge: Cambridge University Press, 1992), pp. 149–96.
2. There are a few exceptions, see, for example: R. Gray, D.L. Owen, and C.A. Adams, *Accounting and Accountability: Changes and Challenges in Corporate Social Reporting* (London: Prentice Hall, 1996), p. 38; cited in S. Moggi, V. Filippi, C. Leardini, and G. Rossi, 'Accountability for a place in heaven: A stakeholders' portrait in Verona's confraternities', *Accounting History* 2:2–3 (2016), 236–62, here 238; also see A. Berry, '"Balancing the books": funding provincial hospitals in eighteenth-century England', *Accounting, Business and Financial History* 7:1 (1997), 1–30.
3. B. Croxson, 'The price of charity to the Middlesex Hospital, 1750–1830', in M. Gorsky and S. Sheard (eds), *Financing Medicine: The British Experience since 1750* (London: Routledge, 2006), pp. 23–39, here p. 28.
4. *Address of the Royal Jennerian Society, for the Extermination of the Small-Pox. With the Plan, Regulations, and Instructions for Vaccine Inoculation. To Which is Added, a List of the Subscribers* (London: W. Phillips, 1803).
5. D. Brunton, *The Politics of Vaccination: Practice and Policy in England, Wales, Ireland and Scotland, 1800–1874* (Rochester, NY: Rochester University Press, 2008).
6. Staffan Müller-Wille has defined paper tools as 'devices made from paper and ink, whether in manuscript or print – that were employed in practices of extracting and processing written information like note-taking, listing, cataloguing, or tabulating'. S. Müller-Wille, 'Names and numbers: 'Data' in classical natural history, 1758–1859', *Osiris* 32 (2017), 109–28, here 116.
7. Berry, 'Balancing the books', 2.
8. R. Porter, *The Greatest Benefit to Mankind* (New York: W.W. Norton & Co., 1997), p. 298.
9. L. Grandshaw, 'The rise of the modern hospital in Britain', in Wear (ed.), *Medicine in Society*, pp. 197–218, provides a brief overview of the process of creating new hospitals in the eighteenth and nineteenth centuries.
10. Porter, *The Greatest Benefit to Mankind*, p. 299.
11. Berry, 'Balancing the books', 2.

12 F. Miley and A. Read, 'Go gentle babe: Accounting and the London Foundling Hospital, 1757–97', *Accounting History* 21:2–3 (2016), 167–84, here 170.
13 J. Maltby and J. Rutterford, 'Investing in charities in the nineteenth century: the financialization of philanthropy', *Accounting History* 21:2–3 (2016), 263–80, here 269.
14 For the ongoing practice in nineteenth-century Britain, see B.M. Doyle's Chapter 5, this volume.
15 Miley and Read, 'Go gentle babe', here 169.
16 U. Tröhler emphasises the importance of new charitable hospitals and dispensaries for the growth of numerical evaluations of therapies, see U. Tröhler, *To Improve the Evidence of Medicine: the 18th Century British Origins of a Critical Approach* (Edinburgh: Royal College of Physicians Edinburgh, 2000), p. 12.
17 J. Lettsom, *On the General Treatment and Cure of Fevers* (London, 1772) in Tröhler, *To Improve the Evidence of Medicine*, p. 31.
18 A. Rusnock, 'Catching cowpox: The early spread of smallpox vaccination, 1798–1810', *Bulletin of the History of Medicine* 83 (2009), 17–36.
19 R.B. Fisher, *Edward Jenner (1749–1823)* (London: André Deutsch, 1991), pp. 91–8.
20 J. Baron, *The Life of Edward Jenner, M.D.* 2 vols (London, 1838), here vol. 1, pp. 570–1; Fisher, *Edward Jenner*, pp. 136–7.
21 Minutes of the Board of Directors of the Royal Jennerian Society for the Extermination of the Small Pox (hereafter RJS), 23 December 1802, Wellcome Library, MS 4302.
22 The Society adopted its regulations at the meeting of the Medical Committee on 14 April 1803, Minutes of the Medical Committee, RJS, 14 April 1803, Wellcome Library, MS 4304.
23 See Fisher, *Edward Jenner*, p. 144 for publication details (20,000 small size printed, 5,000 large size for posting), 15 December 1803. The Board of Directors also agreed to print 5,000 more copies, see Minutes of the Medical Committee, RJS, 15 December 1803, Wellcome Library, MS 4304.
24 Minutes of the Medical Committee, RJS, 10 March 1803, Wellcome Library, MS 4304.
25 For example, Dr J.P. Frank of Vienna attended the 7 April 1803 meeting, Minutes of the Medical Committee, RJS, Wellcome MS 4304.
26 C. Murray, Secretary to the RJS, report to the Annual General Court meeting of the RJS held on 6 March 1805, newspaper clipping (origin unknown), Wellcome Library, MS 5244/99.
27 Fisher, *Edward Jenner*, p. 143.

28 RJS General Meeting Minutes, 15 June 1803, Wellcome Library, MS 4303.
29 'The General Post Office having liberally offered to facilitate the communications of the Society throughout the Empire, the Board of Directors were requested to make, without delay, the necessary arrangements for the Society's availing itself of the offer.' Minutes of the Medical Committee, RJS, 15 December 1803, Wellcome Library, MS 4304. In May 1806, the General Post Office withdrew the franking privileges. Minutes of the Medical Committee, RJS, 1 May 1806, Wellcome Library, MS 4304.
30 Rowland Hill (1744–1833) served as minister at Surrey Chapel (London) and at the church in Wotton-under-Edge in Gloucestershire, see P. Saunders, *Edward Jenner: The Cheltenham Years, 1795–1823, being a Chronicle of the Vaccination Campaign* (Hanover and London: University Press of New England, 1982), p. 147.
31 Minutes of the Board of Directors, RJS, 10 March, 1803, Wellcome Library, MS 4302.
32 The initial members of the Medical Committee included Jenner (President), John Coakley Lettsom (Vice-president), James Sims, John Walker, William Farquhar, Charles Aikin, Astley Cooper, and Henry Cline. Minutes of the Board of Directors, RJS, 15 February 1803, Wellcome MS 4392. For details, see Fisher, *Edward Jenner*, p. 138.
33 Fisher, *Edward Jenner*, p. 141.
34 By June 1804, the hours at the Central House had been reduced to 11:00 am to 1:00 pm, Minutes of the Medical Committee, RJS, 25 June 1804, Wellcome Library, MS 4304.
35 Minutes of the Medical Committee, RJS, 23 February 1803, Wellcome Library, MS 4304.
36 Minutes of the Board of Directors, RJS, 17 March 1803, Wellcome Library, MS 4302.
37 Minutes of the Board of Directors, RJS, 24 March 1803, Wellcome Library, MS 4302.
38 Minutes of the Board of Directors, RJS, 31 March 1803, Wellcome Library, MS 4302.
39 Minutes of the Board of Directors, RJS, 7 September 1803, Wellcome Library, MS 4302.
40 Minutes of the Board of Directors, RJS, 19 May 1803, Wellcome Library, MS 4302.
41 Ibid.
42 Minutes of the Board of Directors, RJS, 7 April 1803, Wellcome Library, MS 4302.
43 Ibid.

44 Minutes of the Board of Directors, RJS, 23 June 1803, Wellcome Library, MS 4302.
45 Minutes of the Medical Committee, RJS, 14 April 1803, Wellcome Library, MS 4304.
46 Minutes of the Medical Committee, RJS, 5 May 1803, Wellcome Library, MS 4304.
47 Minutes of the Medical Committee, RJS, 28 April 1803, Wellcome Library, MS 4304.
48 *Address of the Royal Jennerian Society, for the Extermination of the Small-Pox*, p. 52.
49 Minutes of the Board of Directors, RJS, 19 May 1803, Wellcome Library, MS 4302.
50 Ibid.
51 A. Rusnock, 'Medical statistics and hospital medicine: The case of smallpox vaccination', *Centaurus* 49 (2007), 337–59. For a more general discussion of the use of case histories in medical knowledge, see V. Hess and J.A. Mendelsohn, 'Case and series: Medical knowledge and paper technology, 1600–1900', *History of Science* 48 (2010), 287–314.
52 W. Woodville, *Report on a Series of Inoculations for the Variolae Vaccinae, or Cow-Pox: with Remarks and Observations on this Disease, considered a Substitute for the Smallpox* (London, 1799), here p. 114.
53 Minutes of the Board of Directors, RJS, 17 March 1803, Wellcome Library, MS 4302.
54 Minutes of the Medical Committee, RJS, 26 May 1803, Wellcome Library, MS 4304.
55 Here is the excerpt from the RJS minutes: 'The names of the searchers are Slater and Stracey. Mrs. Slater this morning made the following declaration to our Committee: On being apprized by the Undertaker of the death of Mrs. Brooks she went to the house along with her fellow searcher Stracey, they there examined the corpse in the usual manner, and were informed by a female relation of the deceased who had attended her during her illness, that in her opinion the death was owing to the Inflammation in the breast; in which opinion they (the Searchers) acquiesced, but on returning to the Parish Clerks Office, the Searcher Stracey, who had always expressed herself unfavorable to vaccine inoculation, thought proper to declare it her opinion that the death was occasion'd by the Inoculation, which opinion was supported by the Clerk, Mr. Leman: who however, had never seen the deceased during her illness. It may be proper to add, that the Searchers did not look at the arm of the deceased, and also that Mr. Leman the Clerk of Shoreditch Parish had always opposed the new Inoculation.' Minutes of the Board of Directors, RJS, 24 March 1803, Wellcome Library, MS 4302.

The Royal Jennerian Society and vaccine production   229

56 Minutes of the Board of Directors, RJS, 19 May 1803, Wellcome Library, MS 4302.
57 Minutes of the Medical Committee, RJS, 14 March 1804, Wellcome Library, MS 4304.
58 Minutes of the Medical Committee, RJS, 19 July 1804, Wellcome Library, MS 4304.
59 Minutes of the Medical Committee, RJS, 6 September 1804, Wellcome Library, MS 4304.
60 Minutes of the Medical Committee, RJS, 9 May 1805, Wellcome Library, MS 4304.
61 Minutes of the Medical Committee, RJS, 5 May 1803, Wellcome Library, MS 4304.
62 Baron, *Life of Jenner*, pp. 576–7.
63 Baron, *Life of Jenner*, p. 577.
64 Edward Jenner to Charles Murray, 1 March 1808, Wellcome Library, MS 5244/6.
65 Vaccination Debates Folio, June 1808, Wellcome Library, MS 3662.
66 Fisher, *Edward Jenner*, p. 199.
67 Ibid., p. 211.
68 Edward Jenner's first biographer, John Baron, attributes the decline of the RJS to the activities of the resident inoculator John Walker, who in his practice and writings did not follow Jenner's mode of vaccination. The Medical Board was poised to dismiss Walker in 1806, but Walker resigned, see Baron, *Life of Jenner*, pp. 577–83. Jenner's own comments, however, underline the central importance of funding to the RJS's survival.

9

The industry of clinical trials and the rise of medico-economic accounting: The case of antidepressants, 1970–90

Jean-Paul Gaudillière and Volker Hess

Three processes – pharmaceutical revolution, drug regulation, and new methodologies – radically changed clinical research during the three decades after the Second World War. The existing historiography accordingly highlights two of them: pharmaceutical revolution and drug regulation.[1] We would like to address the shift in the research methodology with special emphasis on accounting.[2] No other story than that of the invention, marketing, and prescription of the first drugs labelled 'antidepressants' can better illustrate the far-reaching interdependencies between the development of revolutionary treatments and the regulative activities of state authorities.[3] This story also provides the point of departure of our own analysis. The methodologies of drug research and development did not only comprise new strategies in drug testing (screening) but also techniques for preparing, proceeding, and editing the data from bedside observation. In effect, the clinical research at hospitals was reorganised in the same way as the research and development in the pharmaceutical companies. In a nutshell, this chapter argues that in the course of this process, we not only faced the mounting role of an invisible industrialist operating in the background of the bench and the bedside, but also see emerging an invisible bookkeeper holding together the domains of knowledge and economy. Accounting – understood as tools of knowledge production – is thus restricted neither to financial transactions nor to any kind of administrative transactions within enterprises, hospitals, and other health organisations.[4] Instead, this chapter extends Hopwood's idea[5] to enlarge the economy-focused concepts of accounting to the domain of knowing in order to understand accounting as the activity of drawing and comparing lists[6] used in a second step for defining and ranking values by ways of counting.

Accounting and counting are indeed closely related, especially in the field of medicine, but they differ in the sense that accounting relies on a balancing mode of counting permitted by the comparison of lists. Medical counting has literally arisen from accounting and did not disappear with the rise of medical statistics. The beginnings of medical quantification are rooted in the seventeenth century.[7] John Graunt, the learned draper and member of the Royal Society, thus applied the techniques used for bookkeeping to the weekly lists of death in London. Calculating the ratios of burials to christenings was not the plus or minus of financial transactions but the gains or losses of God's blessed London community. Some years later, the secretary of the Royal Society again used the same bookkeeping to quantify the benefits and risks of inoculation. And in the nineteenth century, Pierre Charles Alexandre Louis balanced the rate of healed typhus patients treated with and without blood-letting in the form of a table – one column for those who survived the traditional therapy and another yet shorter column for those who survived the expectative therapy (abstaining from any special treatment). Medical quantifying was originally nothing else than bookkeeping medical facts – observations like inoculations or plague death, diseased or deceased patients. The general outcome of such 'merchant's logick'[8] in medical bookkeeping is rating values – money, the public good, medical utility – or, as in the following case, the properties of chemical substances as both therapeutic agent and pharmaceutical product. More specifically, our case study shows how late twentieth-century accounting of drugs originated in and strongly reinforced the blending of values typical of medical science on the one hand, and of the market economy on the other hand.

On the basis of this (enlarged) definition, the chapter's argument discusses two forms of accounting involved in the research and marketing of Ciba-Geigy's antidepressants. The first part focuses on the clinical accounting associated with the organisation and evaluation of clinical research, specifically on a series of technologies that balanced clinical features with the effects of drugs in order to document efficacy and build a hierarchy of putative uses and prescription motives. The second part focuses on the market-based accounting that originated in the development of scientific marketing and that involved a more direct incorporation of data on sales, prescriptions, and market-shares in order to document the commercialisation potential of new products and build a hierarchy of targets and promotional investments.

Geigy had begun developing psychopharmaceuticals in the early 1950s. The case study on Roland Kuhn illustrates how wild clinical trials yielded the first antidepressants.[9] Testing new compounds remained on the agenda when Ciba and Geigy merged in 1970. But assessing new drugs had now become hard paperwork. Clinicians were no longer given blank boxes or white sachets but instead batches of paper detailing the protocol of study. What was exhaustively described there was nothing less than what to investigate and how to do it: duration of treatment, Galenic form, administrative procedures, target population, inclusion and exclusion criteria, guidelines for information and patient consent, prescribed laboratory tests, examination schedules including checklists and protocols for physical observation, definitions of the tested variables (specifying target, add-ons, safety and efficacy criteria), and, last but not least, rules governing every eventuality, from patients dropping out to adverse or fatal events. There was no room for variation or personal contribution, not to mention any ideas for improving the examination. From the 1970s, multi-centre studies no longer provided space for the unforeseen. Clinical trials no longer accepted creative input or ad hoc improvisations. Consequently, testing drugs was less experimental than performative: a good trial performed what had been taken into account in advance. This allowed the domain of both clinical experimentation and industrial research to be combined.

The question we therefore wish to tackle is: why and how was clinical tinkering as a norm of clinical research replaced by accounting? We argue that the answer lies in the changing organisation, purposes, and uses of clinical trials that accompanied their relocation within the industry-based screening machinery. Between 1950 and 1990, clinical research became industrial in the sense that most of the work involved in designing and performing clinical research was done under the leadership and close supervision of the industry, using a linear pipeline model and relying on an increasingly intricate relationship between patient-based investigations, marketing, and prescription. The idea we'd like to put forward is that this change was both rooted in and favoured by specific forms of counting and accounting as well as shared practices of 'aggregation and balancing' that spread within hospital wards, company marketing and finance divisions, and even regulatory agencies.

Clinical research

To understand this transformation, we have to take a closer look at this new way of assessing drug treatment. This section will follow clinical activities to the bedside where clinicians were obsessed, first of all, with paperwork. Unlike Kuhn's wild experimentation, testing in the 1980s meant struggling through a bunch of pre-printed forms.

The so-called Case Report Form (CRF) vividly illustrates the rising paperwork. Introduced in the late 1970s, the CRF had quickly become the heart of any clinical trial. By the 1980s, the CRF was already more than a dozen pages long, and today it can easily swell to doorstop size, comprising all documents needed to inform the patients, to register the test persons, to record the clinical observation, to copy the laboratory readings, to report the adverse drug effects, etc. In the Levoprotiline study, the CRF comprised twenty-three pages, fifteen of them covered by the checkboxes of psychological tests to be conducted for each patient.

The reports themselves were much shorter. Only three pages were devoted to clinicians documenting bedside observations – and only one of them applied to cases of unforeseen events. Starting on page one, the psychiatrist described the patient's disease course at four different observation moments (see Figure 9.1) – at the beginning of the trial and at the end of four consecutive weeks. Observations were recorded in checkboxes, numbers rated the observed symptoms: '1' meant 'no longer present'; '5' stood for 'very severe manifestations'. The 'Depression's severity' was also specified by seven items rated from 1 to 5. On the next page, the clinical investigator evaluated the overall effects ('Globalurteil') using the same grades. The last page was designed for reporting possible adverse drug effects with respect to severity and causality. Schemes for weekly test results, ECG findings, and co-medication rounded out the CRF, as well as a form for diagnostic coding that served to translate nosological categories into a so-called 'syndrome diagnosis'. Recoding meant dedifferentiation. In-house diagnostic entities as well as psychopathologically motivated categories like 'depressive distress', 'mourning reaction', 'endogenous or neurotic depression' were replaced

UNTERSUCHUNGS-ZEITPUNKTE	VOR BEH. BEGINN	nach 1 WOCHE	nach 2 WOCHEN	nach 3 WOCHEN	nach 4 WOCHEN
SCHWEREGRAD DER DEPRESSION	$\mid\frac{4}{8}\mid$	$\mid\frac{3}{9}\mid$	$\mid\frac{3}{10}\mid$	$\mid\frac{2}{11}\mid$	$\mid\underline{}_{12}\mid$
ZIELSYMPTOME					
DEPRESSIVE GRUNDSTIMMUNG	$\mid\frac{4}{13}\mid$	$\mid\frac{3}{14}\mid$	$\mid\frac{3}{15}\mid$	$\mid\frac{2}{16}\mid$	$\mid\underline{}_{17}\mid$
A N G S T	$\mid\frac{4}{18}\mid$	$\mid\frac{4}{19}\mid$	$\mid\frac{4}{20}\mid$	$\mid\frac{4}{21}\mid$	$\mid\underline{}_{22}\mid$
AGITIERTHEIT	$\mid\frac{4}{23}\mid$	$\mid\frac{3}{24}\mid$	$\mid\frac{3}{25}\mid$	$\mid\frac{4}{26}\mid$	$\mid\underline{}_{27}\mid$
H E M M U N G	$\mid\frac{1}{28}\mid$	$\mid\frac{1}{29}\mid$	$\mid\frac{1}{30}\mid$	$\mid\frac{1}{31}\mid$	$\mid\underline{}_{32}\mid$
A P A T H I E	$\mid\frac{1}{33}\mid$	$\mid\frac{1}{34}\mid$	$\mid\frac{1}{35}\mid$	$\mid\frac{1}{36}\mid$	$\mid\underline{}_{37}\mid$
SCHLAFSTÖRUNGEN	$\mid\frac{4}{38}\mid$	$\mid\frac{4}{39}\mid$	$\mid\frac{3}{40}\mid$	$\mid\frac{3}{41}\mid$	$\mid\underline{}_{42}\mid$

9.1 The CRF of the Levoprotiline study: Depressive mood, anxiety, agitation, inhibition, apathy, insomnia, and physical complaints

by the concept of a uniform depression with several degrees of severity. For instance, the given diagnosis 'endogenous depression with obviously hypochondriac manner' was translated into a two-tier number coded by the *Diagnostic and Statistical Manual*.[10] In the Levoprotiline case, the same CRF was used for the twenty clinical trials listed in the final report of the drug examination process carried out in more than sixty trial centres in four countries (NL, CSSR, FRG, GDR) with different methods – from double-blinded and case-controlled trials to unblended, open mono-centred studies.[11]

The form was used not simply for examining the efficacy, tolerance, safety, and side effects in comparison with competing antidepressants, but also for so-called 'special studies'. These mono-centred studies were reminiscent of Kuhn's early trials because the open protocols were not closely related to selected indications. Levoprotiline, for instance, was used to test the effect in patients with anxiety states, panic-syndromes, severe neurosis or social behaviour disorders, and eating disorders of juvenile girls. In other words, adjacent clinical fields were explored in the hope of eliciting further indications beyond those targeted by the actual drug approval process.

The study protocol transformed words into numbers. Quantifying analyses replaced qualitative observations when drug effects were disaggregated into countable units. How this worked is illustrated by the scale that Max Hamilton had introduced in the early 1960s to objectify drug treatment.[12]

The Hamilton Rating Scale for Depression (HRSD) reduced observations to checklists or blanks to be filled in. This made observations 'countable'. Furthermore, the operation at the bedside processed the information in accordance with the designs of the company's R&D department. In effect, the CRF enabled research activities to be divided between the observations on the ward and the interpretations in the company, between the performing actors and those who were designing and interpreting the protocol, between those jotting down numbers and those accounting for their values. Finally, the CRF eliminated the unpredictable. There was no fill-in-slot for the unforeseen – beyond the categories of 'adverse drug reaction' and 'drop-out', no space was available to account for any differences between the observed and the expected.

In effect, the CRF made visible what was wanted. The seven items used for qualifying patient' depression are the best example of this. The list seems innocuous enough. Several meetings were conducted in Basel and Frankfurt and after long discussions, the management in Basel agreed, at least for the selection portrayed (see Figure 9.1), that: 'All studies pursued the same strategy in order to avoid the erroneous assumption of equality in efficacy (beta-risk) as follows': initially, the efficacy is assessed by a kind of '"Ur-Meter" for testing antidepressants'.[13] However, the 'Ur-Meter' was not good enough. The company claimed 'some weakness of method'. For this reason, the R&D department combined the HRSD with an aggregate based on seven items called 'target symptoms' (see Figure 9.1).[14] Although taken from the HRSD, the new assortment didn't cover the original spectrum. Instead, the ratio was designed to reveal the differences between the new compound and other competing drugs. This was a crucial step: picking up a few items and rearranging them changed the psychopathological order of the rating scale to a new, user-defined one. Doing this, the accounts could now be freely combined.[15] Careful selection allowed for shifting the balance of outcomes, increasing small effects, and focusing on particular symptoms – even if the summed scores were equal. Like bookkeeping, the listing juxtaposed debits (less well) and credits (better) in order to calculate the drug's credit for treatment and market potential. Although the CRF also counted the number of cured, improved, or uncured patients, it mainly targeted the relevant effects – as credits in the balance against other competing antidepressants.

This technique had been used in earlier drug trials. When the direct comparison of the antidepressants' ratings showed no recognisable differences, reducing the HRSD to only few single symptoms allowed researchers to scale up effects, which could barely be seen otherwise. In trials of the antidepressant Ludiomil in the 1970s, a member of Ciba's R&D department frankly explained: the clinical data 'have no relevance for medical practice if you don't know how to interpret and communicate them correctly'. He demonstrated convincingly at a conference how 'target symptoms' could be isolated from the HRSD, re-combined, matched anew, and 'correctly explained' in the company's favour.[16] Slight adjustments in the list revealed that competing antidepressants worked not only 'less well' in some respects, but clearly 'worse'.

This way of listing takes two rationalities into account (see Figure 9.2). Translating the counting into qualitative value judgements ('better') merged the clinical outcome registered by the HRSD with the marketing value depicted in the last two lines. Slight qualitative differences were retranslated into discrete numbers.

Defining 'target symptoms' was crucial. In the case of the Levoprotiline study, the CRF was reworked several times according to 'the

Target-Symptom	Imipramine	Amitriptyline	Ludiomil
Insomnia early	less well	better	less well
Inhibition	less well	less well	better
Agitation	better	less well	better
Compulsive symptoms	better	less well	better
Work difficulties & apathy	less well	better	better
better	2	3	5
worse	4	3	1

9.2 Target symptoms shape the efficacy of the CG antidepressant Ludiomil® (Maprotiline). Five items on the Hamilton-Scale affected significantly by the three drugs in different ways.

requests by CGB [Ciba-Geigy Basel] for modifications to the studies'.[17] Considering the final target symptoms, it seems remarkable that just three of them had been classified as core symptoms of any depressive disorder since the diagnosis was invented by Emil Kraepelin in the late nineteenth century.[18] The other 'target symptoms' counted as main symptoms of other psychoses (anxiety; agitation) or were more or less unspecific (insomnia). They were regarded as being far less typical for the clinical entity of depression than the former three. Other HRSD items would have been more specific, for instance 'loss of joy' or 'loss of empathy'. As a result, a patient with agitated anxiety status and sleeplessness was attributed the same pathological weight as a patient with the classical triad of depressive mood, apathy, and inhibition.

To cut a long story short, despite the high degree of conformity, considerable resources were required in order to homogenise the data. When the CRFs were returned to the R&D department, they were checked for two criteria: completeness and plausibility. Local investigators were sometimes asked to submit missing measurements or to check laboratory readings. Computing was also labour intensive.[19] All data were recorded, checked, and calculated using electronic data processing. Some information was only analysed to answer questions unique to a respective trial. Most of the data, however, were assessed in order to open up new possibilities and by using the same technique used to account for the target symptoms. Thanks to the standardised CRF, single parameters could be isolated, rearranged, grouped, and correlated independently of the original trial. This made it possible, for instance, to gather elderly patients from eight clinical trials and to rearrange them to a new group of older test subjects in order to shape the new indication of 'late-life depression'. Recombining and assembling the data enabled researchers to compose and evaluate subsets. Evaluation criteria could be developed and pursued in ways that had been unforeseen at the beginning of data processing.

As a consequence, the evaluation and analysis of bedside observation became more flexible and data collection was further standardised. On the one hand, only what was reported, proved, and properly documented in the specified form could be acknowledged, counted, and accredited. On the other hand, the documented data could be calculated in manifold relations: efficacy was balanced (and rebalanced) by target symptoms, target symptoms grouped and regrouped by indications, and indications shaped and reshaped with respect to competing products. Side-effects were also distributed and reallocated to various categories in order to prove the new drug's advantages over other substances. Patients and the related populations were grouped and regrouped in order to identify specific gains in relation to both the therapeutic indications and the market rates. Increasingly, counting became a way of accounting. The new methodology of the clinical trials (the package of materials and related techniques) established new ways of assessing therapeutic effects, and simultaneously transformed the old benefit–risk ratio into a fine-grained analysis of 'more or less desirable' items; i.e. advantages and disadvantages in comparison with competing drugs were modulated in various respects according to symptoms, diseases, patient groups, indications, etc. Counting the results of the tested drug also accounted its market value. Clinical accounting amalgamated treatment with marketing. In the Levoprotiline case, however, Ciba-Geigy manipulated the data too much. The company was indeed able to shape the superiority of the new compound with respect to a few target symptoms (see above). But German authorities refused approval on account of the entire HRSD scores.[20] The company waived its right to appeal the decision and closed the pipeline. Other derivatives of tri- and quadrocyclic antidepressants also failed to receive approval. Among the drugs of this generation only Paroxetine – a new type of antidepressant based on selective serotonine reuptake inhibition – reached the market. But that is another story.[21]

Marketing

In the late 1960s, Geigy started to purchase information generated outside the firm by specialised agencies. In spite of the cost, which was deemed very high, management had decided to subscribe to the monthly information on pharmaceutical sales that Intercontinental Marketing Services (IMS), a US-based private consulting agency, had begun to produce and sell. Counting the monthly sales rates was closely related to evaluating and reorganising the R&D of new compounds.[22] Market-based accounting involved three levels:

1. Comparing the sales of Geigy's products with their main competitors.

Clinical trials and medico-economic accounting 239

2. Assessing the size of the 'global' psychotropic drugs domain as one single class that included tranquilisers, neuroleptics, and antidepressants.
3. Exploring physicians' motives for prescription, especially the connections they made between products, symptoms, and indications.

The market-based accounting reinforced the basis for strategic planning and shifted the management of products in the direction of therapeutic classes as overarching units of research, development, and marketing. Specific figures aggregating market data and comparing them with various kinds of resources and investments were therefore tabulated in order to objectify the situation of the firm and ease the discussion of strategic choices. Debates on research input, where the research stood, and where it needed to be strengthened or rolled-back illustrate this point. In 1966, the division for neuro- and psycho-pharmaceuticals, established within the marketing department, prepared an overarching assessment of the sector.[23] The paper included two types of aggregated data. First, classical sheets summarised production and sales for Ciba-Geigy products with comments about recent changes. Second, accounting graphs allowed investments in research and development to be compared with the structure of the world market – both of which were specified in relation to diagnostically classified psychotropic drugs. This reference enabled Ciba-Geigy to plan further research efforts and investments. The report showed, for instance, the strength of Ciba-Geigy in antidepressants, its weakness in tranquilisers and – more importantly in the eyes of the authors – 'new fields'. Even if this way of focusing on research investment was new, the accounting was based on very traditional bookkeeping methods that weighed 'costs' (in-house investments) against 'benefits' (existing sales on the global market).

Such discussions led to an internal reassessment of priorities and in particular of the relationship between tranquilisers and antidepressants. By the late 1960s, management had already endorsed the idea that to surpass the success of its own Tofranil and ensure future growth of income and profits, the objective was to lessen the divide between the tranquiliser and antidepressant niches. Given the strength of Roche's products and the very recent failure of direct competition with profiled tranquilisers,[24] such blurring would best be achieved by inventing an antidepressant that targeted the mild mental complaints encountered in general practice.[25]

The second consequence of the 1960s reorganisation was an enhanced and more formal circulation of information between the clinical research and marketing departments. Coordination started to operate at two levels: that of daily promotion and advertising campaigns involving the selection of clinical data and its shaping and transformation into promotional material; and that of long-term planning, selection of market segments, and specific requests for new trials and/or product development.

Specialised committees and tools were established to ensure more coordinated decision-making. At the top level, marketing people were – for instance – invited to the research meetings, like the annual general conference of scientists from Geigy Basel and from its subsidy in the United States. The 1973 conference thus estimated that, in the central nervous area, antidepressants remained a high priority both in the United States and in Europe while tranquilisers, despite their massive importance in global sales, should rank second.[26]

At weekly meetings of a 'working group for medical-pharmaceutical information' (*Arbeitsgruppe pharmazeutisch-medizinische Information*), the heads of both the clinical and marketing departments in Basel discussed products currently on the market, as well as those already in the pipeline. Their memos, which circulated throughout all upper levels of management, summarised major decisions about the surveillance of sales, the production of publicity material, the organisation of campaigns, and the outcome of prioritised trials.

Medical marketing information was actually given so much priority that an entire 'product management information' section was set up. It coordinated the follow-up of trials and the preparation of product-oriented material for medical representatives. It was responsible for writing regular – almost weekly – information sheets for the sales force managers, who would in turn use the material in meetings with their representatives.

The impact of this combination of technologies can be best appreciated using the example of Ludiomil, a new antidepressant that the Ciba-Geigy company introduced in the early 1970s. Ludiomil actually originated in Ciba research. Its preclinical trajectory was comparable to that of Tofranil since it had also been synthesised as an analogue of chlorpromazine. Its transformation into an antidepressant was a product of the merger between Ciba and Geigy.

Market-based accounting was powerfully documented in the material elaborated for this first launch. It occurred at several levels.

1. With attempts to position Ludiomil in relation to Geigy's other antidepressants in order to avoid 'cannibalism', i.e. Ludiomil use resulting in decreased sales of Tofranil and Anafranil; Ludiomil's major clinical assets were in this respect its reduced side-effects and its ability to overlap with the symptoms associated with the use of tranquilisers, i.e. anxiety.
2. With formal comparisons between Ludiomil and its immediate competitors, especially amitriptyline; in addition to these arguments, results emphasising the rapid response and (relative) efficacy in the treatment of all forms of depression were thus mobilised so that Ludiomil could be labelled a quick 'generic' antidepressant.

How were trials and the results of clinical accounting used and reframed in this context of joint work by the clinical research and marketing departments? Two examples will help distinguish between two levels. The first level was the assessment of individual trials. Let's consider the launch of Ludiomil in Switzerland. A marketing information memo circulated in April 1973 included a detailed description of one of the two Swiss clinical trials completed in 1972. The memo was aimed at training representatives and was not designed for external use.[27] The trial compared Ludiomil with Pfizer's Doxepin (Sinequan®). It already included 1,400 patients and involved psychiatrists as well as general practitioners. The summing up table produced a qualitative evaluation through the graphic elimination of 'non-significant differences' and the inclusion of short comments on the respective value of Ludiomil and Doxepin or of the various dosages of Ludiomil. Without sacrificing the complexity of the trial, the table thus provided support for the claim that Ludiomil was better than Doxepin, especially in general practice and when higher dosages were chosen.

The second level of accounting involved comparing trials. In 1972, Geigy organised a major gathering of depression specialists in St Moritz, including its entire network of collaborating psychiatrists, to discuss the status of 'depressive states'. Right after the meeting, an internal memo summarised the discussions with a clear divide between 'the clinical results and their 'value in promotional perspective'. The outcome was a series of quasi-slogans for representatives like: 'Early onset of action, also in severe depression, because of its good tolerance, Ludiomil can also be prescribed at full dosage from the onset of treatment.'

The last stage in the mobilisation and rewriting of research results involved the production of material to be handed to practising physicians. This too involved accounting work grounded in paper technologies. Among the vast palette of tools invented to deliver company-based facts to doctors, leaflets and booklets became increasingly important during this period. For the launch of Ludiomil, one particular series, including six leaflets, adhered to the internal assessments of the 1972 St Moritz symposium. The series reproduced some of the results and focused on visual demonstration, with each leaflet being centred around one graph or one table with few comments. These originated in previously discussed material. Data were isolated and sorted according to the firm's understanding of prescription patterns. For instance, one leaflet was organised around a table taken from the St Moritz volume. That table displayed the effect of Ludiomil on sleeplessness in order to argue that Ludiomil – in contrast to Anafranil – was able to restore sleep throughout the entire night, was comparatively more efficient, and was therefore worth specific promotional investments to enhance prescriptions.

In July 1975, while a new Ludiomil campaign was being prepared in Germany, the information material designed by Ciba-Geigy for its representatives included the following statements:[28]

> Previous key-point in the praxis: indication 'psycho-vegetative disorders'.
> New key-point in the praxis: indication 'masked depression'.
> Rationale: The indication 'masked depression' is a more adequate description of Ludiomil as a general-practice-oriented antidepressant instead of the tranquiliser label 'psycho-vegetative disorders'.
> Argument: When promoting Ludiomil in physicians' practice, we repeatedly stumble across the competition of tranquilisers. [...] The results transmitted by our cartel partner in Germany suggest that the choice made during the first phase of marketing, which was to profile Ludiomil as a small-dosage psychochemical principally for

the indication of 'psycho-vegetative disorders', has presently permitted entry into the market, but one cannot speak of a breakthrough in any sense of the term. To equate Ludiomil with tranquilisers, [...] be it at the profile level or at the indication level, is not the right way. The practitioner must be convinced through our explanatory campaigns that an antidepressant (like Ludiomil) is not an alternative to a tranquiliser and that, in parallel, tranquilisers are not an alternative for the treatment of depressed patients, including patients with masked depression.

The category of masked depression was not entirely new. It had surfaced in the psychiatric literature in relation to atypical cases, such as depressed states in which the typical triad of depression was difficult to identify owing to the emphasis on somatic symptoms that typified such patients' complaints. What led these patients to be targeted by psychiatry was a threefold situation: that their symptoms resisted the inquiries of physicians, that they did not disappear after treatment, and that they could vary considerably during the course of the pathology. Psychiatrists referred to them as 'depression without depression' as opposed to hypochondria or neurovegetative asthenia, since a careful and sustained anamnesis would bring to the surface the signs of a history of altered mood and thus provide grounds for an association with endogenous depression.[29]

The new profiling of Ludiomil as an antidepressant with anxiolytic properties specially designed for the treatment of mild or masked depression in general practice started as a second launch phase in 1973. The strategy was advanced through a second symposium in St Moritz, the entire purpose of which was to discuss masked depression. Once again organised by Ciba-Geigy's clinical-research department, the event juxtaposed contrasting understandings and definitions of masked depression. Participants discussed at great length the definition, boundaries, and putative aetiology of masked depression, as well as its role in what were taken to be simple facts, such as the rising incidence of depressive disorders in general practice and their connection to life in modern industrial societies. In spite of their heterogeneous views on aetiology, nosology, and treatment, all the participants endorsed the term and agreed that the problem had great importance in routine practice.

This type of market-based accounting did not translate 'clinical facts' into 'statements of promotional value', but tried to reveal a new target population, a new need for antidepressants rooted in the existence of a previously invisible (or non-existent) category of depressive patients. The main data for such accounting were therefore not the clinical trials, but rather the market-research surveys conducted by the firm, its inquiries into physicians' activities, their diagnosis and prescription practices.

The representative of Ciba-Geigy thus presented the results of an inquiry the firm had conducted with the psychiatrist Walter Pöldinger documenting psychiatrists' views on 'masked or larved depression'. A majority of the 1,162 specialists surveyed in Switzerland, Germany, and Austria explained that the value of the concept was, above all, educational. As Austrian psychiatrist Walter Walcher powerfully stated:

> [Masked] depression has already entered general practice. Its value resides in the fact that today, more often than in the past, many depressive patients are diagnosed earlier and benefit from a targeted treatment. It thus helps physicians, and of course patients as well, as they have very often been treated at a somatic level with no result, simply because nobody thought of masked depression.[30]

One consequence of this understanding was the agreement that general practitioners needed help in making 'correct' diagnoses. When addressing the issue of how this understanding would be conveyed in the training of general practitioners, the attendees at the St Moritz conference forgot everything about the putative specificity of depression with somatic manifestations. The idea of the mask was to be taken literally rather than metaphorically: a 'real' depression was hidden behind the somatic symptoms, and it had to be unravelled. Ludwig S. Geisler, the one single internist in the audience, thus insisted on the need for a catalogue of questions for the non-specialist: 'He should begin for instance with questions about sleeplessness, and end with questions about the impossibility of enjoying life.'[31]

In 1974, the third St Moritz meeting gathered nearly the same group of specialists to discuss depression in general practice, addressing both diagnosis and therapeutic responses on the basis of a new survey the firm had conducted in Austria, France, Germany, and Switzerland. This time, W. Pöldinger's presentation strongly emphasised that 5 to 10 per cent of general-practice patients were allegedly affected with 'larved depression'.[32]

The St Moritz meetings provided important background for the firm's attempts to strategically position Ludiomil and shape its prescription. The process affected accounting practices both at the level of marketing and clinical research. The impact of marketing-based accounting was more direct and significant. The entire promotion of Ludiomil was swiftly refashioned after the perspective of 'masked depression'. A March 1975 'product information for marketing' Ludiomil, aimed at pharmaceutical representatives, explicitly described the new strategy of promoting the category at the same time as the drug itself:

> Keyword: 'Masked Depression'
> In Switzerland and Germany, according to our evaluation, a third to two-thirds of the cases of this diagnosis should in fact be characterised as 'larved depression,' which is generally handled through psychochemicals (predominantly tranquilizers).
> The time is ripe to replace this pseudotherapy of depressive states with targeted action. Since it is much easier to link the new perspectives offered by larved depression with a new, rather than with an old product, we shall target the treatment of this indication with Ludiomil. [...]
> Marketing concept. Ultimately, it is a matter of convincing the physician that the prescription of tranquilizers for depressive disorders is actually a medical failure. Beyond that, we need to offer him help in diagnosis, which could take the form of three questions he should ask his patient, and if the responses are positive, this should bring up the possibility that a case of masked depression may be at hand.[33]

Using in-house and psychiatrists' surveys of the frequency of symptoms encountered in general practice, marketing thus quantified the great potential of Ludiomil, estimating the frequency of patients affected with masked depression being subjected to 'inadequate' treatment, i.e tranquilisers, MAO-antidepressants, or classical tricyclic antidepressants. The figure summarising this computation was very impressive: Ludiomil could seize a very significant share of the psychotropic market.

On the research side, new trials were launched that integrated either masked depression or depression with 'somatic/vegetative manifestations' as a main category for the inclusion and comparison of Ludiomil with the efficacy of tranquilisers in general practice.[34] By the late 1970s, however, only three trials specifically targeting masked depression had been conducted, all of them in Germany.[35] Rather than providing valuable results on the selective advantages of Ludiomil, the main effect of this direct feedback from marketing evaluation into research was to enlarge the palette of target symptoms in antidepressant trials to include somatic or vegetative pains or disorders, as the case of Levoprotiline would show.

The trajectory of Ludiomil and the rise of scientific marketing at Ciba-Geigy thus reveal several layers of accounting that relied on assessment of the market for psychotropic drugs. The first layer was a derivative of classical bookkeeping since it compared Ciba-Geigy's input in the form of research investments with output in the form of existing global sales. The second layer was a derivative of clinical accounting. It translated the quantitative results of clinical research into worthy promotional investments. This translation assumed that the balancing of symptoms and effects would trigger more prescriptions by physicians, albeit providing no estimate of increased sales. The third layer linked the redefinition of depression with surveys of prescription patterns. It blended clinical and market data in order to calculate the sales potential of this new indication and in turn justify investments in the collective construction of masked depression. What comes to the fore is therefore the critical function market-based accounting played in the firm's strategic planning, namely in its attempts to rationalise research and marketing investments through a series of balancing acts that weighed the properties of in-house drugs against estimated shares of psychotropic drug sales.

Two ways of accounting?

In our two chapter sections, we have seen different forms of accounting. The first part describes accounting as a technique in assessing therapeutic effects, which transformed the old ratio of benefit–risk into a fine-grained analysis of target–symptoms. Marketing concerns drove the balancing of 'wanted' and 'non-wanted' symptoms. The counted symptoms were evaluated in relation to the multiple effects of tested antidepressants. The 'wanted' was defined with respect to user groups, indications, profiles of competing drugs, market segments, and marketing strategies. Evaluating the efficacy in clinical trials using checklists, rating scales, and other quantifying instruments became an ingredient in the company's accounting techniques for balancing effort and success, expenses and incomes. Clinical accounting can therefore not be isolated from the form of accounting described in the second section. Clinically based accounting actually provides the basis for market-based accounting.

As the second part has shown, market-based accounting cannot be reduced to mere balancing of revenues and costs. Even if the question of maximising the former remains at its core, the related techniques seem rather to mobilise clinical accounting results and to make them economically usable. Translating clinical accounting into an account of future prescriptions and sales became crucial for making decisions about both research investments and marketing plans. Market-based accounting thus balances drugs, symptoms, diseases, and populations from the perspective of market shares. This was the backbone of the form of strategic planning that large pharmaceutical firms like Ciba-Geigy developed to manage mounting investments in R&D and marketing. Screening thus turned into much more than the coupling of chemistry and pharmacological testing, becoming an integrated pipeline of actions (and decisions) from chemical synthesis to promotion.

Needless to say, these two forms of accounting were related by drug legislation. State authorities like the FDA used accounting techniques as a control technology. They balanced not the target symptoms, but the side and adverse effects, assessing the molecule as well as its competing products. Some applications failed this balancing act. In the end, Levoprotiline was not approved because the clinical trials showed that it was no safer than other antidepressants. Accounting was not only made to comply with the company's accountability to the law, but also to satisfy the state's responsibilities for public health. These responsibilities did not leave the industrial forms of accounting untouched.

Should we therefore consider more ways of accounting? Before we enlarge our perspective beyond clinical and market-based accounting to the holy trinity of state, medicine, and industry, we should take a second look. It may be analytically convenient to oppose clinical counting and market-based accounting. But it is obvious that these two methods, despite relying on different actors, techniques, and aims, did not develop in isolation. They were rather closely related and played a critical role in companies' responses to the pressure that state authorities exerted to increase the accountability of an industry whose products were supposed to contribute to better health. One may therefore wonder if it is meaningful to distinguish two different ways of accounting for symptoms, effects, populations, and revenues – to consider just the dominant parameters taken into account when conducting, evaluating, and using clinical trials, which in their vast majority were organised and paid for by industry.

We wish to propose in this concluding section that multiplying the ways of accounting makes little sense. Three elements should be taken into account when arguing this case. The first is the blending of activities documented in both parts within this chapter. Blending was not only a matter of transferring statements and accounts between medicine and marketing. It was rooted in a convergence of activities associated with similar (and sometimes identical) techniques of aggregation, reduction, and prioritisation. The second element is that the loops between research and marketing discussed in the second part are not simply feedback mechanisms that provided for an input of clinical facts in marketing or an input of sales and prescription results in research. Instead, these loops relied on a form of integration, i.e. on a multi-faceted and very concrete circulation of materials, techniques, and people between both poles. Third, even if research and marketing may be thought of as two different social worlds with their own actors (physicians versus managers), sites (hospitals versus plants and offices), and values (knowledge versus growth), the world of large and standardised clinical trials emerged out of new organisational boundary structures mostly within the industry, as well outside its walls if one considers the fate of drug applications or the activities of 'key opinion leaders'.

Our proposal is therefore that – in order to analyse this configuration and the specificity of the situation created by the profound reorganisation of pharmacy and medicine which took place during the postwar therapeutic revolution – one needs a broader definition of accounting that encompasses more than just administrative bookkeeping or a mere balancing of monetised costs and benefits. Accounting should be viewed as rooted in counting and aggregation technologies, but also as something neither as broad nor as reducible to these techniques. Accounting is a way of comparing and balancing values as inputs and outputs in order to produce hierarchies that guide, rule, and justify future action. In the context of drug research and development, it plays a decisive role in bringing together 'the counter' and 'the bedside' and managing what are massively private, for profit, investments in research and marketing. The invisible bookkeeper has thus – in most instances – been located within the industry, even if the impact of his/her activities was deeply felt at the sites of clinical encounters, well beyond the boundaries of company headquarters. Things could have been different. For instance, one may reflect upon cancer research, where most clinical trials remained in the world of hospitals and academia, or upon the attempts by the British NHS to develop public health-based accounting. But it remains a matter of fact that the rise of clinical trials was massively predicated on their internalisation by drug companies, on their blending with scientific marketing, and on the absence of alternative producers of drug-related clinical knowledge.

This does not imply that state authorities and administrative regulation played no role in these developments. The contrast between the trajectories of Ludiomil and Levoprotiline readily show the opposite, since the first one passed the regulatory test without difficulties while Ciba-Geigy never convinced German regulators that the second one was efficient enough to be approved. At stake were – of course – the properties of the molecules, but also the changes in legal requirements for evidence, which took place between the early 1970s and the late 1980s with mounting reliance on controlled trials. As argued elsewhere, the ways of regulating drugs in the late twentieth century are many and involve the medical professions and industries, as evidenced here, as well as state bodies and consumers.[36] However, this multiplicity is not without a hierarchy that depends on the drug class, related therapeutic fields, and the scale of diffusion. In this respect, one decisive feature of the 'psychopharmaceutical revolution' is the critical role company-based clinical research came to play in the assessment of utility and efficacy for all actors participating in the regulatory arena.

We therefore see no strong reason why one should consider the various kinds of accounting discussed above as entities belonging to different *regimes* of action. The blending of clinical research and marketing has been a development with major consequences, some of which, like the difficulties in feeding back clinical experience within the screening pipeline, are still with us. We therefore propose to label the one single regime we have identified a *medico-economic mode of accounting*.

Notes

1 The literature about the so-called pharmaceutical revolution is enormous. For a recent overview, see J.A. Greene, F. Condrau, and E. Siegel Watkins (eds), *Therapeutic Revolutions: Pharmaceuticals and Social Change in the Twentieth Century* (Chicago: The University of Chicago Press, 2016). For drug regulation, see A. Daemmrich, *Pharmacopolitics: Drug Regulation in the United States and Germany* (Chapel Hill: The University of North Carolina Press, 2004), pp. IX–XIII, 1–203; D.P. Carpenter, *Reputation and Power: Organizational Image and Pharmaceutical Regulation at the FDA* (Princeton: Princeton University Press, 2010), p. 802; J.-P. Gaudillière and V. Hess (eds), *Ways of Regulating Drugs in the 19th and 20th Centuries, Science, Technology and Medicine in Modern History* (London: Palgrave, 2012).

2 M.L. Meldrum, '"Departures from the Design": The Randomized Clinical Trial in Historical Context, 1946–1970' (PhD Thesis, State University of New York at Stony Brook, 1994). For the prehistory of modern drug trials, see H.M. Marks, *The Progress of Experiment. Science and Therapeutic Reform in the United States, 1900–1990* (Cambridge: Cambridge University Press, 1990); B. Toth, 'Clinical Trials in British Medicine 1858–1948, With Special Reference to the Development of the Randomised Controlled Trial' (PhD Thesis, University of Bristol, 1998); J.A. Greene, *Prescribing by Numbers. Drugs and the Definition of Disease* (Baltimore: John Hopkins University Press, 2007); D. Tobell, *Pills, Power and Policy: The Struggle for Drug Reform in Cold War America and its Consequences* (Berkeley: University of California Press, 2011).

3 D. Healy, *The Antidepressant Era* (Cambridge, MA: Harvard University Press, 1997); L. Gerber and J.-P. Gaudillière, 'Marketing masked depression: Physicians, pharmaceutical firms, and the redefinition of mood disorders in the 1960s and 1970s', *Bulletin of the History of Medicine* 90 (2016), 455–90.

4 A.D. Chandler, *The Visible Hand: The Managerial Revolution in American Business* (Cambridge, MA: Belknap Press, 1977); W. Fong Chua, 'Experts, networks and inscriptions in the fabrication of accounting images: A story of the representation of three public hospitals', *Accounting, Organizations and Society* 20 (1995), 111–45.

5 A.G. Hopwood, 'The archaeology of accounting systems', *Accounting, Organizations and Society* 12 (1987), 207–34.

6 For the technique of listing in general, see J. Goody, 'What's in a list', in J. Goody, *The Domestication of the Savage Mind* (Cambridge: Cambridge University Press, 1977), 74–111.
7 See A. Rusnock, *Vital Accounts. Quantifying Health and Population in Eighteenth-century England and France* (Cambridge: Cambridge University Press, 2002). Further examples can be found in G. Jorland, A. Opinel, and G. Weisz (eds), *Body Counts: Medical Quantification in Historical & Sociological Perspectives* (Montréal: McGill-Queen's University Press, 2005).
8 A. Rusnock, '"The merchant's logick". Numerical debates over smallpox inoculation in eighteenth century England', in E. Magnello and A. Hardy (eds), *The Road to Medical Statistics* (Amsterdam: Rodopi, 2002), pp. 37–54.
9 M. Meier, M. König, and M. Tornay, *Testfall Münsterlingen. Klinische Versuche in der Psychiatrie, 1940–1980* (Zürich: Chronos, 2019), pp. 68–82.
10 Historisches Psychiatriearchiv der Charité Berlin, Patient record file 497/90, discharge summary (proband).
11 V. Hess, L. Hottenrott, and P. Steinkamp, *Testen im Osten. DDR-Arzneimittelstudien im Auftrag westlicher Pharmaindustrie, 1964–1990* (Berlin: be.bra, 2016), pp. 77–8.
12 M. Worboys, 'The Hamilton Rating Scale for depression: The making of a "gold standard" and the unmaking of a chronic illness, 1960–1980', *Chronic Illness* 9 (2013), 202–19.
13 Ergänzung zum Expertenbericht (see below: Expertenbericht), Klinische Dokumentation vom 7. August 1987 (78_20141103 Experten-Bericht Teil 1122257), p. 9, Archive of the Institute for the History of Medicine, Charité Berlin, Arzneimittelforschung DDR (henceforth: IGM B, Arzneimittelforschung).
14 Hamilton Rating Scale for Depression, items 1, 4–6, 7 (apathy for work and activities), 8 (inhibition for psychomotor retardation), 9, 10–11, 12–13.
15 Goody, 'What's in a list'.
16 O. de S. Pinto, S. P. Afeiche, E. Bartholini, and P. Loustalot, 'Internationale Erfahrungen mit Ludiomil', in P. Kielholz (ed.), *Depressive Zustände: Erkennung, Bewertung, Behandlung* (Bern: Hans Huber, 1972), pp. 254–66.
17 Minutes of the workshop of the German company groups at 15 January 1985.
18 M. Schmidt-Degenhard, 'Versteinertes Dasein: Zur Geschichte der Melancholie', *Aus Forschung und Medizin*, 5 (1990), 45–56; G. Greenberg, *Manufacturing Depression: The Secret History of a Modern Disease* (New York: Simon & Schuster, 2010).
19 CGW calculated that twenty-five to thirty workdays of a biometric assistance were needed simply to prepare the data in accordance with the

international requirements (see Minutes of the workshop of the German companies groups at 15 January 1985).
20 Letter CG-W to CG-B on the status of the approval, 1 October 1990, Novartis Archives 45_122 0055349_Levoprotilin_GCP 12 103, A_Korrespondenz (IGM B, Arzneimittelforschung).
21 D. Healy, *Let Them Eat Prozac. The Unhealthy Relationship Between the Pharmaceutical Industry and Depression* (New York: New York University Press, 2004).
22 Novartis Archives, Basel, Geigy Collection, PP 36, Produktion Pharma, Pharmaforschung Quartalberichte, 1965–1970, Geigy Pharmaceuticals, 'Review of Psychotherapeutic Marketing for Marketing/Research', 9 October 1968.
23 Novartis Archives, Basel, Geigy Collection, PP 36, Psycho-Neuropharmaka Standortbestimmung der Ciba-Geigy Produkte 1975–76, Arbeitspapier für die Präsentation vor der EDL, 21 October 1976.
24 L. Gerber and J.-P. Gaudillière, 'Marketing masked depression', 455–90.
25 Novartis Archives, Basel, Geigy Collection, PP 36 Produktion Pharma, Pharmaforschung Quartalberichte, 1965–1970, Der Markt für Psychopharmaka, Report to the production department by A. Fuchs, 3 August 1967.
26 Novartis Archives, Basel, Ciba-Geigy Collection, PH 4.02 Division Pharmaforschung Konzern, Minutes and documents Research Conference Basel-U.S.A., 1973.
27 Novartis Archives, Basel, Ciba-Geigy Collection, PH 7.04 Division Pharma, Präparate und Information, Folder Produktinformation für das Marketing Ludiomil, Supplement zur Marketing Information, April 1973.
28 Novartis Archives, Basel, Ciba-Geigy collection, PH 7.04 Division Pharma, Präparate und Information, Folder Produktinformation für das Marketing, Ludiomil. Supplement zur Marketing Information, July 1974.
29 J. Lange, 'Die endogenen und reaktiven Gemütserkrankungen und die manisch-depressive Konstitution', in O. Bumke (ed.), *Handbuch der Geisteskrankheiten*, Vol. 4 (Berlin: Springer, 1928), pp. 1–231.
30 P. Kielholz (ed.), *Die larvierte Depression. Internationales Symposium, St. Moritz, 8.–10. Januar 1973* (Bern: Hans Huber, 1973), p. 315.
31 Kielholz (ed.), *Die larvierte Depression*, p. 291.
32 W. Pöldinger, 'Zusammenfassende Darstellung der Fragen und Ergebnisse einer Umfrage bei Allgemeinpraktiken und nichtpsychiatrischen Fachärzten in der Bundesrepublik Deutschland, in Berlin, Frankreich, Österreich und der Schweiz', in Kielholz (ed.), *Depressive Zustände*, here pp. 123–39.

33 Novartis Archives, Basel, Ciba-Geigy Collection, PH 7.04 Division Pharma, Produktinformation für das Marketing, Ludiomil, Supplement zur Marketing Information, March 1975, pp. 3–4.
34 Novartis Archives, Basel, Ciba-Geigy Collection, PH 4.02 Division Pharmaforschung Konzern, Minutes and Documents Research Conference Basel-U.S.A., 1979.
35 Ibid.
36 See the contributions in Gaudillière and Hess (eds), *Ways of Regulating*.

10

Accounting for Esther Smucker: The Mennonite church, the US National Institutes of Health, and the trade in healthy bodies, 1950–70

Laura Stark

Esther Smucker had many virtues, but a knack for accounting was not among them. She totalled columns incorrectly, deducted funds from the wrong source, and laboured over the maths.

Yet from the autumn of 1965 to 1966, she was the local accountant for the Mennonite church on the wards of the Clinical Center of the US National Institutes of Health (henceforth NIH). A retired schoolteacher and devout Mennonite, Esther had joined the church's national 'voluntary service' programme along with her long-time friend Mary Warye, also a retired teacher and committed member of their local Mennonite congregation in Liberty, Ohio. Mennonites who joined voluntary service would leave their homes for a year or several months to witness the teachings of Jesus (service, sacrifice, peace) through volunteer work in the United States and abroad in keeping with the principles of this relatively conservative Christian religious tradition.[1] Four times a year, Mennonites from across North America flocked to the national training centre for two weeks of orientation, during which they would select from one of a dozen placement options depending on where they wanted to work and what they wanted to do – farm labour or office work, for example. Esther and Mary decided they wanted to serve as 'normal control' research subjects at the NIH located in Bethesda, Maryland just outside of Washington, DC. Upon this decision, they also accepted the job of 'unit leader' for the Mennonite contingent going to the NIH Clinical Center (Figure 10.1). The job of unit leader required that they keep the local accounts. Esther took the lead.

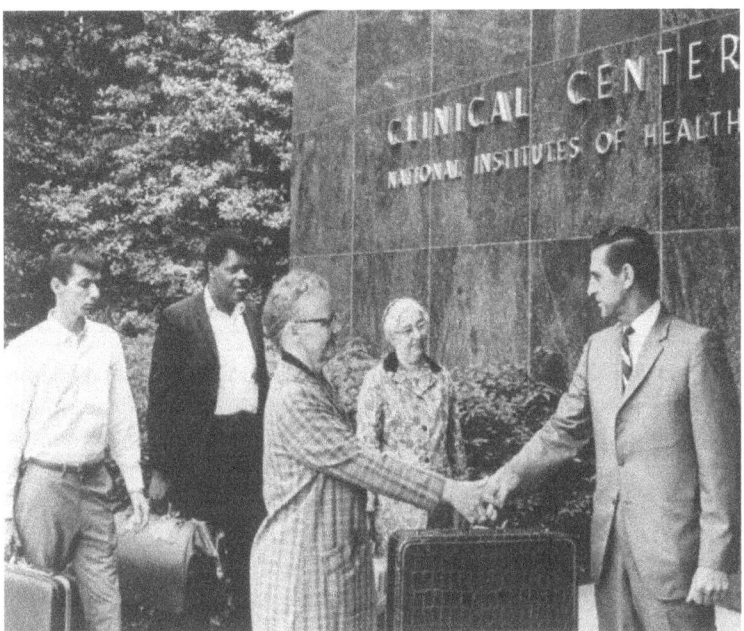

10.1 Esther Smucker and Mary Warye were admitted to the NIH Clinical Center in September 1965. Delbert Nye was director of NIH's Normal Volunteer Patient Program, which Esther and Mary joined to serve as 'normal control' research subject for the Mennonite church. They agreed to be the unit leaders for the Mennonite Voluntary Service group placed at the Clinical Center, which involved serving as the church's local accountants. This staged arrival scene, dated nine months after their actual admission, was likely photographed for publicity, though it was never ultimately used in promotional materials. The original photo caption reads: 'Esther Smucker shakes hands with Mr. Delbert Nye, director of the normal control patient program. Mary Warye watches in the background.'

If maths was not her forte, Esther nonetheless had other virtues to recommend her as the church's local accountant. She was responsible and fastidious; punctual and politically quiet at a time when many younger volunteers were active in the US Civil Rights movement that was emerging in the streets of segregated Washington and the offices of

Capitol Hill. Plus, the church had to take what it could get. Accounting was a necessity of the modern bureaucracy that the Mennonite church exemplified.[2]

This chapter follows the travels of Esther and Mary across land and through ledgers using archived and unprocessed materials from the Mennonite Central Committee and the NIH, along with published scientific articles and my publicly available 'vernacular archive' of former NIH research subjects and the scientists who studied them.[3] In doing so, this chapter documents how they were accounting and being accounted for – by NIH budget offices, clinical researchers, the Mennonite church, and themselves. First, Mennonites appeared literally in the legers of NIH. They were essential research materials whose time was being purchased in a given quantity for a given price, and I examine, how accounting helped the NIH and the Mennonite church temporarily to align their missions. Their alignment through practices of accounting allowed a moral market in healthy civilian bodies – at the time, ethically questionable and legally unprecedented – to emerge and become routine in law and lived experience (see section *Aligning*). Second, as part of this moral market, Mennonites were enrolled in experiments, including studies of metabolism, a field with a long tradition of accounting as a research technique. For metabolic researchers, bodies were *in vivo* accounts through which they could record input and output to understand how bodies balanced. Comparing how accounting operated as a mode of attention clarifies when and how categories such as age, gender, and race, were made real (see section *Figuring*). Third, Mennonites – including Esther and Mary – were doing the physical work of bookkeeping on the wards. They walked, talked, and took note of other Mennonites' comings and goings around the Clinical Center to get an account of their time. As a result, accounting operated as a form of surveillance and discipline in the hospital. The labour of accounting – though carried out by church volunteers and directed towards each other – enforced the embodied discipline that clinical researchers capitalised upon without them needing to assert it directly (see section *Surveilling*).

This chapter documents that accounting in medicine was used in multiple, simultaneous modes and considers the effects. Ultimately, attention to accounting in medicine demonstrates that any power accorded to late modern medicine is an ongoing accomplishment, not an inherent quality of the field, given its dependence on other institutions for necessary resources and much-needed discipline. More broadly, I argue that by requiring an explanation of the past and a forecast of the future, accounting shapes the epistemic possibilities of medical knowledge itself. Thus, attention to accounting in medicine is distinctively well suited to show how practices seemingly ancillary to medicine can alter both organisational and human bodies, and the ways available for living in each.

Aligning

'Judging from the size of this place, one would expect an impersonal atmosphere,' Esther and Mary agreed, 'but this is far from the case.' They had arrived at the NIH Clinical Center days earlier during the warm mid-Atlantic autumn of 1965. Inside the brick building they had seen from a distance poking above Bethesda's suburban skyline, they had been assigned to a shared hospital room. They unpacked their luggage and sent news of their happy arrival to Bruce Harder, the staff director of the Mennonite Voluntary Service programme. 'Each wing of each floor is a separate unit in itself', they marveled. 'Everyone seems to put forth so much effort to make things as plasant (sic) for us as possible. Our contacts with the patients and the personnel has (sic) been very pleasant and we are thoroughly enjoying the experience.'[4]

The Clinical Center had opened a decade earlier and was the US government's premier research hospital (Figure 10.2). Researchers were employees of the government as part of the NIH's 'intramural' programme; they were not employees of other institutions receiving federal grants as part of the NIH's 'extramural' programme. As such, intramural researchers were distinctive – and their encounters with sick and healthy patient-subjects all the more important to study – because federal laws and policies were designed around the local needs and habits of the scientists that the NIH employed directly. For example, federal regulations on research with 'human subjects' were extended from the local policies of the NIH Clinical Center to all institutions in the US and abroad that received federal grants.[5] Moreover, the NIH's intramural scientists were unusually influential in shaping international and extra-national rules for research in the postwar decades.[6] The NIH's

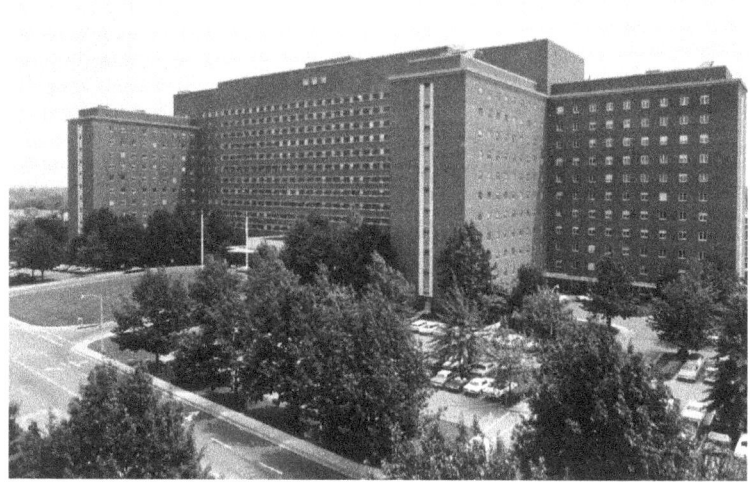

10.2 The NIH Clinical Center opened in 1953 on the agency's main campus in Bethesda, Maryland, and started a new programme, the Normal Volunteer Patient Program, to get essential research material for scientists: healthy human subjects for medical experiments. Esther and Mary, like other 'Normals', lived in hospital rooms for weeks, months, or years alongside sick patients.

intramural accounting practices are important to examine, not (only) because they followed the broad contours of other medical facilities, but because they created the moral and legal conditions of possibility for research at other sites.

Congressional funding for the Clinical Center as a specifically research-oriented facility presumed that scientists had access to an essential resource: namely, human subjects.[7] The place was unusual in that anyone admitted to the facility was required to be part of medical studies. They would not be admitted exclusively for treatment. When the Clinical Center opened in 1953, sick people were readily available. But healthy people were another matter. Why would a healthy person check herself into a hospital? Prior to the Second World War, many Western medical researchers tapped state institutions (such as prisons and the military) or turned to intimate relationships (such as students and family members) for healthy human subjects to use in their experiments. But researchers at the Clinical Center needed a sizable and steady source of healthy civilians to live long-term in the facility. The practice of using healthy civilians – much less, white middle-class people – was legally unprecedented and morally unacceptable in the 1950s. In the years after the Second World War, NIH administrators were well aware of the dubiousness of proposing such a practice.

Exacerbating the problem, NIH required legal contracts to purchase research materials, including human subjects. At the time the Clinical Center opened, the NIH conventionally used 'procurement contracts' as the legal instrument through which it exchanged money for goods. NIH administrators extended this existing procurement-contract infrastructure to the purchase of healthy civilians, technically their 'man-time', to solve the problem of acquiring healthy humans. As the Clinical Center was about to open in 1953, administrators negotiated with national leaders of the Historic Peace Churches, which included the Mennonite church, in hopes of acquiring healthy human subjects from a pool of religious conscientious objectors – by definition all men. Church leaders encouraged them to broaden their imagination. They suggested that the NIH's new Normal Volunteer Patient Program could be integrated as a placement option into the churches' existing Voluntary Service programmes, which included both men and women, civilians as well as conscripts.[8] In 1954, an NIH lawyer reported to agency directors on the results of the negotiations: 'I proposed arrangements under which I felt we could "purchase" service from the organization on a man-month basis.' The peace-church leaders had 'received the proposal very well and agreed to cooperate.'[9] The NIH agreed to pay the church organisations a 10 per cent 'administrative fee' for each volunteer who joined the programme, which was calculated by the NIH's Office of Procurement using the agency's new 'man-month' metric. The NIH also deposited in church accounts the monthly stipend that each volunteer earned from their service.

The 'procurement contract' documented an agreement that had until then only been spoken and written informally, not manifest in a legally binding instrument. In doing so, the procurement-contract mechanism, now broadened to humans, allowed the exchange to materialise. Starting in 1954, the mechanism created an infrastructure through which NIH contracted with dozens of non-government organiations in the 1950s, 1960s, and 1970s to provide healthy, rights-bearing civilians as human subjects.[10] NIH administrators' extension of the procurement contract to human subjects allowed the government agency to operate within an existing procurement infrastructure that required it to pay organisations rather than individuals, which muted any clamour from the questionable act of paying individuals directly for the use of their bodies (Figure 10.3).

Accounting practices were among a suite of activities that allowed the organisations' seemingly unrelated interests to align.[11] The procurement contract set the legal terms of the transaction, but the everyday practice of accounting allowed money and bodies to be exchanged. In the transaction, the bodies were refigured from medical human subjects to religious service workers, thus legitimising the movement of money and bodies. The conventions – and conventionality – of accounting helped to solve the postwar puzzle of how to gain access to an essential resource for medical research, legally and morally.

The account books aligned the two organisations and, by allowing money to change hands, they brought the activity into being as a lawful activity, in turn reforming people's moral sensibility. The money's awkward passage through space makes this apparent. Esther and Mary lived on NIH property and inside an NIH building. They could have walked within minutes to the budget office on the NIH campus where their stipends originated. Yet the NIH sent the money from Bethesda, Maryland to Goshen, Indiana, the headquarters of the Mennonite church, which then authorised unit leaders back at the Clinical Center in Bethesda to pay individuals living there – that is, to pay themselves with NIH funds using a church-issued chequebook. This arrangement could hardly be described as efficient. It dramatises the fact that the NIH was restricted from directly paying individuals it 'procured'. Through its translocation, the money moved organisations and turned potential wages into a stipend, foreclosing any suggestion of employment rights.[12] Even though individuals received the money for time spent and activities carried out for NIH scientists, the money

No.	Item	Institutes	Contract No. S4-43-ph	Company	Period
61	Repair Ultra Centrifuge	NCI-MRA MHI-NMI NIAMD	513	Spinco Division Beckman Instrument Company	7-1-55/6-30-56
62	Photo Processing Service	OD-SRB Roy Perry	519	District Photo Service	7-1-55/6-30-56
63	Radioisotopes	NIMDB Dr. Shy	626	Abbott Laboratories	7-1-55/6-30-56
64	Motion Picture Film Processing	All NIH	643	Byron, Inc.	7-1-55/6-30-56
65	Tutoring Service	CC & All Institutes	646	Montg. Co. Board of Educa.	7-1-55/8-31-55
68	Casework Data, N.Y.	NIMH	679	Research Founda. for Mental Hygiene	7-1-55/6-30-56
73	Cats and Kittens	Dr. Gay Bldg. 14A	684	James Anthony	7-15-55 thru 6-30-56
78	Pellets, Monkey	OS	712	Dietrich & Gambrill	8-15-55 thru 6-30-56
79	Eggs, fertile	NMI Dr. Uts	697	Duckworth Hatchery	8-1-55/6-30-56
RENEWAL CONTRACTS:			SAPH		
101-55	Volunteer Service	All NIH	59542	General Brotherhood Board	7-1-55/6-30-56
103-55	Volunteer Service	All NIH	59586	Mennonite Central Comm.	7-1-55/6-30-56
66-54	Elevator Service	DMB-OD	59507	Otis Elevator Service	7-1-55/6-30-56
46-55	Service and Maintain RCA Microscopes, Vacuum Units, and Defraction Units	All NIH	60971	RCA Service Co., Inc.	7-1-55/6-30-56
47-55	Service and Repair Spectrophotometers	NCI-NHI NIAMD	60975	Perkin-Elmer Corp.	7-1-55/6-30-56
48-55	Service and Repair I.E.C. Centrifuges	All NIH	60972	International Equipment Co.	7-1-55/6-30-56

10.3 To get healthy human subjects for scientists' research in the Clinical Center, the NIH established a legal instrument for buying research supplies from vendors: the 'procurement contract'. The second line item under 'renewal contracts' in the NIH's 1956 inventory of contracts is contract 103-55, 'Volunteer Service' from Mennonite Central Committee.

became a stipend from the church rather than wages from the NIH. Thus, accounting was the means through which two large, bureaucratic organisations coordinated their actions. In the ledgers, their goals and ontologies came temporarily into alignment.

In the process, accounting naturalised bodies as an item of exchange. Far from a sacred object protected from market exchanges, bodies were inserted into familiar accounting practices, enabling a new 'moral market' to emerge. Cultural historians of economies argue that money is not inherently corruptive, and instead ask scholars to consider what meanings are associated with money, how those meanings are established and managed, and which instruments and techniques enable monetary exchange of sacred materials.[13] At the Clinical Center, Mennonite bodies slid into preexisting accounting routines established for non-human materials.[14] Thus, a new and potentially morally uncomfortable practice was possible because it was folded into a set of existing legal instruments: procurement contracts and account books.

By routinising the procedure, the organisations brought into being a legal market that also gradually reshaped moral sensibilities towards experimentation. For Mennonites, including Mary and Esther, pain and deprivation were not inimical to their voluntary service; suffering for Jesus was the reason and reward for their participation.[15] From the staff office of the church's voluntary service, Bruce Harder admired the Mennonite disposition of virtuous suffering and then awarded praise to individual Mennonites who exemplified it by allowing themselves to be experimented upon. 'I know the doctors are happy that you, Esther and Mary, are sacrificing of yourselves for such an interesting and important research project', he told them.[16] Accounting made available a new disposition towards non-therapeutic research on healthy people because voluntary service workers qua human subjects gave religious meaning to their experiences.

Attention to accounting practices shows the specific ways in which the seeming power of the NIH depended on the Mennonite church and how the NIH was able to enroll the church organisation in garnering its own strength. Working towards different missions with different vocabularies, ledgers aligned in such a way that the organisations could accomplish a consequential shift in the legal, scientific, and experiential possibilities of human experimentation. Accounting and the alignment it afforded were essential to open these new possibilities.

Figuring

When Esther and Mary selected the Clinical Center as their placement for voluntary service, they knew they would be 'normal control' research subjects. It is unlikely, however, that they knew which studies would enroll them. They soon learned.[17] 'We are participating in a Metabolic Balance Study', they explained to Harder:

> This consists of a very carefully planned constant diet which we will have for the duration of the study – probably thirty days. In this study after they have our diets stabilized and fixed according to our tastes, we are given doses of isotopes, sometimes orally in milk and sometimes intravenously, at which time the calcium is traced by a very intricate machine. At the beginning of each cycle on the day the dose is given, we are 'counted' by the machine for 6 hours and [for the] 5 days following for 20 minutes per day. This same cycle is repeated about every two weeks, allowing an interval between for the count to become normal again.[18]

By early October 1965, they had each been through one cycle and were preparing for more. 'We are the first female normals in this age bracket that they have been able to find for this study', they bragged. 'Since the disease (osteoporosis) which they are studying, occurs only in older people, they were eager to find someone (sic) of our age group.'[19] The metabolic researchers were interested in how bodies absorbed nutrients, especially calcium, so they put Mary and Esther on strictly controlled diets.[20] The pair, considering themselves vernacular experts on the domestic-industrial elements of the Clinical Center, were especially attentive to the meal experience. 'Our food is all weighed many times in tenths of grams and only the choice, U. S. Fancy Grade of meats and canned goods are used', they explained. 'Everything for the duration of the diet has to be from the same place and the same day's run to maintain even quality and food content.' To comply with research protocol, they often put their faces to the plate, licking their platters clean. Thanksgiving dinner at the Clinical Center was an amusing disappointment for Mary, who was on study. The existence of multiple contexts of time – the scientific study versus the cultural world – was apparent on such occasions.

In addition to the calcium tracer studies, the metabolic researchers ran additional experiments through their bodies. One would swallow bags of mercury stuck in their noses or mouths, or would have bits of their intestine clipped for analysis – an unpopular procedure among the normal volunteers over the years. Meanwhile, the other would continue with the tracer study, guzzling distilled water and having blood drawn after researchers administered radioisotope-tagged calcium through an IV or a glass of milk. The tracer study underscores the importance of the NIH's role in broader US government efforts to rehabilitate the reputation of atomic research. New medical technologies were essential to this effort as US bombs continued to be tested and protested.[21] Mary and Esther marvelled at the science and the scientists, blushing at their own humble part in the enterprise. Back at Mennonite headquarters, Harder shared their awe. 'You really lost me on that word osteoporosis!!!??'[22] he exclaimed from the Mennonite main office. Mary noted in December, 'Esther is ready for the third cycle in this study, but there will be no isotopes available until next week.' She explained to Harder: 'The doctor told us that it takes three years to make an isotope and they come from Oak Ridge, Tennessee.' Their foresight was commendable. 'Considering the fact that they must anticipate the need so far in advance, they have done an excellent job of supplying the demand.'[23] Indeed, anticipation was a key disposition in human-subject research that accounting required and instilled.[24]

The techniques of clinical science, and especially metabolic research, have long drawn on practices of accounting to study the body as a ledger. Esther and Mary were a case in point. The church and the NIH urged all of the Voluntary Service members to do a second form of volunteer work through a 'career assignment'.[25] Esther and Mary had intended to work in the Patient Recreation Department, where as 'healthy patients' they had been making latch-hook rugs. Instead, the metabolic researchers snagged them for their free labour. 'They are going to train Esther to operate the calculating and the counting machine which have to do with our study', they enthused.[26] (Meanwhile, they put Mary to work typing.) As religious volunteers, they were counting themselves as clinical data.[27]

The similitude of monetary and metabolic accounting draws attention to the ways in which their ledgers differed, and particularly how they made the same thing (a person) legible in different ways. Esther and Mary were rendered under two modes of accounting: that of the metabolic study, which rendered human subjects, and that of church personnel lists, which rendered the same people as religious volunteers. By reading historical records against each other it becomes apparent what traits were considered real and relevant for each organisation. As a methodological approach for historians, the comparative study of accounting practices under different modes can indicate the priorities of organisations, in this case a religious and a medical organisation. Metabolic research and religious service figured the same bodies very differently, and this observation throws into relief the specific terms in which each organisation imagined people – and how they might have imagined them otherwise.

The only traits formally recorded in church personnel lists were name, address, and the volunteer's branch of the Mennonite church (there were many). For metabolic researchers, however, chronological age was essential because they imagined age as a biological reality with physical thresholds that registered in the body. For the church, chronological age was irrelevant, even if a person's moment in life, in a social sense, was a factor. In the 1950s, the Mennonite Voluntary Service was clipped from its original association with 'alternative service' for (young, male) conscientious objectors. The programme allowed Mennonites to volunteer at a time in their lives when they had funds and flexibility to get away from home for a year or a few months. Fresh out of high school or college-aged seemed the perfect time. However, older people also often fit the profile of the ideal voluntary service worker: no work, no family constraints, and lots of time.

Like chronological age, a person's gender was an essential category for researchers, but when rendered as a volunteer by the church, it disappeared.[28] By accounting for gender, metabolic researchers enacted the category as biological fact. At the same time, researchers depended on the sociality of their human subjects in order to then render them as gendered, molecular individuals. 'They would appreciate having more older volunteers', Esther relayed to church administrators after chatting with researchers. 'We promised to try to recruit some of our teacher friends this summer if we can.' This remark shows that it was far from random how Mennonites were distributed across the various placement sites for voluntary service. Researchers' demand for what they regarded as biological data actively patterned the distribution of Mennonites into the variety of voluntary service placements the church had on offer. The fulfilment of researchers' demands relied upon the social networks of people as religious volunteers at the same time researchers were figuring them as human subjects.

Reading how people were rendered under different modes of accounting also shows how, despite their differences, these modes of accounting reinforced shared biases. Importantly, race went unmarked in the accounts of both metabolic research and voluntary service. Race could be made invisible because both Mennonite volunteers and experimental patients at the Clinical Center were overwhelmingly White – the unmarked racial category. Far from a postracial setting, the Clinical Center (and like other sites of US medical research generally at this time) should be understood as an intensely racialised space because of its site-specific racial homogeneity. It is no coincidence that in clinical research designed to learn about 'normal' bodies, White people were enrolled. Black Americans were present inside the Clinical Center, to be sure, but were working as janitors, technicians, and nurses. Thus, what might seem to be an ethical choice in the 1960s (to avoid research on Black Americans) is best seen as evidence of the production of whiteness as a social-biological norm. Furthermore, the *clinical* studies of White Americans as representatives of biological normality magnified White medical privilege. Clinical studies were carried out most extensively on diseases that largely affected the White middle-class electorate[29] and the NIH had an interest in ensuring (White) patients' social comfort: to be served by Black Americans in the Clinical Center was one thing, but to share a hospital room (including bathroom) for several months was another matter.[30]

When researchers did study Black Americans, they tended to carry out field research on pathology, as the Tuskegee Studies most tragically attest.[31] As a result, it was impossible for researchers to query their own race-based conclusions because of the overlay of the categories of clinic/field, White/Black, and normal/pathological. At a time when the US Civil Rights movement was at a fever pitch, the bodies of Black Americans were missing from clinical research on normalcy, allowing conclusions based on racially homogenous spaces to persist unchallenged. The NIH's turn to the Mennonite church as a supplier of 'normal controls' reinforced the implicit racial biases of each organisation.[32]

From inside their own bodies, Mary and Esther accounted for themselves as religious volunteers above all – even, perhaps especially, when their bodies were on metabolic ledgers. 'We have had the same food every day now for six weeks', they reported in early winter. This was not a complaint: 'Believe it or not, we are enjoying it as much now as we did in the beginning.' To be sure, they did not find the procedures or the restrictions pleasant. But discomfort was the point. Indeed, they aspired to witness the suffering of Jesus and physical pain mapped onto this agenda. They understood their medical experiences in religious terms. 'After Christmas we'll be trading our ordeals', they reported, referring to the Christian tradition of trial by ordeal. When researchers needed them to repeat a study, they reported 'we have agreed to go through the ordeal again.'[33] The more daunting and bizarre the study, the better. They made for better stories and tougher tests of commitment and courage over which they could prevail. In March of 1966, they got a vacation from the studies and dashed off a note from the road: 'We are looking forward to getting back in the harness.'

When they had arrived at the Clinical Center, Esther and Mary had intended to serve there for a few weeks before moving on to another placement site. But in the course of being measured and weighed, inspected and injected, they watched researchers assign value to their bodies and in the process Esther and Mary noticed that their aged female bodies had value.[34] By the spring, Mary and Esther felt 'pretty much like permanent fixtures', and requested that the church allow them to continue their placement as normal controls, explaining, 'the doctor informed us yesterday that they would like for us to stay the whole year. They seem to think that we are valuable because they have very few female normals in our age group. He said they are not nearly through with these calcium studies and they have further plans of loaning us to some of the other institutes for different studies later on.'

Accounting produced its own continuation and lent inertia to activities already being accounted for in the terms set by the ledgers – such as age, gender, and race. Attention to this process offers a cautionary tale. By juxtaposing the ways that the same people were accounted for in metabolic studies and religious service, it is possible to see the multiple realities they produced: worlds in which people might be nodes in networks or molecular individuals. Importantly, the different ways of imagining people that the accounts revealed and produced, also allowed the organisations to engage and ultimately lock together for the long term. Metabolic researchers had to project their need for normal controls, which anticipated its own fulfilment. Church leaders forecasted their organisation's income and available bodies, accounting for scientists' demand, which in turn encouraged the church to channel prospective volunteers to the NIH placement site. The NIH was a particularly lucrative and reliable placement for the church compared to other sites. By the 1960s, administrators of the Mennonite Voluntary Service Program and the NIH Normal Volunteer Patient Program had friendly professional relationships that both groups were eager to maintain. The seemingly independent choice of Mennonite volunteers about which placement option to select would be better described as an interdependent decision. Witness Esther and Mary's joint decision to go to the Clinical Center and their efforts to recruit more NIH volunteers through their intimate networks. In the process of recording and predicting, marking and occluding, accounting practices sustained political biases built into the transaction.[35]

Surveilling

Mary and Esther were 'normal control' research subjects as a condition of their placement at the Clinical Center. But they were also the local accountants for the Mennonite church as a result of accepting the official position of 'unit leaders'. As a profession, the field of accounting had long since formalised methods to educate, credential, and license its own members, and, in so doing, to narrow the market for services. By linking the virtues of objectivity with techniques of quantification, accountants sought to distinguish the 'legitimate' from the merely skillful and thereby to protect their exclusive claim to expert knowledge and their market position.[36]

Yet accountants manqué did not go away. Instead, informal accountants like Esther and Mary continued to keep the books outside of offices and diffused into unexpected places, such as homes or hospital wards. Far from quashing vernacular accountants, the professionalisation of the field had the effect of expanding rather than narrowing practices of accounting and increasing the need for bookkeepers beyond office buildings. Professionalisation also made vernacular accountants more difficult to locate in the historical record because accounting came to be synonymous with the formal practice, a bias that archives can reproduce.

In church records, however, Esther and Mary take shape as they carried out the everyday work of accounting, just like other unit leaders who came before and would come after. As local accountants, the pair were issued four chequebooks from the church with Esther's name printed on them. They paid stipends to themselves and to other volunteers, covered travel expenses, and allotted funds for approved recreational expenses, like attending Sunday worship at Hyattsville Mennonite Church. They filed administrative reports, kept balance sheets, and calculated income and expenses.[37] They submitted reimbursement for collective unit expenses – the cost of admissions to galleries and shows, the outlay for a tank of gas to ferry Mennonites to church or to visit friends, and other acceptable adventures. They projected unit costs, requested advances, and conferred by phone with the main church office.[38]

As the church's local accountants, they had discretion and were encouraged to use it.[39] 'Esther, will you please handle Arlene's finances just as you do for the other unit members?' Harder asked when a new young Mennonite was set to join the Clinical Center placement unit. 'Arlene should receive the regular $15 monthly allowance and I think she will also want to be reimbursed for traveling expenses from Telford to NIH. Please handle this as you see fit.'[40] Just as often, they sought counsel from the church budget offices on whether expenses were allowable, revealing the hierarchical structure of the church bureaucracy (Figure 10.4). When one Mennonite volunteer got sick and could no longer be used as a healthy human subject, they wondered whether to pay him. 'Bill Lehman's status has been changed from a normal to that of a patient', they reported to the church's main office. 'Should his allowance be continued?' (The answer: 'Definitely'.) Esther and Mary did not relish the accounting work.[41] But they filed their reports fastidiously and even sought out a typewriter at the NIH to file financial records with the church. 'I would guess that you studied the Unit Leader's Handbook since you did an excellent job of completing the financial report', Harder eventually praised. 'The report was in A-1 shape!'[42]

Their balance sheets did not stand alone. They were among a set of paper tools and homespun methods that comprised accounting practices. In two-page monthly reports, Esther and Mary gave an account of the lived space and time that the numbers indexed. They attached

                                    SUMMER   SERVICE
Mennonite Central Committee   Report No. 1 - 2 -③- ⓐ
Akron, Pennsylvania   (Circle Correct Number)

                        REPORT OF UNIT INCOME AND EXPENSES
Unit __NIH__   Reporting Period From _Aug 1_ to _Aug 30_
Report Prepared by __Marilyn Brown__   Date _____

CASH ON HAND BEGINNING OF PERIOD --------------------------------$ _94.00_

                        RECEIPTS   170.00 cash advance
Received from Akron:
    Date _____   --------$ _____
    Date _____   --------$ _____
Contributions from Other Sources
    Where _____   --------$ _____
    Where _____   --------$ _____

                                        TOTAL RECEIPTS --$ _____
                                        TOTAL CASH AVAILABLE --$ _94.00_

                        DISBURSEMENTS
Unit Expenses for Operation and Administration   F5-2   121.85
    Unit Postage, telephone, telegraph --------$ _.10_   9J 1-3(NIH)
    Transportation ---------------------------$ _11.10_   170.00
    Other (list) _____ -----$ 48.15
                 _____ -----$ send receipt
                                    TOTAL-----------$ _11.20_   9/2/64 cm

Unit Expenses for Religious Life (list)
    _____ -----$ _____
    _____ -----$ _____
    _____ -----$ _____
                                    TOTAL-----------$ _____

Unit Expenses for Education and Recreation (list)
    Costs Dinner (9 at $3.85)   -----$ _34.65_
    _____ -----$ _____
    _____ -----$ _____
    _____ -----$ _____
                                    TOTAL-----------$ _34.65_
                                    TOTAL DISBURSEMENTS ---$ _45.85_
                                    CASH ON HAND END OF PERIOD ---$ _48.15_

10.4 The Mennonite church and the Church of the Brethren signed the first contracts with the NIH for healthy human subjects, which were recruited through the churches' 'voluntary service' programs. The NIH paid the church organisations the cost of a stipend for voluntary service workers and a 10 per cent 'processing fee'. The churches also reimbursed voluntary service workers at NIH for their additional expenses, such as 'education and recreation' activities, and 'operation and administration' costs including phone and postage for church business. From among the group of voluntary service workers living at the Clinical Center, the churches assigned a 'unit leader', who worked as a vernacular accountant for the church to manage its local finances.

the stable numbers on the page to a story unfolding within a social context. They revealed the flow of time as experienced, while they also rendered time in the account books as a stable 'present'. To do so, they plotted numbers into narrative structure – featuring visits from friends, tours of monuments, and many misadventures while navigating Washington's streets. Rather than urge them to stick to the bullet points, the main office praised their novel bureaucratic style. 'Thanks once again for a most interesting administrative report!' Esther and Mary sent postcards, Christmas greetings, and notes in round cursive script, as Harder encouraged them along. In short, they adapted their jobs as bookkeepers to the documentary forms they already knew, letters rather than memos, for example. 'Your administrative report was really "warm and homey"', Harder commented.[43] By encoding quixotic stories of derring-do and morality tales, local accountants like Esther and Mary innovated on the documentary practices of accounting.

In the process of keeping the books, they accomplished even more. The diffusion of accounting responsibilities to informal practitioners created an intimate discipline inside the Clinical Center. Specifically, accounting operated as a form of surveillance and produced a religiously grounded, embodied restraint on the ward level. Local accountants literally sought people out to get an account of their time, to enquire whether the time was profitably spent, and, depending on the answer, to pay them. 'When you see the financial report, please don't think we went to church just once in August', they urged Harder. 'We went, but others provided the transportation for a change.'[44] Similarly, they accounted for another volunteer's absence from church and subsequent lack of request for travel reimbursement. The young woman, a bit more spry and elastic than Esther and Mary, had been enrolled in fever studies at the Clinical Center and was extremely contagious. In addition to explaining time spent, Mary and Esther surveilled other volunteers and judged their actions in the name of bookkeeping. When two young Mennonite volunteers rented a limousine to tour Washington – somehow inadvertently – Esther and Mary refused to reimburse the boys. Ultimately, they passed the line item on to Harder to decide. It was an innocent mistake, he wagered, and told them to pay the bill.

For one year, Esther and Mary tracked down other volunteers, assessed their use of time, and reported on their activities as well as their own. The practical tasks associated with quantifying and economising medicine were carried out by the human subjects themselves.[45] In the process, NIH researchers profited from the discipline that the church's local accountants instilled. Researchers could extract clinical data without protest or query because their human subjects, though living inside the Clinical Center, were part of another organisation that oriented their experience of the hospital and that enforced a form of obedience sympathetic to researchers' needs. Discipline in medical research was accomplished through church labour and its accounting practices.

In the postwar period, the work of medical administration carried out in separate offices and by specially trained accountants was itself 'outsourced' beyond the medical organisation, and yet physically back into the space of the wards. Esther and Mary show us how the *experience* of accounting functioned to sustain medical research. Human subjects' financial recording and reporting on the wards maintained them in a web of local connections and held them in regular ongoing relationships with the distant organisation that arranged their stay, namely the church. Financial recordkeeping and reporting functioned, in a Foucauldian sense, as the means whereby human subjects disciplined and accounted for themselves both morally and statistically.

Conclusion

When they left the Clinical Center in the fall of 1966, Esther and Mary handed off the account books to the new unit leader. They passed on bank statements, chequebooks, and the previous year's financial reports to the next Mennonite, who would likewise record and produce the accountable behaviour of the religious volunteers. 'I have already delivered the goods to Victor', they confirmed with the Mennonite headquarters in September. As local accountants, Esther and Mary had filled a role that others had served before them and others would fill after. They were replaceable by design, embedded as they were in the modern bureaucracies of church and state.

As the story of Esther and Mary makes clear, attention to accounting in medicine is important because it is a world-making enterprise. During the 1950s, NIH administrators and church leaders created a new moral market for healthy civilians to serve as human subjects – people who were perfect strangers to researchers, were in perfect health, and had no debt to the state. Accounting practices had allowed the NIH and churches to align, which created and sustained new legal and moral possibilities for human experimentation. In turn, these possibilities channelled the things that came to be known, as well as those things left unimagined, in the name of medicine. Until 1960, the only people who were enrolled as healthy human subjects at the Clinical Center were Anabaptist voluntary service workers. The arrangement with churches eventually encouraged and enabled the NIH to establish long-term reliable sources of human subjects with additional organisations including colleges, civic groups, and labour unions. By the 1970s, this new market for healthy human subjects was well established, to the extent that the US regulations on human-subjects research passed in 1974 functioned not to dismantle the market but to protect it by setting rules that presumed its acceptability.[46]

The practice of accounting also performed the future by requiring both NIH researchers and church staff to forecast budgets, which in turn required researchers to forecast their demands for 'normal controls'. Researchers had to anticipate and thereby to plan their future studies, which brought into being research questions crafted around the (human) materials at hand, making those studies a possibility, and even a priority, on the horizon of time. The imperatives of projecting and hypothesising meant that accounting in medicine served to create the goals of researchers – goals that in turn drove the choices of future 'normal controls' *prior to* their arrival: Mennonite leaders guided voluntary service workers to join the NIH placement in order to satisfy researchers' demand. This dimension of accounting – forecasting and budget planning – knits together with shifts in research design both in the clinic and in field research. For example, accounting can be considered alongside new forms of longitudinal research, which would yield the concept of the 'risk factor' and the investments in 'preventative thinking' that it enabled.[47]

Furthermore, the practice brought into being accountable bodies. Local accountants for the church, such as Esther and Mary, produced pliant human subjects for researchers through surveillance and discipline for the purposes of church bookkeeping. Incidentally but importantly, they prepared bodies for the discipline that the experimental system expected and reinforced. Simultaneously, church groups disciplined researchers. The pliant religious volunteers taught researchers how to comport themselves with their normal controls (for best results:

be friendly, intimate), and the church's religiously accountable bodies prompted researchers to imagine what they could expect from their research materials. Trained on the specific examples of normal controls from Anabaptist churches, researchers would be surprised to find that those normal controls were unusual – that is, unusually compliant. The specificity of Mennonites as human subjects only came into focus when the NIH expanded its 'procurement contract' infrastructure to include secular organisations, such as colleges and labour unions. They sent less tractable souls to serve as human subjects at the NIH, on whom the NIH enforced the behavioural expectations set by Anabaptists.

In turn, accounting functioned to make political categories legible as biological realities, such as age, gender, and race. Innovations in the NIH's established accounting system, through which the agency extended the 'procurement contract' mechanism beyond hardgoods to humans, allowed the US government to carry out large-scale basic research on new groups of people, particularly women and older people, in addition to the conventional demographic of younger men used as stand-ins for healthy bodies.[48] Thus, the Mennonites who came to the Clinical Center affected what studies researchers pursued and the questions they later asked – in turn channelling the answers they received toward questions of health: molecular or contextual, genetic or structural. Steven Epstein has documented how race as a social-historical category became naturalised as a biological essence through (well-intended) postwar research regulations.[49] Likewise, I suggest that the alignment of state and church via their accounting infrastructures allowed the NIH the practical ability to do research on civilians – which added to medical settings new social beings to be understood in biological form and asserted at the molecular level that to be normal in America was to be White. Accounting techniques were used in multiple ways, and so they both entrenched and made apparent the occlusions, emphases, and shared biases of the different organisations. Not only 'medical discovery' but the contingencies of financial administration contributed to the commitment to biologically based notions of political concepts, specifically gender and race.

Overall, my research suggests how organisations beyond the field of medicine structured the market for human subjects and the practice of medical knowledge-making through accounting techniques. Practices that had been ethically and legally impossible, such as exchanging humans for money, were assimilated into existing practices of non-medical organisations, such as the Mennonite church's 'voluntary service' programme and the accounting practices the organisation had in place. These seemingly ancillary organisations promoted specific habits of self-discipline and provided a narrative for the experience of serving in experiments, such as virtuous suffering; these habits and narratives were necessary for researchers to have access to essential research materials: healthy human bodies. The legal, moral, and social infrastructures that supported research in turn channelled the possibilities for gendered and racist knowledge-making.

Medical organisations are often assumed to have substantial power to shape policy and discipline bodies in late modernity.[50] Attention to accounting practices shows the extent to which any power attributed to medicine as an institution depends on its alignment with organisations conventionally thought of as 'outside' of the field. Medical organisations may indeed have political and epistemic authority. But as Esther and Mary demonstrate, that power is always incomplete and dependent upon a pre-emptive faith in the power of medicine, which is required to bring new bodies – and bodies of knowledge – into being.

Notes

1 B.W. Redekop and C.W. Redekop, *Power, Authority, and the Anabaptist Tradition* (Baltimore: Johns Hopkins University Press, 2001).
2 J.A. Aho, *Confession and Bookkeeping: The Religious, Moral, and Rhetorical Roots of Modern Accounting* (Albany: State University of New York Press, 2005).
3 This chapter is one piece of my broader project on the first generations of healthy human subjects who served at the US National Institutes of Health through its Normal Volunteer Patient Program. The 'Vernacular Archive of Normal Volunteers' (VANV) is an online publicly available repository at the Harvard University Countway Library of Medicine. Stark, Laura. 2017. 'Vernacular Archive of Normal Volunteers (VANV), 1954–2017 (inclusive).' https://doi.org/10.7910/DVN/OD6DVW, https://doi.org/10.7910/DVN/GUAZDH, and https://doi.org/10.7910/DVN/WFFS4W. Harvard Dataverse, V1. Collection H MS c464, Harvard Medical Library in the Francis A. Countway Library of Medicine, Boston, MA.
4 Administrative report by Smucker and Warye, 6 October 1965, Folder: National Institutes of Health, Mennonite Service Unit, 1965, Series MCC IX-6-3, Mennonite Central Committee Archive, Goshen, Indiana (hereafter MCC).

5 L. Stark, *Behind Closed Doors: IRBs and the Making of Ethical Research* (Chicago: University of Chicago Press, 2012).
6 S.E. Lederer, 'Children as guinea pigs: Historical perspective', *Accountability in Research* 10:1 (2003), 1–16; N. Chorev, *The World Health Organization between North and South* (Ithaca: Cornell University Press, 2012); R.M. Packard, *A History of Global Health: Interventions into the Lives of Other Peoples* (Baltimore: Johns Hopkins University Press, 2016).
7 R. Mandel, *Beacon of Hope* (NIH, undated). www-dev.ors.od.nih.gov/medart/Stetten/becon_of_hope/founding_years_Pg2.htm.
8 L. Stark, 'Contracting health: Procurement contracts, total institutions, and the problem of virtuous suffering in postwar human experiment', *Social History of Medicine*, 31:4 (2018), 818–46.
9 Ladimer to Shannon, Memo 'The Use of Conscientious Objectors', 21 September 1953, Document 023221, INTRA 2-1-9, National Institutes of Health.
10 Stark, 'Contracting health'.
11 A.M. Preston, 'The birth of clinical accounting: A study of the emergence and transformations of discourses on costs and practices of accounting in U.S. hospitals', *Accounting, Organizations and Society* 17:1 (1992), 63–100.
12 L. Stark, 'Work, welfare, and the values of voluntarism: Rethinking Anscombe's "Action under a description" in postwar markets for human subjects', *American Journal of Cultural Sociology* 5:1–2 (2017), 181–224.
13 M. Fourcade, 'Cents and sensibility: Economic valuation and the nature of "Nature"', *American Journal of Sociology* 116:6 (2011), 1721–7; D. Akyel, 'Qualification under moral constraints: The funeral purchase as a problem of valuation', in J. Beckert and C. Musselin (eds), *Constructing Quality: The Classification of Goods in Markets* (Oxford: Oxford University Press, 2013), pp. 223–46.
14 M. Fourcade and K. Healy, 'Moral views of market society', *Annual Review of Sociology* 33:1 (2007), 285–311; S. Quinn, '"The miracles of bookkeeping": How budget politics link fiscal policies and financial markets', *American Journal of Sociology* 123:1 (2017), 48–85.
15 Harder to Smucker and Warye, 7 October 1965; see also Braun to Friesen, 4 February 1965, MCC.
16 Harder to Smucker and Warye, 7 October 1965, MCC.
17 It is unclear whether they signed consent forms because researchers did not consistently or uniformly use signature-based forms during the 1960s, despite NIH lawyers' pleadings to adopt the practice to safeguard against legal liability, see Stark, *Behind Closed Doors*.
18 Administrative report by Smucker and Warye, 6 October 1965, MCC.

19 Ibid. An additional older Mennonite, Mr. Kehn, was also on metabolic studies at this time.
20 S.J. Birge, W.A. Peck, M. Berman, and G.D. Whedon, 'Study of calcium absorption in man: A kinetic analysis and physiologic model', *Journal of Clinical Investigation* 48:9 (September 1969), 1705–13.
21 A.N.H. Creager, *Life Atomic: A History of Radioisotopes in Science and Medicine* (Chicago: University of Chicago Press, 2013).
22 Harder to Smucker and Warye, 7 October 1965, MCC.
23 Smucker to Harder, 2 December 1965, MCC: 'We are still plodding away on our Metabolic Balance Study with a few slight changes. Mary is drinking glass after glass of distilled water, giving blood samples, and absorbing I. V.s, and Esther is swallowing tube after tube via the nose and mouth interchangeably. Today she had a bag of mercury tied on the end of it to weight it down. After Christmas we'll be trading our ordeals.'

Harder to Smucker, 14 December 1965, MCC: 'I actually wish I could have joined you for your Thanksgiving Day meal. I'd give anything to sit down and enjoy, just once, a Thanksgiving Day meal which did not have turkey on the menu. On the other hand, please don't write and inform me what you were able to eat on Thanksgiving because I probably wouldn't have wanted that either. I certainly hope that drinking glass after glass of distilled water was not the extent of Mary's Thanksgiving feasting.'
24 I. Hacking, *The Taming of Chance* (Cambridge: Cambridge University Press, 1990).
25 This phrase shows that voluntary service was designed with younger Mennonites in mind – where idle time sowed mischief and disgruntlement – rather than retirees like Esther and Mary. In the early 1960s, the church introduced the 'older service' programme in which Esther and Mary participated.
26 Administrative report by Smucker and Warye, 6 October 1965, MCC.
27 L. Stark, 'The bureaucratic ethic and the spirit of bio-capitalism', in J. Bangham, J. Kaplan, and X. Chacko (eds), *Invisible Labor* (London: Rowman & Littlefield International, forthcoming). For an indispensable analysis of clinical labour, see M. Cooper and C. Waldby, *Clinical Labor: Tissue Donors and Research Subjects in the Global Bioeconomy* (Durham, NC: Duke University Press Books, 2014).
28 J. Butler, *Gender Trouble: Feminism and the Subversion of Identity* (New York: Routledge, 2006); K.M. Barad, *Meeting the Universe Halfway: Quantum Physics and the Entanglement of Matter and Meaning* (Durham, NC: Duke University Press, 2007).
29 A. Nelson, *Body and Soul: The Black Panther Party and the Fight against Medical Discrimination* (Minneapolis: University of Minnesota Press, 2011).

30 P.P. Reynolds, 'The federal government's use of title VI and Medicare to racially integrate hospitals in the United States, 1963 through 1967', *The American Journal of Public Health* 87:11 (1997), 1850–8.
31 J.H. Jones, *Bad Blood: The Tuskegee Syphilis Experiment* (New York: Free Press, revised edn, 1993); S. Reverby, *Examining Tuskegee: The Infamous Syphilis Study and its Legacy* (Chapel Hill: University of North Carolina Press, 2009); A. Brandt, 'Racism and research. The case of the Tuskegee syphilis study', *Hastings Center Report* 8:6 (1978), 21–9; K. Wailoo, *How Cancer Crossed the Color Line* (Oxford: Oxford University Press, 2011).
32 H.L. Brown, *Black and Mennonite. A Search for Identity* (Eugene: Wipf and Stock Publishers, 2001).
33 Administrative report by Smucker and Warye, 2 January 1966, MCC: 'Mary is no longer on the metabolic diet, but gets her meals from the regular kitchen. Although it is a constant diet and all must be eaten, it is not weighed quite so accurately, so she doesn't have to be quite so particular about licking the platter clean […] Esther is still on the metabolic diet (low calcium and low phosphorus) but will probably be changing to a high phosphorus diet next week after a few more tests. She had an intestinal biopsy last Friday and Mary had one today.'
34 Administrative report by Smucker and Warye, 6 October 1965, MCC: 'At the beginning of each cycle on the day the dose is given, we are "counted" by the machine for six hours and five days following for twenty minutes per day. This same cycle is repeated about every two weeks, allowing an interval between for the count to become normal again.'
35 M. Strathern, *Audit Cultures: Anthropological Studies in Accountability, Ethics and the Academy* (London: Routledge, 2000).
36 T.M. Porter, *Trust in Numbers: The Pursuit of Objectivity in Science and Public Life* (Princeton: Princeton University Press, 1995).
37 Administrative report by Smucker and Warye, 3 November 1965, MCC: 'at the present time our bank balance is $29.35 and, as you will see in the financial report, our October expenses are $70.53'. They also reported that Mr. Kehn was owed $40.
38 Administrative report by Smucker and Warye, 1 March 1965, MCC. Esther spoke with Harder around 1 March 1966. Since Harder spoke with Esther, rather than Mary, it implies that she was understood, of the pair, to be the unit leader although reports were often signed with both names. Harder addressed Esther in most of his obligatory but personal replies to the administrative reports to acknowledge he received them. For example, Harder wrote to Esther: 'Please send my personal greetings to Mary and all the boys at NIH.' Harder to Smucker, 7 March 1966, MCC.

39 Administrative report by Smucker and Warye, 10 October 1965, MCC: 'Mr. Kehn is also on a metabolic diet and is on the east wing of our floor. He has been assisting in the metabolic laboratory for some time.'
40 Harder to Smucker and Warye, 7 October 1965, MCC.
41 Administrative report by Smucker, 1 September 1966, MCC: 'I [Esther] have already delivered the goods to Victor, including the past year's financial reports, bank statements, and checks. I told him he could write the next reports, so this will be the last one from us. We've enjoyed the contacts but not the writing.'
42 Harder to Smucker and Warye, 7 October 1965, MCC.
43 Ibid.
44 Administrative report by Smucker, 1 September 1966, MCC.
45 D. Bouk, *How Our Days Became Numbered: Risk and the Rise of the Statistical Individual* (Chicago: University of Chicago Press, 2015); S.E. Igo, *The Averaged American: Surveys, Citizens, and the Making of a Mass Public* (Cambridge, MA: Harvard University Press, 2007).
46 Stark, *Behind Closed Doors*.
47 R. Aronowitz, *Risky Medicine: Our Quest to Cure Fear and Uncertainty* (Chicago: University of Chicago Press, 2015); J.A. Greene, *Prescribing by Numbers: Drugs and the Definition of Disease* (Baltimore: Johns Hopkins University Press, 2007).
48 G. Kutcher, *Contested Medicine: Cancer Research and the Military* (Chicago: University of Chicago Press, 2009); E. Welsome, *The Plutonium Files: America's Secret Medical Experiments in the Cold War* (New York: Dial Press, 1999).
49 S. Epstein, *Inclusion: The Politics of Difference in Medical Research* (Chicago: University of Chicago Press, 2007).
50 P. Starr, *The Social Transformation of American Medicine* (New York: Basic Books, 1982); D.P. Carpenter, *Reputation and Power: Organizational Image and Pharmaceutical Regulation at the FDA* (Princeton: Princeton University Press, 2010); D.A. Tobbell, *Pills, Power, and Policy: The Struggle for Drug Reform in Cold War America and Its Consequences* (Berkeley: University of California Press, 2011); M. Foucault, *The Birth of the Clinic: An Archaeology of Medical Perception* (New York: Vintage Books, 1994).

Part IV
Polity

11

States of healing in early modern Germany: Military health care and the management of manpower

Sebastian Pranghofer

The century after the end of the Thirty Years' War (1618–48) is usually characterised as a period of accelerated state formation within the Holy Roman Empire.[1] During this period, the close proximity and imbrication of civil and military medicine reshaped notions of military manpower as one of the key assets of the early modern state. Individual soldiers and their bodies were transformed into populations that could be measured and managed on a large scale.[2] Such developments fit with broader processes during the period, when population emerged both as a theoretical concept and a field of political intervention.[3] This culminated in the mid-eighteenth century in new evidence-based and statistical approaches to policy and politics.[4] Military health care and the management of manpower played a key role in this process. I argue that eighteenth-century military populations were considered to be assets and that their value was primarily based on their utility (*Nutzen*) in waging war. And within the context of cameralism, that utility can be interpreted in terms of a military economy of the body. To maximise the usefulness of military manpower, other principles such as order (*Ordnung*) and frugality (*Sparsamkeit*) had to be taken into account as well.

Lists and tables that were used in war offices, regiments, and field hospitals to account for soldiers and their physical state, and that are now discussed as 'paper technologies',[5] had the long-term epistemic effect of establishing the notion of the military population as a dynamic factor. To examine the relationship between military medicine and the management of military manpower, this chapter focuses on the Electorate of Hanover and the Kingdom of Prussia from the 1680s to the 1760s.[6] In both states, the connections between military reform, the institutionalisation of public health, and changing notions of individual and collective bodies can be traced in the administrative and medical practices of the military administration and field hospitals. These are documented in reports from companies, regiments, and field hospitals, officers' compensation claims, and the settlements over hired troops.

The serial and tabular format of many of these documents illustrates how numerical accounts of military personnel were the basis on which medical practitioners developed a quantitative view of patient populations. In order to place these documents in a political and institutional framework, the first part of this chapter sketches the development of Hanoverian military medicine and its administration from around 1680 to the end of the Seven Years' War. The second part will introduce the main tools used to administer manpower in the military and to account for sick and wounded soldiers. The increasing involvement of the state, growing armies, and an expanding bureaucracy required sophisticated administrative tools to ensure the exact measurement and efficient use of human resources. The third part discusses mid-eighteenth-century statistics in military medicine and how they affected medical knowledge. The final section will show how those statistics fundamentally reshaped medical notions of the body and conclude that the medical and accounting practices of early modern militaries created a specific economy of the body.

Accounting for care and provision in Hanoverian military hospitals

Although standing armies had already begun to take shape in the Guelph territories during the Thirty Years' War, their closer integration into the state only came with the military reforms of the second half of the seventeenth century. In the principality of Calenberg, a war office (*Kriegskanzlei*) was created in 1680, centralising administrative responsibility for the army. New standing orders were released in 1683, which introduced a consistent hierarchy and chain of command for the army and tied it more closely to the state by implementing a system of military justice, whose representatives were appointed as civil servants.[7] The army grew continuously during the last two decades of the seventeenth century. When the future king of Great Britain, Georg August of Brunswick-Lüneburg (1660–1727), inherited the principality of Lüneburg-Grubenhagen with its army in 1705, the Hanoverian army of 22,000 men was one of the largest military forces in the Holy Roman Empire.[8]

As part of the military reforms in the Guelph territories, efforts were made to improve care for the soldiers. While a hospital for invalids was established in the principality of Lüneburg-Grubenhagen in 1679 with an endowment from Prince Georg Wilhelm (1624–1705), the first hospital arrangements in the principality of Calenberg were made in 1695. In Celle (Lüneburg-Grubenhagen) the money was used to build a hospital and cover the costs of lodging invalids, while in Calenberg the towns of Eldagsen, Pattensen, and Springe were, in lieu of billeting, subsidised to provide housing for invalid soldiers.[9] Control over the hospital's economy was exercised by commissaries from the war office and their secretaries.[10] They had to account for larger groups of servicemen outside the regimental economy and to settle bills with other departments, suppliers, local authorities, as well as the regiments, where contributions to the hospital coffers were regularly deducted from soldiers' pay.[11] Hospital officials also had to keep track of sick and wounded soldiers and make sure that, in case of recovery, they were struck off the hospital lists and their regiments notified. According to the 1728 instructions for the hospital secretaries, they also had to keep receipt books to document and justify pensions and other payments and submit annual accounts of the hospital's income and expenses.[12]

The hospitals for invalids provided support and care for soldiers permanently unfit for service. Soldiers suffering from acute diseases or injuries, however, were looked after during peace time by their company surgeons, the regimental surgeon, or local town physicians, who were often responsible for the garrison. Sick and wounded men were usually treated in their quarters and soldiers on leave who fell ill had their medical expenses reimbursed from the regimental medical coffer.[13] During campaigns, this system was routinely expanded and the care for sick and wounded soldiers was provided in camp by the company and regimental surgeons as well as in temporary field hospitals.[14] The administrative practices and control mechanisms in the field hospitals were similar to those in the Hanoverian hospitals for invalids. The director of the field hospitals and his secretaries also had to keep patient lists that were checked against regimental lists.[15] The hospital administration was responsible for the patients' well-being and settled its accounts with the commissariat. While the fiscal responsibility for the field hospitals lay with the director and commissariat, medical care was supervised by the physician and surgeon general, who were responsible to the commanding general and the war office.[16]

During the late seventeenth century and at the beginning of the War of the Spanish Succession (1701–14), field hospitals would usually be set up by the state or authority on whose payroll the Hanoverian regiments were fighting. During the wars against the Turks in Greece in the 1680s, for example, contracts required the Republic of Venice to care for the sick and wounded Hanoverian soldiers in its pay.[17] During the war of the Spanish Succession, Hanoverian troops in English pay and fighting with Marlborough's army were treated in the English hospital, which was run by an English contractor.[18] The Hanoverian regiments operating in the Netherlands in Dutch pay were treated in Dutch hospitals, which were also run by contractors – albeit with some involvement from Hanoverian doctors, such as the court physician Ernst Christoph Wolff (1674–1737), who were responsible for providing general medical care and supervising the hospital.[19]

The hospitals in the Netherlands during the War of the Spanish Succession were supervised by a commissary, did not cause visible frictions, and seem to have operated smoothly during the first years of the war. However, from 1709, the war office in Hanover, its commissary in the Netherlands, Johann Georg Craushaar (1657–1734),[20] the commanding generals Friedrich Johann von Bothmer (1658–1729) and Cuno Josua von Bülow (1658–1733), as well as the Hanoverian ambassador in The Hague, Elias von Klinggräff (d. 1717), began to discuss the possibility of establishing independent hospitals for the Hanoverian troops in the Netherlands. After concerns had been raised about the losses and poor quality of care in Dutch hospitals, in January 1710 the government in Hanover instructed Bothmer to raise the issue with the Dutch government and discuss the possibility of field hospitals in the Netherlands under the direct control of the war office.[21] In a letter to Bothmer, the war office made it clear that 'we are, for a better conservation of those people [i e. sick and wounded Hanoverian soldiers treated in Dutch hospitals], prepared to take them away from the Dutch hospitals and establish a hospital of our own troops'.[22] Bothmer was further instructed to approach the Dutch government with the suggestion of establishing field hospitals in the Netherlands under the control of the Hanoverian commissariat. The war office seemed to be confident that, given more efficient hospital administration and accounting, it could provide hospital care more cheaply than the Dutch contractors. In negotiations with the Dutch, it hoped that by promising to charge them only two-thirds of their previous expenses, the government in The Hague would agree to a field hospital under Hanoverian control.[23]

New arrangements were agreed over the summer of 1710 that allowed the Hanoverian war office to establish its own hospitals. To cover the costs, the war office would receive a daily rate from the Dutch for each sick or injured soldier treated in the hospital.[24] There is no direct evidence of how the daily rates were calculated for the Hanoverian hospitals in the Netherlands, but in the English hospital during the War of the Spanish Succession the rates were roughly based on the current costs of food.[25] During its first year of operation, the Hanoverian field hospitals incurred higher expenses than the war office expected and was plagued by organisational problems. In a memorandum from 1711, the commissary Craushaar complained about logistical problems resulting from an inadequately equipped hospital train, about problems recruiting qualified personnel, and about sloppy bookkeeping.[26] However, inaccurate accounting was not simply caused by incompetence or negligence, but also by an attempt to defraud the Dutch government.

According to another memorandum, Craushaar first complained in April 1711 that the Hanoverian army in the Netherlands kept many sick and wounded soldiers with the regiments instead of sending them to the hospital. At the same time, these men were put on the hospital lists in order to elicit payment from the Dutch.[27] Craushaar worried that the Dutch might detect this attempt to defraud them, warning that their civil servants were highly skilled in accounting and dealing with hospital bills. These worries were confirmed when the Dutch initially refused to accept the Hanoverian hospital bills, and a renewal of the contract for the Hanoverian hospitals in the Netherlands for the campaign year 1712 almost failed due to prolonged negotiations over the settlement of outstanding bills.[28] Craushaar's worries that the Dutch administrators might detect the attempts from Hanoverian commanders to defraud them were not unfounded. The problem of fraudulent manpower accounting was widespread and a common theme in early modern military handbooks.[29] In particular, officers often accounted for more men than actually served under their command and soldiers frequently sold equipment and then claimed expenses for its loss.[30]

Embezzlement was also a problem in military hospitals. In the case of the Hanoverian field hospitals in the Netherlands during the war of the Spanish Succession, the former hospital clerk Nieport accused the physician general Wolff of fraud. In a letter to the war office from April 1711, he claimed that after he had been unfairly dismissed from the hospital Wolff had cheated him by retaining part of his salary. Nieport also claimed that Wolff had repeatedly channelled hospital funds into his own pocket and was an incompetent accountant and administrator.[31] After returning from the Netherlands, Nieport raised further concerns about Wolff's behaviour, accusing him, the entrepreneur Ruffini, and the abbess of Byloque in Ghent, of having cheated the war office by claiming payment for more sick and wounded soldiers in the hospital at the monastery of Byloque than had actually been treated there in 1707.[32]

New hospital regulations, including detailed rules for the accounting of daily rates, were a direct response to such disputes. Significantly, in both the previous contract with the entrepreneur and the new hospital regulations from July 1711, only the daily rations were directly related to the classification and medical treatment of patients, with different diets being prescribed for patients able to enjoy full portions and for weaker ones requiring a special diet.[33] Standard arrangements were also required for the logistics needed to transport patients and supplies, as well as for hospital administration and personnel, for which the physician general Wolff and the surgeon general Kannengießer were responsible. Although targeting very different subjects, these regulations reflected the financial concerns of the war office and its interest in the cost-efficient management of manpower and the prevention of losses. The aim was essentially to prevent fraud and avoid unnecessary expenses, but still to allow hospitals to provide adequate medical care for sick and wounded soldiers.

Practical issues concerning the hospital's daily business, such as supplies and medical treatment, remained in the hands of doctors and administrators. Successive regulations for Hanoverian field hospitals during the Wars of the Austrian Succession (1740–48) and the Seven Years' War indicate that field hospitals were growing in size and complexity.[34] The regulations governed a growing number of officials with specialised responsibilities, set out administrative processes in increasing detail, and provided detailed instructions on the use and maintenance of hospital equipment. However, responsibility for practical measures – such as transporting sick and wounded soldiers, arranging hospital wards, or treating patients – were left to hospital staff.

Accounting practices and the management of manpower

When the war office in Hanover assumed control over the field hospitals in the Netherlands during the War of the Spanish Succession, the bodies of sick and wounded servicemen became directly subject to state power. To manage this human asset, a whole range of administrative tools, similar to those used in bookkeeping and accounting, were put to use. At different levels within the military, from the war office down to the field hospitals and military units, information was collected about soldiers. For example, casualty lists were kept for Hanoverian regiments that fought with Marlborough's army during 1704 and 1705. They classified battle casualties into 'wounded' (*Blessierte*) and 'badly wounded' (*hart Blessierte*),[35] but generally gave no further hints as to the nature of the injuries. Only two lists from the de Luc infantry regiment, compiled after the battles of Schellenberg and Blenheim in July and August 1704, provided details about soldiers' injuries, distinguishing between those who had been killed on the battlefield, those who had died from their wounds in hospital, or those who were badly wounded or just wounded. Most casualties and deaths in the category 'badly wounded' resulted from gunshot wounds in which bullets had gone through or were lodged in the body. The majority of injuries in the third category 'wounded' seem to have come from minor traumas or shots that had only grazed the soldiers.[36] However, the main purpose of the categorisation was not to gather information on the frequency of different types of injuries, but to calculate compensation. According to an aggregate table of compensation costs, badly wounded soldiers were paid twice their monthly pay, while other wounded soldiers were compensated simply in the amount of their monthly pay.[37]

The administrative tools used in the field hospitals for financial purposes had their origins in the economy of late medieval and early modern municipal hospitals, where admission lists and accounting books were used to balance the costs of board and treatment against revenues.[38] In early modern field hospitals, such lists were kept because the expenses associated with sustaining and treating sick and wounded soldiers would be covered by the war chest and no longer by the soldier's regiment. During the War of the Spanish Succession, the hospital lists recording soldiers from the Bothmer and Bernstorff regiments were used to calculate the expenses for soldiers treated in the hospital based on the number of days during which board and medical treatment were provided.[39] These were collected together with other accounts of the field hospital's income and expenses.[40] In the process of negotiating hospital payments between the British government and the Hanoverian regiments, the hospital accounts would have provided important information to settle outstanding bills.

However, the collection and processing of data on military manpower was not only of financial value, but of moral value as well. Standardised accounting for soldiers was an important administrative tool for controlling costs because expenses for provisions could only be claimed for men who were effectively present. Military handbooks advised administrators how to make sure that the number of men was correct. They were to check the returns and, in cases of suspected fraud, visit the suspicious units.[41] There is evidence that, at least since the Thirty Years War in Germany, standardised documents and procedures were used to account for manpower in the armies.[42] Commissaries and war secretaries were expected to keep 'reliable lists and accounts of manpower [...], complete the same weekly or at least monthly from the special lists of the muster secretaries [...], and attach the same so that we can see each time how strong our army is'.[43]

By the mid-eighteenth century, recordkeeping and submitting returns were standardised procedures during campaigns and were used for operational and strategic planning.[44] Regimental administrators were required to submit monthly returns detailing casualties and differentiating them by rank, type of loss, and including both men and horses; these in turn were based on regular reports from each company.[45] The returns formed the basis for monthly tables that provided an overview of the army's effective strength. At least since the mid-eighteenth century, such lists and tables had come to be regarded as providing vital information about military manpower. The war office in Hanover, for example, collected all available monthly tables from May 1744 to February 1748 into a series and copied them into a journal of important documents and information related to the War of the Austrian Succession (Figure 11.1).[46] Such data made manpower trends visible and

Military health care and the management of manpower 291

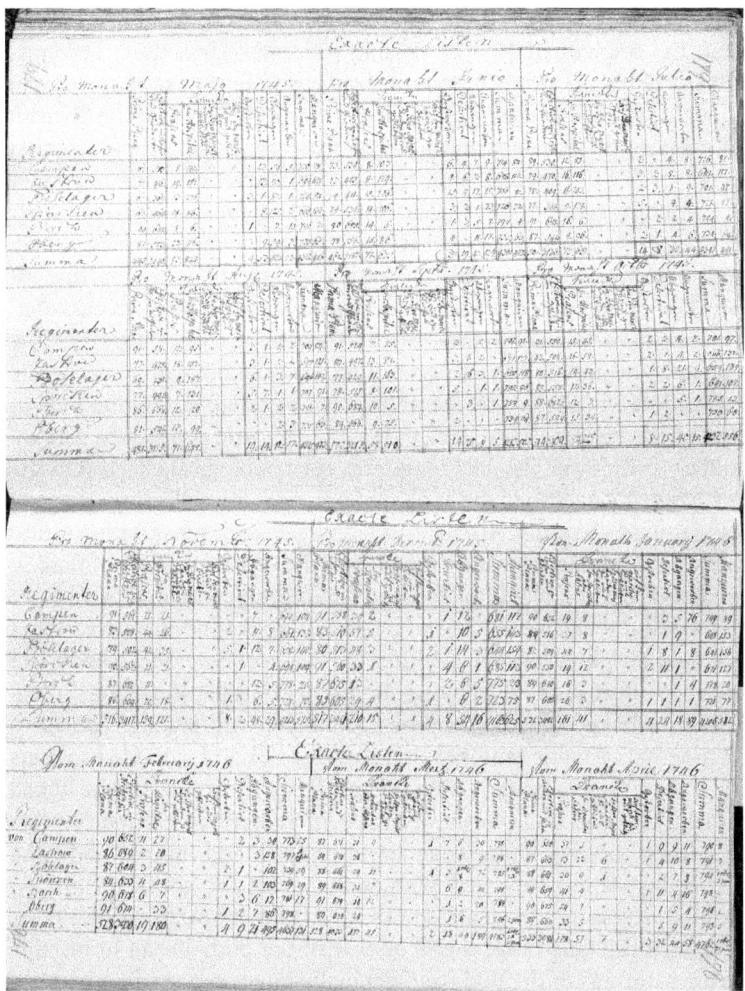

11.1 Aggregate manpower tables of the Hanoverian regiments in the Netherlands from May 1745 to April 1746.

potentially allowed medical officers and military commanders to relate them to particular developments and events during the war.[47]

The administrative tools used to manage manpower in early modern armies reflected the bureaucratic and economic interests shared by military administrators, field commanders, and the state. They facilitated the implementation of reliable processes for settling accounts and efficiently managing manpower and funds. For the principalities of Lüneburg-Grubenhagen and Calenberg during the War of the Spanish Succession, the casualty and hospital lists also recorded information about other data, such as hospital bills. Such practices were necessary in a military economy in which commanding officers managed their companies and regiments in order to extract profit and thereby sustain their own livelihood as military entrepreneurs. For the government in Hanover, tighter control over the military and greater accountability were used to justify subsidies and ensure a regular income. The financial and moral aim of accounting for military manpower was a well-ordered military and the prevention of fraud, all for the benefit of the early modern state. However, collecting and processing data on military manpower also had long-term epistemological effects. On the one hand, it established the tools and practices for collecting relatively standardised quantitative data on a large scale and transforming it into viable information. On the other hand, the representation of data in serialised lists and tables made trends in military manpower visible.

During the eighteenth century, the military's administrative offices and field hospitals became key sites for this economy of the body and began to affect medical thinking. In the field hospitals, soldiers' compensation linked together military, economic, and medical concerns. Regimental casualties and hospital costs for sick and wounded soldiers had to be compensated for. Medical and disability expenses were linked to field hospitals and pension funds, which ascribed monetary value to soldiers' bodies. Knowledge about the sick and injured body, the probability of recovery, and predictions about the course of disease were all necessary to calculate both military manpower and the costs of war. In the long term, this economy of the body began to reshape medical notions of the body and gradually integrated medical practice into the management of manpower. From the 1740s there is growing evidence that medical officers began to use data and observations gathered during military campaigns and from hospital records to describe and understand epidemiological and aetiological correlations.

One of the first and most influential medical authors to use such methods was the physician general to the British Army during the War of the Austrian Succession, John Pringle (1707–82).[48] In his *Observations on the Diseases of an Army*, Pringle first gave a general description of the environment and endemic diseases in the Netherlands, followed by an account of the conditions under which the army operated, and its morbidity and mortality rates during the campaigns of 1742 to 1748. For example, Pringle observed that morbidity rates in 1742 had been twice as high (about 18 per cent in July) for the two companies billeted in a lower and damper part of Ghent, as compared to the rest of the garrison, where he estimated morbidity at between 8.4 and 9 per cent. This situation quickly improved when the affected troops were moved to new barracks in better conditions.[49] In the following year, the British army suffered from several outbreaks of infectious diseases and was worst affected by a dysentery epidemic after the Battle of Dettingen on 27 June 1743. Over the summer and autumn, the army had suffered continuously from dysentery and 'remitting fevers' caused by bad weather, which led to an unusually high mortality rate of almost 50 per cent in the hospital at Feckenheim and left the army as a whole with a morbidity rate of 23 per cent at the end of the campaign. Under more favourable conditions in the following year, morbidity rates were down to 17 per cent at the end of the campaign.[50]

In the second part of his book, Pringle claimed that based on his empirical observations he was not only able to classify diseases and to identify their causes and propose preventive measures, but also to calculate 'what number of men may be relied on for service, at different times of the year'.[51] He related the general health of soldiers to their environment (hot, cold, wet or dry), living conditions, and personal behaviour (air, diet, rest and motion, sleep, cleanliness).[52] Based on these observations, he suggested preventive measures to improve conditions in garrisons, camps, and field hospitals, for example by instituting better sanitation and ventilation as well as healthier diets and moderation in the physical strain put on soldiers.[53] Pringle also made general claims about morbidity in the British army and observed, for example, that an early start of the campaign in April resulted in morbidity of about 3.7 per cent after one month, which was on average about 25 per cent higher than morbidity in years when campaigning did not start until May. Furthermore, he drew conclusions about seasonal variations of morbidity and the prevalence of specific diseases, for example, with dysentery in decline in the autumn but remitting fevers still increasing until the first frost.[54]

Pringle's statistical observations conformed to widely held views about the prevalence and course of diseases in early modern armies.

Indeed, contemporaries routinely identified dysentery and fevers as the most common conditions in the field.[55] His aetiology and therapeutic approach were deeply rooted in humoral theory and the idea of the *sex res non naturales*.[56] His focus on environmental factors and preventive measures against the outbreak of infectious diseases had long been adopted by medical authors writing on military medicine.[57] However, unlike his predecessors, Pringle used quantitative data to describe the outbreak and course of diseases. Moreover, he not only calculated the relative morbidity of an army, but also correlated it with environmental factors and advanced claims about typical variations in morbidity during campaigns. However, in the second and third part of his book, where Pringle discussed the diseases that most commonly afflicted an army, he provided no statistical information on the effects of preventive measures and medical treatment. While Pringle was able to offer an epidemiology based on the statistical interpretation of morbidity and mortality in relation to environmental factors, his traditional views on disease causation prevented him from developing an approach that directly related outcomes to specific preventive measures and therapeutic interventions.

Changing views on patient populations

Medical officers like Pringle kept their own medical journals in which they collected information on morbidity and mortality, but also on other aspects of military life that might have affected the health of an army.[58] In the British and other armies, observations on sick and injured soldiers were made largely in field hospitals. The collected information was based on both military records and traditional forms of medical note-taking such as medical diaries and case histories,[59] like those published by leading surgeons and physicians of the Prussian army during the Seven Years' War.[60] In addition, ward journals provided further information on the diagnosis, treatment, and history of each hospitalised patient. Such journals were mandatory (for example in the Charité hospital in Berlin, which also served as a teaching hospital for military surgeons) and were used in Prussian field hospitals at least from the Seven Years' War.[61]

From the middle of the eighteenth century, the wide availability of data and new approaches such as Pringle's statistical interpretation

11.2 Monthly return from the Prussian field hospitals in Saxony during the Seven Years' War for the period from 6 November to 2 December 1760.

of wartime morbidity and mortality began to change clinical knowledge and practice. This is particularly evident in the case of Prussia, where army surgeons and doctors used data on morbidity and mortality in the field hospitals to predict convalescence and make decisions about medical treatment. Initially, most Prussian measures designed to maintain soldiers' health – as well as Hanoverian regulations on camp hygiene, winter quarters, and hospitals – were based on common practice, while the recording of patient numbers was motivated economically and not by any desire to understand epidemiological causes and effects. However, in Prussia, routine hospital reports began to change notions about hospital patients (Figure 11.2).

Hospital returns usually gave no details about how many patients died from injuries, let alone from disease or from what kinds of disease. Most of the time they merely accounted for patients in two categories – officers and men – at the beginning and at the end of the reporting period, as well as convalescents, invalids, and the deceased.[62] The hospital returns were usually accompanied by a letter in which the physician general or director of the field hospital recounted extraordinary events in the hospital and commented on rates of morbidity and mortality. For example, in the letter accompanying the return from Torgau for November 1760, the physician general of the Prussian army,

Christian Andreas Cothenius (1708–89), not only cited improved conditions in the field hospital to explain higher recovery rates, but also predicted the number of convalescents. Based on his observations and barring the outbreak of a fever epidemic, he would be able to send another 2,500 men currently suffering from injuries back to the army within the next month, another 1,500 men within three months, as well as a further 650 men currently suffering from illnesses over the next two months.[63] Cothenius did not correlate specific conditions and their treatment with overall morbidity and mortality. Instead, he used the data and his observations in the field hospital to describe developments in the past and make predictions about future recoveries, all the while taking into account the possibility of future epidemics. Counting bodies was a part of Cothenius's medical practice that increased his and his commanders' knowledge of manpower and their ability to act upon that knowledge.

Others, like the surgeon general to the Prussian army during the Seven Years War, Johann Ulrich Bilguer (1720–96), drew on their experience in field hospitals and on statistics to support their case. In his book on treating wounds by avoiding amputation, he claimed that radical amputation led to higher mortality rates than conservative treatments that paid careful attention to patients and regularly cleaned and dressed their wounds.[64] Bilguer supported his claims not just with case histories, but also with numbers. To provide his readers with more context, he included the number of recoveries and deaths in the field hospital in Torgau, where he had served. During its existence, the hospital treated 6,618 patients, of whom 84 per cent recovered and 9.9 per cent died. Of those patients who died, 38 per cent had been treated for injuries. Bilguer claimed that with his treatment, seriously wounded soldiers had a 50 per cent chance of survival, while only a third of patients who had undergone an amputation survived. According to Bilguer, this was even more remarkable because among the 245 patients in Torgau who had purportedly died of injuries, some might have died from fevers rather than their wounds.[65]

This example illustrates how medical knowledge about the treatment of serious wounds emerged under specific wartime conditions. Bilguer's argument was based on an aggregation of numerous case histories. And the therapeutic success of his conservative treatment was measured and related to the outcome of amputations and to data on overall mortality in the field hospital. While Bilguer used numbers to support his claims about the better outcomes of his treatment, he did not statistically correlate the effects of his treatment with general morbidity and mortality in the field hospital. This was partly because an understanding of the advanced methods of medical statistics that would have enabled practitioners to make such connections was only in its infancy.[66] This also explains why Bilguer failed to provide data to correlate observations on general morbidity and mortality with the different survival rates claimed for patients who received conservative treatment as opposed to those who had undergone amputation.

When Bilguer used numbers to argue for his more conservative approach to the treatment of battle injuries, he was not only making a point about the efficiency of medical treatment, but also following an economic rationale. When he differentiated between half and fully invalid soldiers, recovered and deceased soldiers, his valuation of the body was based on its monetisation and accountability within the economy of the military and state bureaucracy. Just like Pringle and Cothenius, Bilguer subscribed to a quantitative view of medicine and the body. From their perspective as surgeons and physicians general, they looked beyond the individual patient's body and focused on specific large populations. This seems to indicate a major development in mid-eighteenth-century military medicine, when medical practices became part of a larger economy of the body within military administration. Beyond the treatment of injured soldiers, medicine and the calculation and prediction of hospital reports became more important for military administrators, while medicine in turn began to integrate the economic rationale of managing manpower into medical practice. In theory, military medicine now had the ability to correlate preventive measures and therapeutic interventions by exploiting the manpower calculations used by military and state administrators. Therefore, it was now possible to move away from an economy of the body focused on the costs of writing off losses, and towards an economy of the body in which the cost-efficiency of treatment could potentially be factored into a budget.

Body economy, military health care, and the management of manpower

During the late seventeenth and early eighteenth centuries, an economy of the body was established in the Hanoverian military based on the ability to monetise manpower losses. It conformed with the economic values of cameralism in both a financial and a physical sense. While field hospitals were expected to return soldiers on a regular basis without unduly taxing scarce resources, soldiers' bodies were valued based on their condition, recoverability, and fitness. Gathering and cross-referencing data fundamentally changed the notion and valuation of soldiers' bodies. From a constant factor that had to be written off completely, they became a variable factor that could be classified as fit for service, sick, invalid, wounded in hospital, dead, or deserter. Such differentiations made it possible to estimate future military manpower (by evaluating hospital or regimental returns) and improve the strategic planning and management of that manpower.

While the motivation for collecting and processing quantitative manpower data might initially have been primarily economic and embedded in the bureaucratic rationale of a centralised military administration, there is evidence that from the mid-eighteenth century such information began to change how medical practitioners perceived hospital populations. Field hospitals were the main site for this change. Medical officers developed a sense of the dynamic nature of hospital populations that allowed them to identify quantifiable trends in morbidity and mortality and relate them to hospital arrangements, hygienic conditions, and treatment. Drawing on case histories, ward journals, and other records, patient figures were aggregated to larger populations and information about patients' injuries and treatment was transformed into quantifiable data and contributed to further developments in vital and medical statistics.

The paper technologies used to record and account for soldiers' bodies in early modern military administration and field hospitals created a specific notion of the body and reflected the desire of administrators to ensure a comprehensive overview and control of the military. As technologies of power, they shaped a view of the body as a calculable entity and were at the heart of the formation of 'bio-power' in the eighteenth century.[67] As the cases of Hanover and Prussia have shown, such policies were not just motivated by the consolidation of territorial rule and the increase of military force, but also dependent on economic factors. Thus, the quantification and monetisation of soldiers' bodies constituted an economy of the body in a very literal sense and can be regarded as the foundations of a larger bio-economy, in which individual bodies as well as whole populations were subjected to a utilitarian economic rationale and turned into military assets.

Acknowledgments

A previous version of this chapter was presented at the research seminar of the History Department at the University of Saskatchewan (Canada). I would particularly like to thank Matthew Neufeld, James Kennaway and my colleagues in Hamburg, Jutta Nowosadtko, and Kai Lohsträter, for their patience and helpful comments on this chapter in its different developmental stages.

Notes

1 J. Burkhardt, *Vollendung und Neuorientierung des frühmodernen Reiches 1648–1763* (Stuttgart: Klett-Cotta, 2006), pp. 25–54, 170–208. For a critical discussion of the teleological implications of paradigms such as state formation, military revolution, and the fiscal-military state, see S. Pranghofer, 'The early modern medical-military complex: The wider context of the relationship between military, medicine, and the state', *Canadian Journal of History* 51 (2016), 451–72, here 452–6.
2 E. Charters, 'L'histoire de la quantification: La guerre franco-anglaise et le développement des statistiques médicales', *Dix-huitième siècle* 47 (2015), 21–38; M. Neufeld, 'The biopolitics of manning the Royal Navy in Late Stuart England', *Journal of British Studies* 56 (2017), 506–31.
3 J. Nipperdey, *Die Erfindung der Bevölkerungspolitik: Staat, politische Theorie und Population in der Frühen Neuzeit* (Göttingen: Vandenhoeck & Ruprecht, 2012).
4 L. Behrisch, *Die Berechnung der Glückseligkeit: Statistik und Politik in Deutschland und Frankreich im späten Ancien Régime* (Ostfildern: Thorbecke Verlag, 2016), pp. 42–56.
5 V. Hess and J.A. Mendelssohn, 'Case and series: Medical knowledge and paper technology, 1600–1900', *History of Science* 47 (2010), 287–314.
6 In 1692, Ernst August of Brunswick-Lüneburg, reigning duke in the principality of Calenberg since 1679 and the father of George I, was raised to the status of elector. However, the principalities of Calenberg and Lüneburg-Grubenhagen were not united until 1705, after the death of his older brother, Georg Ludwig of Brunswick-Lüneburg. When I speak of Hanover in this chapter, I am usually referring to territories under the rule of the electorate of Brunswick-Lüneburg in their different configurations and sub-divisions as well as their predecessors. Only when necessary will I

differentiate between the different principalities under the rule of different Guelphic dynastic lines.
7 R. Pröve, *Stehendes Heer und städtische Gesellschaft im 18. Jahrhundert: Göttingen und seine Militärbevölkerung 1713–1756* (Munich: Oldenbourg, 1995), pp. 16–19.
8 P.H. Wilson, *German Armies: War and German Politics, 1648–1806* (London: Routledge, 1998), p. 162.
9 C.-H. Colshorn, *Die Hospitalkassen der hannoverschen Armee: Ein Vorläufer der Sozialversicherung seit 1680* (Hildesheim: August Lax Buchhandlung, 1970), pp. 16–17.
10 Ibid., pp. 77–9.
11 Ibid., pp. 47–9.
12 Ibid., pp. 142–4.
13 H. Deichert, *Geschichte des Medizinalwesens im Gebiet des ehemaligen Königreichs Hannover* (Hanover: Hahnsche Buchhandlung, 1908), pp. 298–9.
14 Niedersächsisches Landesarchiv Hannover (hereafter NLA Hann) 47 I, Nr. 354/1–6, six boxes with personnel files and other documents from the Hanoverian field hospitals during the Seven Years' War, 1756–63.
15 NLA Hann, Cal. Br. 16, Nr. 771, hospital regulations for the Hanoverian hospitals in the Netherlands from July 1711, fols 143r–144v; NLA Hann, Hann. 47 I, Nr. 354/1, regulations for the field hospital of the Hanoverian army, 29 March 1744, fols 4r–14v.
16 Deichert, *Geschichte des Medizinalwesens*, pp. 306–9.
17 Contract with the Republic of Venice over the provision of auxiliary troops, 3/13 December 1684, in A. Schwencke, *Geschichte der hannoverschen Truppen in Griechenland, 1685–1689: Zugleich als Beitrag zur Geschichte der Türkenkriege* (Hanover: Hahnsche Buchhandlung, 1854), pp. 181–91, especially p. 185.
18 E. Gruber von Arni, *Hospital Care and the British Standing Army, 1660–1714* (Aldershot: Ashgate, 2006), p. 112.
19 NLA Hann, Cal. Br. 16, Nr. 771, instructions for the court and field physician Wolff, 19 March 1711, fol. 254r–261r, here fol. 254r–254v. Evidence showing that medical care was provided by the power on whose payroll the Hanoverian regiments were fighting is implicit in the contracts with the Dutch and the British governments over the provision of subsidiary and auxiliary troops, see A. Schwencke, *Geschichte der Hannoverschen Truppen im Spanischen Erbfolgekriege 1701–1714* (Hanover: Helwingsche Hofbuchhandlung, 1862), pp. 269–74 (contract with the Netherlands, 18 May 1701, here p. 270) and pp. 275–9 (contract with Great Britain, 10 July 1701, here p. 276).
20 The war commissary Craushaar played a key role as controller and administrator in the service of the Hanoverian war office in the field. In early

modern armies, the commissaries represented the interests of the government vis-à-vis the military, especially when on campaign. They were involved in all decisions about the management of armies, especially the mobilisation and distribution of financial and other resources. On the commissariat in general, see O. Hintze, 'The commissary and his significance in general administrative history: A comparative study', in O. Hintze, *The Historical Essays of Otto Hintze*, edited with an introduction by Felix Gilbert (New York: Oxford University Press, 1975), pp. 267–301. The war commissariat in the field has so far received little attention from historians, see K. Saito, 'Der Kriegskommissar der bayerischen Armee während des dreißigjährigen Krieges', *Militär und Gesellschaft in der Frühen Neuzeit* 17 (2013), 117–23.

21 NLA Hann, Cal. Br. 16, Nr. 771, letter from the privy council in Hanover to the general von Bothmer in The Hague, 24 January 1710, fol. 14r–17r.

22 '[S]o sind wir zur beßeren Conservirung solcher Leut gewillet selbige aus den Holländischen Hospitälern wegzunehmen und ein eigenes Hospital unserer Trouppen aufzurichten' (author's translation), NLA Hann, Cal. Br. 16, Nr. 771, letter from the War Office in Hanover to general von Bothmer in The Hague, 24 June 1710, fol. 14r–17r, here fol. 14r–14v.

23 NLA Hann, Cal. Br. 16, Nr. 771, letter from the War Office in Hanover to general von Bothmer in The Hague, 24 June 1710, fol. 14r–17r, here fol. 15r–17r.

24 NLA Hann, Cal. Br. 16, Nr. 771, contract between the States General of the Netherlands and Hanover on financing the field hospitals, 17 October 1710, fol. 54r–54v.

25 Gruber von Arni, *Hospital Care and the British Standing Army*, pp. 122–3.

26 NLA Hann, Cal. Br. 16, Nr. 771, memorandum by the commissary Craushaar for the War Office in Hanover concerning the Hanoverian field hospitals in the Netherlands, undated [between April and September 1711], fol. 104r–107v.

27 NLA Hann, Cal. Br. 16, Nr. 771, memorandum by the commissary Craushaar for the War Office in Hanover concerning the Hanoverian field hospitals in the Netherlands, 10 April 1711, fol. 76r–80v. Hospital lists from the War of the Spanish Succession have not survived for the hospitals in the Netherlands, but they have survived for the Hanoverian soldiers treated in English hospitals, see NLA Hann, Celle Br. 13, Nr. 212, lists of sick and wounded soldiers from the Hanoverian regiments Bothmer and Bernstorff in the hospital in Nördlingen, 6 July to 30 October 1704, fol. 3r–6v.

28 NLA Hann, Cal. Br. 16, Nr. 771, letter from the commisary Craushaar in Antwerp to the War Office in Hanover, mid-December 1711, fol. 101r–102v.

29 F. Redlich, *The German Military Enterpriser and His Work Force: A Study in European Economic and Social History*, 2 vols (Wiesbaden: Franz Steiner, 1964–65), here vol. 1, pp. 368–71.
30 P. Burschel, *Söldner im Nordwestdeutschland des 16. und 17. Jahrhunderts: Sozialgeschichtliche Studien* (Göttingen: Vandenhoeck & Ruprecht, 1994), pp. 120–9.
31 NLA Hann, Cal. Br. 16, Nr. 771, letter from Nieport in Hanover to the War Office in Hanover, 16 April 1711, fol. 95r–98v.
32 NLA Hann, Cal. Br. 16, Nr. 771, extracts from a memorandum by Nieport for the War Office in Hanover, May 1711, fol. 222r–222v.
33 NLA Hann, Cal. Br. 16, Nr. 771, contract with the entrepreneur Ruffini concerning the provisions for sick and wounded Hanoverian soldiers in the hospitals, 1 June 1708, fol. 4r–5r; and NLA Hann, Cal. Br. 16, Nr. 771, hospital regulations for the Hanoverian field hospital, July 1711, fol. 143r–144v.
34 NLA Hann, Hann 47 I, Nr. 354/1, regulations for the field hospital of the Hanoverian army, 29 March 1744, fol. 4r–14v.
35 NLA Hann, Cal. Br. 16, Nr. 726, lists of losses and other documents related to the campaign of 1704 during the War of the Spanish Succession.
36 NLA Hann, Cal. Br. 16, Nr. 726, list of losses during the battle of Schellenberg from the regiment de Luc, 2 July 1704, fol. 28r–28v; and NLA Hann, Cal. Br. 16, Nr. 726, list of losses during the battle of Schellenberg from the regiment le Luc, 13 August 1704, fol. 38r–39v.
37 NLA Hann, Cal. Br. 16, Nr. 726, overview of the compensation costs for wounded officers and soldiers from 1704, fol. 14r–16r.
38 M.T. Sneider, 'The treasury of the poor: Hospital finance in sixteenth- and seventeenth-century Bologna', in J. Henderson, P. Horden, and A. Pastore (eds), *The Impact of Hospitals 300–2000* (Oxford: Peter Lang, 2007), pp. 93–115; B.S. Fleck, 'Quellen zu Insassen westfälischer Hospitäler im 15. und 16. Jahrhundert', in G. Drossbach (ed.), *Hospitäler in Mittelalter und Früher Neuzeit, Frankreich, Deutschland und Italien. Eine vergleichende Geschichte* (München: Oldenbourg, 2007), pp. 25–39; F. Dross, 'Their daily bread: Managing hospital finances in early modern Germany – a microhistorical approach', in L. Abreu and S. Sheard (eds), *Hospital Life: Theory and Practice from the Medieval to the Modern* (Oxford: Peter Lang, 2013), pp. 49–66.
39 NLA Hann, Celle Br. 13, Nr. 212, lists of sick and wounded soldiers from the Hanoverian regiments Bothmer and Bernstorff in the hospital in Nördlingen, 6 July to 30 October 1704, fol. 3r–6v.
40 NLA Hann, Celle Br. 13, Nr. 212, hospital accounts for the regiments Bothmer and Barnstorff for the treatment of their sick and wounded soldiers in the hospital in Nördlingen, 1704.

41 A. Pisetzky von Kranichfeld, *Kriegs-Secretarius, in welchem alle vorfallender Belegenheiten übliche, und bey denen Kriegs-Cancelleyen gewöhnliche Concept, viel zu dieser Materie gehörige Fragen, Anmerckungen und practicirliche Stratagemata zubefinden, denen Regiments-Secretariis, Kriegs-Concipisten, Musterschreibern, und anderen Kriegs-Bedienten höchst nöthig* (Nürnberg: Johann Hoffmann, 1683), p. 77.

42 Kranichfeld, *Kriegs-Secretarius*, after p. 70, sample table for a regimental return dated 4 January 1644.

43 '[Z]uverläßiger Rollen und Beschreibungen der Mannschaft [...], dieselbe wöchent- oder zum wenigsten monatlich, aus der Musterschreiber bey den Compagnien eingegeben Special-Rollen zuergäntzen [...] und beyzulegen, damit wir, wie starck sich unser Kriegs-Heer befinde, iedesmahl wissen könten.' (author's translation) Kranichfeld, *Kriegs-Secretarius*, pp. 64–5.

44 E. Charters, *Disease, War and the Imperial State: The Welfare of the British Armed Forces during the Seven Years' War* (Chicago: University of Chicago Press, 2014), pp. 103–9.

45 Kranichfeld, *Kriegs-Secretarius*, pp. 64–8.

46 NLA Hann, Hann. 41 III, Nr. 16, aggregate returns from the Hanoverian regiments in the Netherlands, May 1744 to April 1748, fols 176–181.

47 For example, the battles of Fontenay in May 1745 and Rocour in October 1746 were followed by an immediate peak in the number of losses, while over the years a regular increase in morbidity rates during the summer was followed by a regular decline of morbidity during the autumn and winter.

48 S.C. Craig, 'Sir John Pringle MD, early enlightenment thought and the origins of modern military medicine', *Journal for Eighteenth-Century Studies* 38 (2015), 99–114; E. Weidenhammer, 'Patronage and enlightened medicine in the eighteenth-century British military: The rise and fall of Dr John Pringle, 1707–1782', *Social History of Medicine* 29 (2015), 21–43.

49 J. Pringle, *Observations on the Diseases of the Army in Camp and Garrison* (London: A. Millar, D. Wilson and T. Payne, 2nd edn, 1753) [1st edn 1752], pp. 12–13.

50 Ibid., pp. 19–33.
51 Ibid., p. 71.
52 Ibid., pp. 72–93.
53 Ibid., pp. 94–117.
54 Ibid., pp. 118–20.
55 At least by the end of the seventeenth century, the prevalence of infectious diseases and seasonal variations were commonplace among authors of military handbooks. See, for example, W. Dillich, *Hochvernünfftig gegründete und auffgerichtete, in gewisse Classen eingetheilte, bisher verschollen gelegene,*

nunmehr aber eröffnete Kriegs-Schule, 2 vols (Frankfurt: Johann Daniel Zunner, 1689), here vol. 2, pp. 49–53.

56 R. Knoeff and J. Kennaway (eds), *Lifestyle and Medicine in the Enlightenment: The Six Non-Naturals in the Long Eighteenth Century* (Abingdon: Routledge, 2020).

57 See, for example, R. Minderer, *Medicina Militaris. Seu Libellus Castrensis. Euporista ac facile parabilia Medicamenta comprehendens. Id est: Gemaine Handstücklein zur Kriegs Artzney* gehörig (Augsburg: Andreas Aperger [printer], 1620); H. Screta, *Kurzer Bericht fon der allgemein ansteckenden Lagersucht* (Schafhausen: Onofrinus von Waldkirch, 1676).

58 Pringle, *Observations on the Diseases of the Army*, p. vi.

59 M. Stolberg, 'Medical note-taking in the sixteenth and seventeenth centuries', in A. Cerolini (ed.), *Forgetting Medicines: Knowledge Management Evolution in Early Modern Europe* (Leiden: Brill, 2016), pp. 243–64; G.B. Risse, *Hospital Life in Enlightenment Scotland: Care and Teaching at the Royal Infirmary of Edinburgh* (Cambridge: Cambridge University Press, 1986), pp. 296–301.

60 E.G. Baldinger, *Von den Krankheiten einer Armee* (Langnsalza: Johann Christian Martini, 1765); J.L. Schmucker, *Chirurgische Beobachtungen*, 2 vols (Berlin: Friedrich Nicolai, 1774).

61 V. Hess, 'Formalisierte Beobachtung: Die Genese der modernen Krankenakte am Beispiel der Berliner und Pariser Medizin (1725–1830)', *Medizinhistorisches Journal* 45 (2010), 293–340; Baldinger, *Von den Krankheiten einer Armee*, pp. 18–20.

62 Geheimes Staatsarchiv Preußischer Kulturbesitz [Prussian Privy State Archives] (hereafter GStA PK), HA I, Rep. 96, Nr. 85 E e 3, Monthly return from the Prussian field hospitals, 2 December 1760, fol. 19r.

63 GStA PK, HA I, Rep. 96, Nr. 85 E e 3, Letter from Cothenius in Breslau, November 1760, fol. 43r–43v, here fol. 43r.

64 J.U. Bilguer, *Abhandlung von dem sehr seltenen Gebrauch, oder, der beynahe gänzlichen Vermeidung des Ablösens der menschlichen Glieder, aus dem Lateinischen übersetzt und mit noch einigen Wahrnehmungen vermehrt* (Berlin: Arnold Wever, 1761), pp. 101–5.

65 Bilguer, *Abhandlung von dem sehr seltenen Gebrauch*, pp. 147–50.

66 See A. Rusnock, *Vital Accounts: Quantifying Health and Population in Eighteenth-Century England and France* (Cambridge: Cambridge University Press, 2002).

67 Neufeld, 'The biopolitics of manning the Royal Navy', esp. 506–7. See also C. Stein, 'The birth of bio-power in eighteenth-century Germany', *Medical History* 55 (2011), 331–7.

12

Miners' chest: How performative accounting forged the ills of industry

J. Andrew Mendelsohn

Clink. Clink. Clink. One after another, each man dropped a penny through the slot in the top of a large iron canister (Figure 12.1), its lid secured with three separately keyed locks. This happened every week on payday. This was their collective bank account, a way of meeting current needs and saving for future ones. Collectively they monitored credits – the pennies. They deliberated debits – medical costs. And they did their best to balance the two, making sure not to run out. Thus the penny box operated as an account. This made it a machine defining harm. The harm it defined was 'mining disease' and, more broadly, the human cost of the world's prototypical organised, capitalised industry. The penny box rendered human destruction integral rather than peripheral to material production. It sustained both, for centuries.

Occupational health, *Arbeitsmedizin*, industrial hygiene, *médecine du travail* – these are variations on a theme that has often seemed evident to medicine, science, and societies, their public understandings and histories. The theme is simple. Some forms of work are detrimental to health. Study can yield effective intervention and regulation. Hence the existence and development of a special field of inquiry, knowledge, and application.

Yet none of this has been self-evident. Consider 'silicosis', a modern nosological incarnation of dust-related chronic respiratory disease. This diagnosis first appeared in the twentieth century when sandblasting and power tools entered heavy industry with a consequent leap in exposure to mineral dust inhalation. Equally important to the creation of

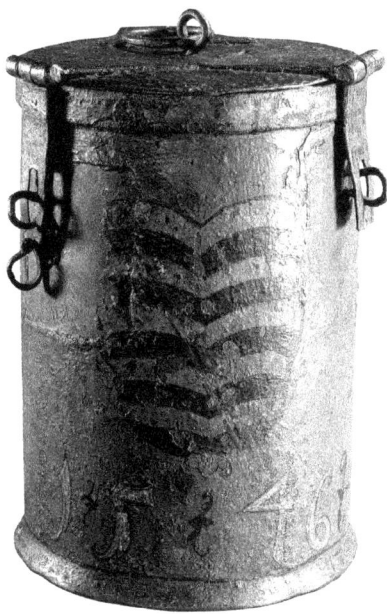

12.1 'Penny box' of a smelters' society (Hüttenknappschaft Freiberg), showing the date 1546 and a version of the Saxon coat of arms.

the disease concept and the politics and practices around it was that 'symptoms were often ambiguous' yet seemed clearly 'rooted in work and factory production' with 'enormous social and economic implications'. Yet 'by the 1950s, silicosis was virtually forgotten'. Symptoms that had indicated 'an occupational history of work in the dusty trades' now indicated 'asthmas, emphysema, or other nonoccupational lung conditions'.[1] The ill effect of work on those doing the work turns out to be both obvious and ambiguous or made ambiguous; put together and taken apart again in multiple ways by diverse actors over time; and contested at scales ranging from conflicting expert opinions in a single case of worker's compensation to controversy over the meaning of statistical information – or methods of assessing danger or risk – to legislative debate or struggle between management and labour.[2] What makes this significant for the history of knowledge and health care, industry, economy, politics, and government is that disease identities and explanations are at stake throughout and stand in a mutually determinative relation with policy, law, intervention (or lack thereof), and the fates of affected groups and individuals.

This chapter concerns an earlier time, from the fifteenth through the eighteenth century. Production-related diagnosis surprisingly lacked this modern instability and contest. It evidenced an emerging system that enabled those modern developments to occur. This happened especially around mining. This was not because mining and its effects on health needed no definition. From chipping away solid rock to supervising up and down ladders and hoists, from pounding ores in the open air to smelting them in huts, from manning winches and pumps to pulling carts, what was mining work? What were its ailments, their forms and causes, and were these specific to mining or generic far beyond it? Whose bodies counted and which influences on them – from the personal to the meteorological, the individual to the collective, the environmentally to the humanly caused, the occupational to the nutritional, the inevitable to the hygienic, from the usual Hippocratic 'airs, waters, places' to the four elements, so highly concentrated in mining, earth, air, fire, and water, and the variety of metals that mining itself made manifest? None of this was given. Yet mining grew a stable system of identifying work-caused illness and treating it, guiding how to prevent it, and caring for those affected and their dependents. This chapter explores the conditions that made that possible. They involve a relationship between two histories hitherto separately told and understood: the economic history (miners' societies and sick funds as the earliest form of social insurance) and the medical history (expertise on miners' diseases as the earliest form of occupational health).[3] Accounting, I shall argue, constituted each in relation to the other. There is one problem, however: a 200-year gap in documentation. Medical *knowledge* around mining took shape on paper in the sixteenth century. Medical *accounts* around mining date from the eighteenth century. The books of bookkeeping are largely missing; or missing medical content. Back to the box.

Accounts performed; ailments defined

Payday was Saturday. Miners gathered for this, generally at noon, in a mining company house or a miners' canteen. Hands and purses opened to receive coins from the shift master with foremen in attendance. The 'penny box' (Figure 12.1) stood by. It belonged to the miners themselves as a fraternity (*Bruderschaft*) or, in later parlance, a society (*Knappschaft*). The jingle of pay was followed by the clink of duty, the penny dropped into the box. These were credits heard rather than written, each penny as though an entry in an iron book, adding up by weight, collectively witnessed rather than clerically and bureaucratically vouchsafed.[4] No one could be missed without missing his pay. And the next week's pay was docked for failing to contribute, or worse, non-contributors were barred from work. A form of both solidarity and discipline, at once moral and material, this was accountability of each for the well-being of all. Accountability for the whole, too, was built into the box: opening separately keyed locks required assembly of independent officers.[5]

Goslar, a major trading and artisanal town in the Harz Mountains, boasted the oldest miners' fraternity or brotherhood. The Bishop of Hildesheim chartered it in 1260. High-medieval cities abounded in church-chartered fraternities; Cologne had eighty in the 1400s. Members of trades or social ranks thereby defined themselves as a group. They also acquired indulgence privileges. Alms-giving and funding a chapel or altar were spiritual credits against debits, their sins, in the final accounting, the Last Judgement of their souls. Dozens more mining fraternities followed Goslar's in the fourteenth and fifteenth centuries, one for each mining town or district (*Revier*) in the major mining areas of Europe. Besides the Harz, these were the Carpathian and Tyrolian mountain regions, under Austrian and Hungarian control, and the Ore Mountains (*Erzgebirge*) of Saxony and Bohemian lands. These had their richest periods through silver lodes but also produced lead, zinc, and copper, some iron and tin, and rare metals like cobalt. Whereas fraternities in general gave alms outside their memberships, mining brotherhoods provided specifically for their members in need. Need usually meant incapacitation for work. Thus, the mining fraternities are viewed as the world's oldest health and social insurance organisation, or 'friendly society'. Over time, funds kept in the penny box or a larger chest mainly for indulgences in the Christian accounting of sin and repentance around the soul became ever more purely funds for the body.[6] Funds were used to care for sick, injured, or ailing miners, later also to support their dependents in case of death. Care could entail a stay in a miners' hospital funded by the brotherhood and usually attached to a church, as was the case in Goslar probably as early as the thirteenth century.[7] The mining brotherhood of the major Tyrolian mining centre Schwaz built a *Bruderhaus* with its own hospital in 1510 (Figure 12.2).[8] Beginning around this time, members' penny contributions were used to pay practitioners' fees.[9]

Debiting the miners' chest was as formalised and public as crediting it. When in the 1530s, for example, the Goslar miners' society members affirmed the already venerable procedure of contributing a penny from wages, they also affirmed a procedure for deciding claims to use the money, including for medical practitioner fees. The 'elected heads [of the miners' society] shall inspect the damage' of anyone 'incapacitated by mining'.[10] Thus, when governments began mandating penny boxes in mining ordinances (*Bergordnungen*), they confirmed and appropriated an existing income/expense practice.[11] This was simple and imperfect accounting practice. But simple accounting could organise attention

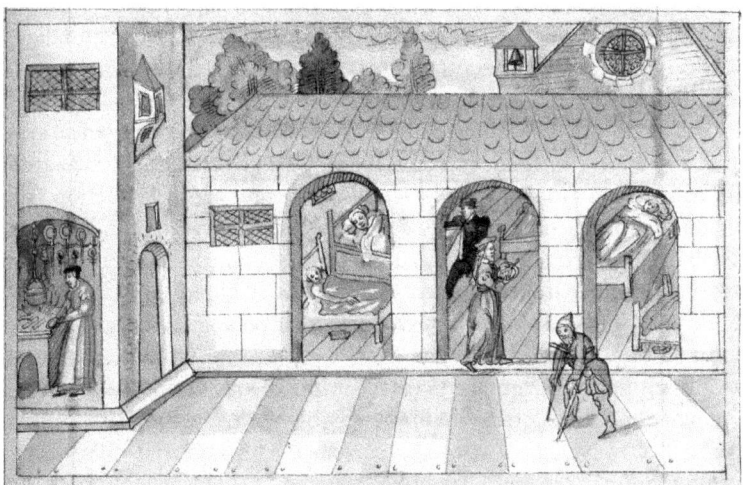

12.2 House of the Mining Brotherhood, Schwaz, Tyrol, showing hospital and sickbeds, c. 1510–50.

no less than complexity could, and its failings focused attention as much as its workings did.[12]

The penny box held together a system of behaviours, values, and relationships both moral and material: pennies *in* from work; pennies *out* for what work did to health. Read with a period eye, the scant documentation suffices to characterise the evaluative aspect of practice. Two keywords reveal its substance and scope. So does inference from other sources.

The first keyword is 'examine' or 'inspect'. It belonged to a whole special vocabulary: *besehen, Besehung, besichtigen, Besichtigung, Schau,* all given in Latin as *inspectio*. These terms meant much more than having a look. They referred to procedures of close visual examination and judgement according to known criteria and standards. These often included tests of various sorts, and the language of inspecting occurs together with that of testing or assaying (*probieren*), notably in mining and minting, but also across the guilds and in medicine and surgery. Medieval and early modern usage is well known for human bodies (leprosy, wounds), mining (ore assay, shaft inspection), and forestry.[13] The annals of public medicine abound in *Schau*. Sixteenth-century civic medical certificates show office-holders and relief applicants negotiating inspection results in more or less standardised descriptive and diagnostic terms. So do fifteenth-century leprosy inspection certificates; supplications by the sick for funded care; and, closest to our subject here though only beginning to be studied by historians, supplications by ailing miners or their wives for relief.[14] '*Bergbau*' in the literal sense of production in the mountains was *the* nexus for these inspection and judgement practices, not only because of the high value of metals, but also because, as the name suggests, it required complex building works, above and below ground, subject to strains of all kinds; constant movement and management of rivers-worth of water; and the use of fire underground and in smelting above. *Bergbau* subjected both land and people to the most capital-intensive, arduous, long-term, and destructive work and therefore to intensive scrutiny.[15] 'Inspecting' (*besichtigen* and collectively: '*alle ... besichtigen sollen*') appears in 1490s Saxon mining ordinances for evaluating progress made through rock by hewers; for assessing rock newly laid bare and any mineral deposits, as well as the condition of ladders, chains, ropes; yet also for determining something like risk to health: degree of 'dangerousness' (*ferlicheit*) and specifically 'danger from water' (*wassersnodt*) and 'noxious atmosphere' (*bosem wetter*) in order to factor these into the wages of those working underground compared to those working above ground 'in the field'.[16] In 1544, six years after the assembled members of the Goslar miners' society decided that their annually elected heads must inspect bodies – '*den schaden besehen*' – to decide claims on the sick fund, more rules were introduced requiring, among other things, that every four weeks four expert men tour underground 'to inspect the construction works in the mines, so that no one [comes] to harm and so that nothing is built too close to ore and copper fumes'[17] – a remarkable mix of attention to the human frame, the built framework of the mines, and the relation between the two.

Thus, both mining and wider contexts of practice and meaning strongly suggest that the undocumented *besehen* of sick, injured, or ailing mining-society members was empirical, methodical, and witnessed according to public expectations about inspection. Debiting the fund belonged to a wide empirical and rational culture of evaluation that (a) certainly took nothing for granted about the condition of bodies in sickness and health; and (b) specified physical rather than moral criteria, like the need or worthiness familiar in poor relief and charitable care. Such practices determined mining ailments just as they did 'pox' or 'leprosy' and with at least as much, if not more, diagnostic ambiguity to navigate.

The second keyword in the sample passage quoted above is *Schaden*, translatable as 'damage'. It indicates a wide scope of inspected and evaluated ailments. This very general term applied beyond physical injuries to a whole range of bodily conditions as well as to things gone awry in the mines (and to be avoided by regular inspection). *Schaden* occurs multiple times in Central European mining ordinances, as does *Gebrechen*, a term applied to the mining works and typically to human ailment and infirmity.[18] Applied to bodies, language of injury and damage did not specify acute as opposed to chronic. Miners' societies clearly recognised the need to support both. A miner's 'chronic rheumatic pain in the right side' belonged in bills to the sick fund as much as acute injuries did.[19] Rather, *Schaden* specified an occurrence or condition to which a claim could be attached – exactly as claims could be made for *Schaden* to a mining operation through negligence or error. *Schaden* thereby asserted unity in the diversity of symptoms and causes. Whatever combination of age, individual constitution, and type of work each case presented, funded care defined bodily condition as the product of employment in the mining industry.

The third interpretive point requires inference from other sources. How knowledgeable was miners' inspecting and judging of bodies for claims on the sick fund? Only when state mining authorities and companies began employing official mining doctors, mainly in the seventeenth century, did examination pass into medically trained hands and eyes.[20] How can we possibly approach this question if no miners, foremen, or even literate mining administrators in the fifteenth and sixteenth centuries wrote tracts on either mining or its health affairs, nor produced any records of these examinations? The short answer is: via physicians. Reading patient experience through doctors' writings is methodologically hazardous. But in this case it is surprisingly straightforward. Physicians used terms that they clearly did not invent and that can be regarded as folk terminology. One of these was '*Bergsucht*', for respiratory wasting illness, after which the first book on the subject was titled, *Von der Bergsucht und anderen Bergkrankheiten*, composed in the 1520s–30s by Theophrastus von Hohenheim, already gaining fame as the radical doctor styling himself Paracelsus.[21] Ailing miners and their wives used the term '*Bergsucht*' in relief supplications.[22] An ailing miner with no hope of being able to work again was *bergfertig*: done-in by mining, literally 'finished by the mountain'. Another term was '*Hüttenkatze*' – literally, 'hut cat' – for a condition associated with the fumes of smelting (hence '*Hütten*') and especially with lead exposure; its namesake symptom was the feeling that one's entrails were alive with a wriggling scratching cat.[23] It is scarcely conceivable that these miners' disease concepts – which were both clinical (*Katze, Sucht*) and aetiological (*Hütten, Berg*) – were not in use when decisions were made about spending pennies from the miners' chest. *Bergsucht, Hüttenkatze,* and the like were not only 'popular medicine' or folk knowledge, but categories that allowed the collective to debit the account.[24]

The point here is not that medical knowledge came 'from below', but rather that the miners already used it to run a health system of diagnosis and resource allocation based on nosological and aetiological concepts. Popular language was technical language. Folk terminology comprised not oral 'culture', but oral accounting – even oral accounting bureaucracy in so far as the miners' societies divided roles among several kinds of elected or appointed officer and had formal procedures of impersonal judgement, all of which became integrated with municipal and state administration in the seventeenth and eighteenth centuries. Though preserved mainly because doctors wrote it down, this language would have resounded in the collective 'inspection' of claimants' bodies; in the collective act of opening the separately keyed locks to debit the chest for spending on members' health; and finally in an annual assembly for what was called a 'reckoning', when members gathered to 'inspect' any written income and expenses of the brotherhood and to hear medical needs.

Altogether this was live accounting, interwoven with collective life – and matters of life and death. At the level of individual contributions and benefits, it was far more performed than written. This did not make it simply an oral tradition. Like any other economic – and spiritual – collective of the time, mining brotherhoods were hardly unaware of the biblical account book metaphor and of basic household bookkeeping practice. Brotherhoods began keeping general account books as early as 1515.[25] Only in the eighteenth century, as we shall see, did they begin recording medical expenses. Meanwhile, in the preceding centuries, though far from the sophistication of early modern merchants' double-entry accounts and audits, income was collectively heard weekly in the clink of pennies into the box, expenses for members' health heard regularly in the scrape of three different keys to open the chest, and both heard annually as an auditory 'reckoning' in a general assembly. This accounting without books, or for centuries with few and general ones, was witnessed in the act, thus more transparently kept than any books could ever be. It was audited not by outsiders, expected to be impartial, but by all parties, in the assembly of everyone who had an interest in what went into the box and what was taken out of it.

Unlimited funds, or no fund at all, would have meant no such activity. Solidarity created the need to allocate finite collective resources and to maintain them for what tomorrow might bring. Balancing the box, whatever its vicissitudes over the centuries, created collective attention to injury and illness, standards and criteria for differentiating among cases and attributing causes. Goslar's so-called mining or miners' society ordinance offers a rare early documented glimpse of such attention. The source is in fact a record of three annual assemblies of miners following the dissolution of their fraternity early in the Reformation. At the first of these, in 1532, they considered the hazards and ailments of their work and resolved to return to their old practice of contributing a ha'penny weekly – now a penny biweekly – to care for their own. They also resolved to keep a 'reckoning' (*reckenschop*) of this income and expense. Evidently they did so. Four years later, at an annual assembly in 1536, they held an audit – also called a 'reckoning' – and discussed whether to improve care and recovery by providing for doctors' fees. Evidently their reckonings showed them that this expense could not be met on the current income arrangement. So they held a survey ('*ummefrage*') to hear the views of every member and thereupon resolved to double the fund by requiring weekly rather than biweekly pennies.[26] These actions assumed that a useful if rough idea of medical need and cost could be achieved collectively through the views of all members and thus that they were more or less informed on such matters. This was balancing the box for health.

By the seventeenth century in Saxony, registers were being kept of miners' 'box pennies' owed in arrears, evidently to ensure they eventually were paid in.[27] By the eighteenth century in a wide variety of mining areas, rules on spending 'from the box' began requiring official medical certification 'that the ailment came from work' or was not 'pretended' (malingering) and had been immediately reported, as this would enable knowing whether it had happened through work.[28] Accounting for expenses to miners' society sick funds became so detailed in the Harz in the 1700s that prescriptions for each patient were listed with costs – 5 Groschen for a 'mixture', 2 Groschen for a 'powder', 6 for the mixture again, and so on, amounting to as many as a dozen medicines listed per patient – here for one Joseph Brettschneider – per financial quarter.[29]

Why does the creation and sustaining of the fund out of miners' pay matter to the argument? Surely 'mining disease' would be defined simply by agreeing on allocation criteria. Where the money came from would not affect this. It did, however, and in several ways. First, the penny contributions were not charity. They were taken from work – and not just any work, but this kind of work, what each man was paid for his chiselling underground or smelting, and moreover directly, on the very day of pay for work. To use that money was therefore to relate care and hence ailment to the work – rather than to a benefactor or to a wider community, a Christian or civic ethic.[30] It was also to separate care, ailment, and its (work) conditions from those of the rest of the population and its health, wealth, and environment. Poor relief or other parish or municipal support would not have justified separate medicine for miners, nor contributed to the framing of mining disease. When ailing miners later came to communicate in writing with fund administrators, they attested to incapacitation 'through' their 'occupational work in the mining operation', even using the modern (and Lutheran) concept of a 'calling' rather than a trade or art. Damage through *Beruffs Arbeit*, as this Freiberg miner put it in the early 1700s, justified recompense from the 'brotherhood of dear God'.[31] This framing of ailments was especially meaningful because, although 'mining' and 'miner' imply a coherent industry and occupation, the forms of work were extremely diverse; and those involved often had an additional livelihood, usually in agricultural labour.[32] Finally, sick-fund contributions came from everyone, including foremen, and eventually from shareholders and even administrators in some areas. This meant that injuries and ills were not framed by differentiation into parties, one of which could be at fault (whether the worker or the supervisor or the shareholders or the regulating government), but rather as intrinsic to mining. Unlike charity and poor relief, contributing money did not perform inequality and dependency. Every Saturday it stated, with a clink, the vulnerability of all at work – despite differences in immediate environment and exposure – to being incapacitated for work by work and thus also the coherence of ills across all this diversity: ills, therefore, not of trades or environments, but of industry, of production.

These regularly repeated scenes of communication about illness and incapacitation necessarily transcended personal bodily experience and individual cognition to generate, refine, and perpetuate collective knowledge of health and disease. Moreover, this was not a whole mining town's knowledge of *all* illness and health in their midst. There was plenty. Writers in early modern mining areas chronicled leprosy, scurvy, rheumatic fever, *Schnarrpickel*, the French disease, the Hungarian disease, plague, English sweating sickness, dysentery, hectic fever (consumption) – and those were only the more notable kinds.[33] A collective fund meant an identity for whatever ailed the men in so far as they and their peers could agree that it had to do with being 'on the mountain' (*uppe deme Rammelsberge* or on whichever other one it was) toiling for ore and metal, rather than anything else debilitating about their individual constitutions, habits, diet, family history, living conditions, environment, or other livelihoods. Clearly, all of that did not belong in their meetings and the 'reckoning'.

From mining account to medical knowledge

The penny box was a disease-defining account. Necessarily poised between differentiation and ambiguity, it had to split respiratory illness into mining and non-mining forms. It split disease-inducing climate into mining and non-mining airs, waters, places, effluvia – the 'weather' above ground from the 'weather', as miners called it, underground. The account also lumped together the hazards of hut and tunnel, of hewing and smelting, dust and fumes, as well as metals of all sorts – indeed the pathologies of all four elements: earth, air, fire, and water – into mining disease, *Bergkrankheiten*, ills of an industry.[34] Because the sick fund was theirs and not an employer's or state's or insurer's, this could happen in a stable and cumulative manner, without the contests over fault or pre-existing condition and the erasures of aetiology that became typical when in the nineteenth and twentieth centuries sick funds came to belong not to those at risk of getting sick but to employers, investors, states, insurance companies – opposing interests. The workings of the brotherhood and its sick fund defined ailments as incapacitation for work and incapacitation as what work did to bodies. If it did this for miners, it did so for miners' doctors, too. For they were paid from the fund.

Or they were paid directly by mining companies. The coverage of doctors' fees for mining 'workers' was written into law as early as 1518. In the sixteenth century, mining expanded into new areas of the Saxon, Bohemian, and Harz regions and then into other political territories, from Brandenburg to Trier to Württemberg. Miners' societies, community chests, and penny boxes were established wherever they did not already exist. Moreover, beginning with the new mining district of Joachimsthal in the Bohemian region of the Ore Mountains in 1518, local lords and territorial rulers decreed in mining ordinances that companies (*Gewerke*) pay miners their wages and medical practitioner fees for eight weeks following incapacitation.[35] This benefit was presumably meant to attract experienced miners from long-established Bohemian districts and from adjacent Saxony and the Harz. It seems also to have attracted doctors: Joachimsthal quickly became the earliest epicentre of writing on mining and health. The medical benefits article in the Joachimsthal mining ordinance specified injured limbs, but also more vaguely *Schaden*, which we shall see from doctors' writings and later invoices were as likely to be respiratory, rheumatic, or ulcerative. The Joachimsthaler article was widely copied in new and revised mining ordinances from the sixteenth to the eighteenth centuries.[36] It was also expanded to require fixed regular contributions from the mining companies to the miners' society sick fund and to spell out a complementary relationship between short-term medical benefits and long-term penny-box support or 'alms' for incapacitation.[37]

Since antiquity, no one doubted that the fumes of heated metals were bad to breathe. Yet until the sixteenth century, they were held to cause *morbi metallici* or dangers to goldsmiths and other metalworkers. 'Mining diseases' was a different construct involving the human price of a whole industrial sector. Thus, it was no coincidence that, as the arts of mining and assaying metals began to be written down in handbooks for the first time around 1500 and especially by doctors, the earliest and most reprinted medical chapter in such general handbooks was no treatise on mining disease, but a medical guide for goldsmiths and other metalworkers. Its author was Dr Ulrich Ellenbog, who had little or no contact with mining, but much with the rich urban trades of fine metalwork. Written in 1473, and probably never intended for wide circulation and publication, his brief regimen and guide against noxious fumes was addressed to the master goldsmiths – 'subtle and fine craft' – of the Imperial City of Augsburg, where he had been appointed physician to the prince-bishopric. Years later, printers appended it to the first mining and assay manuals, doubtless hoping to boost sales.[38] All that soon changed.

Around 1500, physicians began living and working in mining towns and publishing on all aspects of mining. They clearly relied on the miners, a dependency reflected in the dialogue form they chose for such tracts. Doctors seldom wrote in dialogue, usually sticking to the genres of *historia*, regimen, and *consilium*. But the Freiberg civic doctor Ulrich Rülein of Calw wrote his much-reprinted *Bergbüchlein* (1505) in dialogue form, as did Joachimsthal civic doctor Georgius Agricola his *Bermannus* of 1530, an early version of his celebrated *De re metallica*.[39] Physicians conversed intensively with miners, not only as doctors, but as humanist scholars writing on nature and the practical arts, as administrators in the capacity of official town physician or civic doctor, as mining investors themselves, and even as Bürgermcisters of mining towns. Rülein, a Leipzig medical graduate and mathematics teacher, was all of these in the centuries-old Saxon mining capital Freiberg around 1500 and even drew up the plans for building a new mining town, Annaberg.[40] Agricola came to hold all of these interactive positions and more during his career in Joachimsthal and Chemnitz in the 1520s–50s. Numerous sixteenth-century German, Bohemian, Hungarian, and Tyrolian doctors spent some or all of their careers in mining towns and areas. Many were physicians in civic office. Paracelsus' father would have treated miners as the civic doctor of Villach in the mining region of Carinthia.[41]

The first such doctor to publish guidance at length was Magnus Hundt. It was a job bid. In 1529, he addressed a ninety-page booklet directly to the Bürgermeister, Council, and Miners' Society of newly booming Joachimsthal, asking to be appointed its civic doctor (the post Agricola was about to leave), citing a patronage relationship with Joachimsthal's territorial lord and referring to his prior 'seven years of medical practice in your community'.[42] Accordingly, and although cited in the twentieth century as a pioneering work of occupational health, Hundt's *A Useful Regimen Including Remedies* was a household manual for common ailments of men, women, and children of Joachimsthal, especially chest illnesses including cough and heaviness of breath, but also headache, dizziness, and gout, from which 'many good friends in the valley' suffer. The manual's ninety pages alternate between detailed recipes and the Galenic physician's typical moralising attribution of illness to 'evil ways' or intemperance in using non-naturals, particularly food and drink, and so were clearly also written for a Count and Council interested in public order and labour fitness in the sixteenth century's quintessential silver-rush boomtown.

Buried in these ninety pages of regimen and recipes are three pages giving Hundt's only descriptive account of disease. Tellingly, this was an ailment mainly affecting 'people in mining' exposed to the fumes of sulphur, lead, and mercury, steam, and noxious 'weather' underground. A sufferer felt

> as though his breath wanted to leave him ... if he sits or gets up somewhat, he feels as though something [*etwas*] is lying upon his chest as though the amount of air is not drawn sufficiently to breathe, he must therefore draw often ... as though he had been running ... anxious as though something [*eppes*] is lying on his chest and wants to suffocate him, [he] cannot lie down, must sit ... a heavy pain, as though one was drawing [breath] harder and harder, and [it] wanted to strangle him.

This reads nothing like the well-redacted disease *historia* beginning to be penned in the sixteenth century by learned physicians. The disease history goes round and round the same symptoms a dozen times. Scraps of patient narrative (how it feels) rather than doctor's description (what is seen) recur in varying language and simile, the formal slipping into the colloquial (*etwas, eppes*). Hundt evidently compiled miners' voices – and valued each.[43]

Other writers on mining disease were not physicians, but Reformed clergy. The Lutheran Reformation began in mining areas. Luther himself came from a mining family, his father being a hewer who worked his way up to shareholder and then to city councilman in a major mining town. Among the early published thematic collections of Protestant sermons was a book of sixteen mining sermons given by Luther's friend Johannes Mathesius, schoolmaster and then pastor of Joachimsthal.[44] Like doctors, pastors were nodes of communication in their localities, and Mathesius knew in detail from miners about their ills.

In short, we should not imagine pastors and doctors mainly at bedsides and walking around 'observing' mining conditions and disease in miners. Case histories – *observationes* – featuring mining disease are scarce.[45] Nor until the eighteenth century did doctors use the opportunity mining regions afforded for producing pioneering histories (*historia*) of disease in a specific environment. Instead, they wrote down what the miners – foremen, brotherhood elders, officeholders

– had determined from running their own medical system and what that system paid for. Here was a world of lay diagnosis structured over decades or centuries by organised funded care around the penny box and now also the company. This, I suggest, is how physicians were able to arrive on the scene and produce a novel medicine of mining in the absence of a classical tradition on the subject and without producing a literature of case observations or medical geography.[46] Accounting had already done the work.

True to their differences, Paracelsus and Agricola did this in contrasting ways and yet, true to the organisation of attention and practice around the penny box, in underlying agreement. Paracelsus, the restless revolutionary who extolled the knowledge of common folk over that of scholars, adopted miners' names for their ailments, such as *Bergsucht*, in various spellings from oral vernacular. Agricola, the humanist who mobilised Greek and Latin classics for pragmatic ends, as in his erudite book on weights and measures, did not adopt folk disease names. Instead, as humanists generally did when confronted with naturalia (does what the herb woman shows me match what Dioscorides describes?), he looked for classical medical terms that matched what he learned from the miners. Thus, the dustiness of work in dry mines 'produces difficulty in breathing, and the disease which the Greeks call ἄσθμα [asthma]'. When corrosive, this dust 'eats away the lungs, and implants consumption [*tabes*] in the body'.[47] Agricola thus opened a place in learned medical knowledge for miners' ailments by elevating them into the terminology of Hippocratic medicine, yet did so entirely without applying its aetiological concepts. He used ancient Greek and Latin terms as shorthand descriptors of conditions whose causation remained mining dust and its corrosive forms rather than the behavioural, constitutional, or climatic conditions that medical authors adduced to explain asthma or *tabes*. Agricola thereby framed a mining identity and aetiology of conditions that could nonetheless be described as much more general phenomena – such as asthma or *tabes* – having nothing to do with mining.

Unlike the twentieth-century physicians who diagnosed 'asthmas, emphysema, or other nonoccupational lung conditions' *instead of* looking for 'an occupational history of work in the dusty trades',[48] Agricola used 'asthma' and 'tabes' to help make clinical sense of a condition he clearly represented as occupational, resulting from work in an industry. Thus he adopted the industrial identity of disease. The fact that Paracelsus did the same in an entirely different, vernacular way, and that he and Agricola were about as different as two major sixteenth-century Central European physicians could be, testifies to the power of the mining context. And this, we have seen, involved more than experience. It had been created around the miners' chest.

Viewed in terms of anatomical seat, affected organs, pathological process, clinical course, and apparent aetiological agent, the ailments that qualified for support from the sick fund, appearing as the *Bergkrankheiten* in Paracelsus and in six or seven unsystematic categories in Agricola's *De re metallica*, had nothing to do with each other: for example, asthma from dust; consumption from corrosive dust; progressive ulcers from a specific mineral (black pompholyx); acute or chronic poisoning from fumes, which Paracelsus differentiated by smelting speciality; rheumatism or other joint problems from cold and humidity.[49] Moreover, mining was heterogeneous in its types of work and physical conditions. Chiselling underground and smelting at the surface were as different as the dust and fumes they produced. Yet they also overlapped by type of ore in a given mine or area. Sixteenth-century Lutheran pastors noted this variety of work and exposure. They represented it back to mining communities in detailed sermons describing illnesses and proper protective gear for each job.[50]

Finally, who was a miner anyway? Only the adult males underground and in smelting huts or also the wives and children who toiled over ores outside? Especially in periods of lower yield, the men, women, and children involved in mining survived by agricultural work. Those other conditions and forms of work also affected their health. Yet counteracting these nosologically disintegrative forces was the fact that mining workers of all kinds – 'foremen, captain, hewer, hauler, machine operator, ore pounder and sorter, ore washer, smith, donkey driver'[51] – united themselves in the brotherhoods and their sick funds. They thus created a unity that the diversity of their occupation and its hazards and of their observable ailments would not predict: namely, miners' diseases. '*Bergkrankheiten*' and '*Bergsucht*' did not even refer to mining, but to the mountain on and in which life and work took place. Thus did organisation around a community chest make mining and its ills cohere. Moreover, states' formalisation and unification of all aspects of mining in the sixteenth and seventeenth centuries brought hewing and smelting together under ever-more comprehensive ordinances and administration, against the grain of modernising processes of occupational differentiation.[52]

Physicians' involvement in mining was the opposite of the main way in which learned medicine underwent empirical Renaissance in the fifteenth and sixteenth centuries: individualisation. Medical practice at princely courts, or for civic or church patrons, individualised disease and thus personalised medicine. Practice for sick-fund members collectivised disease. Mining solidarity and its fund turned the individualising genre, the *consilium*, into a generalising one, like the *Consilium peripneumoniacum* published by Annaberg civic doctor Martin Pansa in 1614. This was the first standalone practical and theoretical guide on mining disease since Paracelsus and the mining sermons of Mathesius. No highly original observer, Pansa drew synthetically on the writers before him.[53] They had written down the nosology and aetiology generated by mining's oral medical system around the penny account. This necessarily combined ways of differentiating with recognition of an ambiguous spectrum. Pansa's version strove to distinguish mining *Bergsucht* from mining *Lungensucht* and both from 'common' *Lungensucht*. When, in the eighteenth century, the system and its physicians became still more nosological about disease in the mining context, they generated repetitively differentiating, yet overlapping ambiguities and combinations of generic descriptive terms.[54] Retrospective diagnosis and classification by occupational health experts and historians in the twentieth century did the same.[55] Mining disease has never had a straightforward existence.

The box in the book

The accounting performed around the miners' chest made doctors participants in defining the bodily effects of mining. But what about physicians' and surgeons' *own* accounting? What role if any did it play in this process? Exploring this question will take us forward into the eighteenth century, when such documentation came into regular use.

Physicians learn from medical practice. Yet what they learn, and how, differs according to the milieu of practice and observation. A common form of recordkeeping used by medical practitioners in a variety of times and places was the register of patients and whether they had paid.[56] As late as the nineteenth century, this could be as simple as a ledger of patients, with each treatment listed and then crossed out when paid. An example from the Harz region in the 1830s shows this being done conscientiously over 946 pages for a period of eight years.[57] Such a record might include information about the remedies prescribed, especially if provided at cost by the doctor, but did not necessarily include much or indeed any information about the illness of each patient. Or if so, this information was as various as were the patients and their ailments in a typical medical practice. Patterns and conclusions could emerge only through transfer into other forms of organisation on paper, forms such as 'commonplaces', compiling and indexing case reports, extracting from them, or rearranging them to make them countable.[58] The illness variety in typical payment-motivated recordkeeping can be seen, for example, in the 'medical register' of an eighteenth-century Thuringian practitioner and civic doctor:

> On 4 January 1753 the beltmaker from Grimmelshausen, first, received a bandage on his lower back, second, he should apply ... tincture to it daily. He suffers from gouty flux, a severe flux on the chest and strong pains. At first he had it over his heart. He **paid** in full. Additionally, he should apply a bandage to his calves, [the gouty flux] is all in his leg and calf. All this, too, he **paid**.
>
> On the 4th came the carpenter's wife from Kühndorf. She should take two doses of alum spirits four times daily. For a year she has a constant menstrual flux and does not sweat. She **paid**.[59]

Now compare payment-motivated documenting of cases in a nearby mining context at around the same time:

> Specification of the internal medications that had to be given to impaired workers [*verunglückte Arbeiter*] ... of the Honourable Zwitterstock Mining Company [*Gewerckschaft*] in Quarter Crucis 1750
>
> Johann Fredrich Grundig ... in the mine, became ill **because of** inhaled poisonous fumes
>
> Ernst Gottfried Behrer ... hurt himself while checking the stores, **which caused** pain in the side

Carl Gottfried ... fell into the water during a flood, **which caused** through alteration stiffness in all limbs

Johann Heinrich ... in the mine hit his right thumb against a wall, **thereby** injuring the main blood vessels

George Ernst ... in the mine, became ill **because of** inhaled poisonous fumes

Johann Christoph ... in the mine, injured himself in the head, **which caused** a large wound with severe contusion[60]

Documents like this show practitioners submitting quarterly reports to mining companies in the form of bills (Figure 12.3). In contrast to typical medical registers, like the nearby Thuringian one quoted above, the entry for each patient summarises not only his condition, but also its causation. The causal attributions in these brief casenotes within an invoice for medical services were meant to show that the treatment costs were incurred as a result of mining work rather than for some unrelated ailment. This logic, as we saw, had been decreed in mining ordinances as early as 1518. Aetiology as payment justification reduced causation to this one question. This was causality as accountability (of mining operations to miners for their health) and sustainability (of mining operations by miners' fitness and familial reproduction). Moreover, practitioners in mining areas saw a wider range of cases (miners with unrelated illnesses, patients not in mining at all). Invoicing the sick fund framed certain cases as mining related and selected them out from a myriad of other cases into a single document. Such documentation accumulated into a file of focused experience.[61]

In the marketplace of practitioners, each kept his own accounts. In the mining world, accounts belonged to a larger whole – comprised of miners' societies, mining companies, administrative polity, and its medical public servants. Medical accounting in the mining context was therefore general rather than particular: that is, generally about mining, work, and industry. It was general *because* it was limited. This generality meant that accounting was tantamount to knowledge of disease – aetiological and nosological.

The shareholders of a mining company included investors, sometimes workers themselves, and always the territorial lord. The company's operations were thus integrated with those of state administration, such that in the seventeenth and eighteenth centuries practitioners

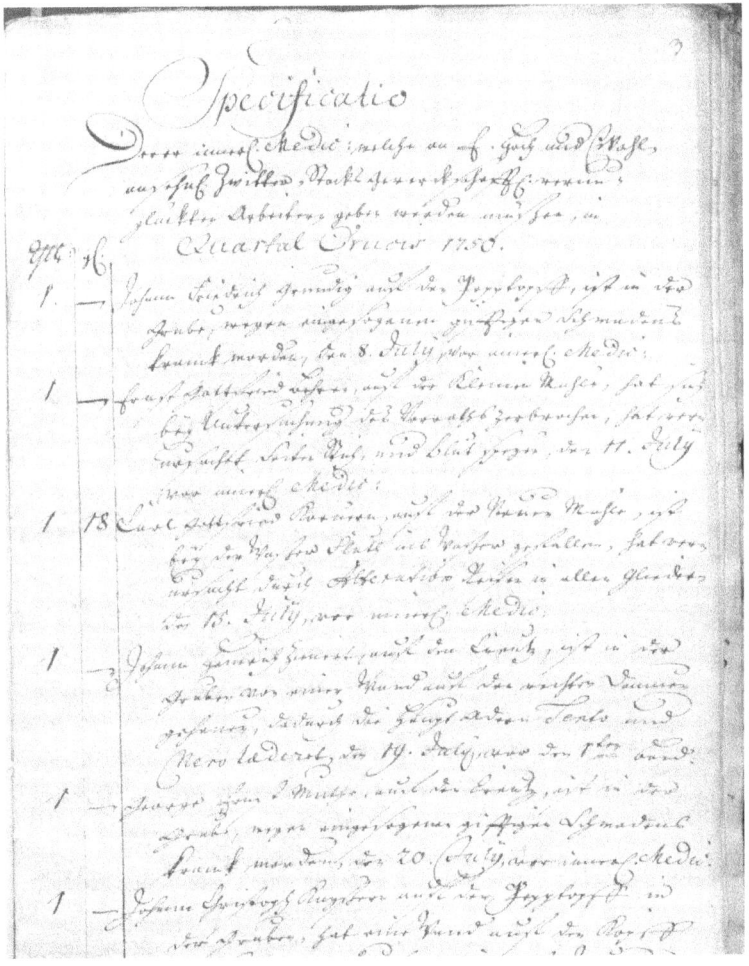

12.3 Quarterly invoice for medications given to miners, 1750.

providing care to miners competed for positions as official mining doctors (*Bergarzt, Bergchirurg, Bergmedicus*) on contract with a salary. States in the eighteenth century generally began requiring quarterly or annual reports from physicians. These took the form of observations of disease and climate together with topography of natural resources. In contrast, the annual report of a mid-eighteenth-century mining doctor or surgeon consisted of numbered mini-case-histories, each justifying the corresponding expenses. Judging such cases – in or out of the account, effectively – was not called diagnosis, but official inspection: '*Besehung*', that keyword we met in sixteenth-century miners' society regulations for debiting the miner's chest.[62] The annual or quarterly report-as-bill shows practice strikingly shaped by the sick fund of a miners' society or mining company and these, in turn, becoming part of state administration. Occasional longer case reports seem like intrusions of another genre (*curatio* or *observatio*), yet were no exception to this pattern. The complications, for example, of one 1734 Marienberg mining injury burst the bounds of summary in the usual quarterly invoice. Yet the case did not turn juridical, as could happen in the nineteenth century. Its two long reports ended in an invoice to the mining authority, only deepening the accounting relationship between case, cost, and work.[63]

The annual audit by oral 'reckoning' in the members' assembly was replaced by an auditor's eye reading page after page of mini-case-reports submitted by mining surgeons and doctors as quarterly accounts of expenses (Figure 12.4). Foreman Pählert's wound, auditor W.G.E. Becker jotted in the margin, 'does not belong [here] for [payment by] this institution'. This was easy to spot. The doctor himself had noted in the mini-history: 'wounded himself at home and not in the mine'.[64] Most cases were not so obvious. Being able to audit these accounts required intimate knowledge of the medical history, over months at a time, of hundreds of miners working in different mines. Becker evidently had this knowledge as a *Bergmeister*.[65] Only thus could the auditor exclude cases where no such notes had been made.[66] Less straightforward cases, whose costs made them stand out from the regular accounts, were by the eighteenth century subject to quasi-juridical examination – '*in Augenschein zu nehmen*' – and evaluation 'of costs' by official mining doctors.[67] Thus, paper and ink grew accounting exactitude and capacities immensely, but the structures were already there. This has wider historical implications.

Conclusion

The power of accounting to structure and enable capitalism or science or states is usually seen to depend on the power of paper techniques.[68]

How performative accounting forged the ills of industry

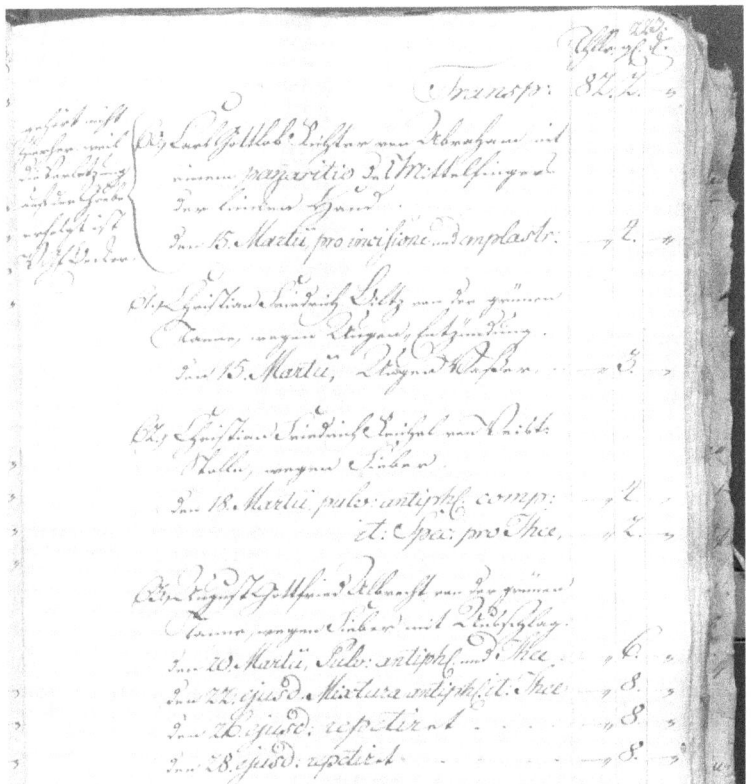

12.4 Quarterly register of medications given to miners, with auditing annotation at bracket in the upper left margin, 1806–11.

Double-entry bookkeeping is the breakthrough technology in these big histories. This chapter has sketched a different, complementary history. Books did what boxes had done. Both were simple. Neither had the sophistication of double-entry and other complex advances in accounting technology. This invites reflection on the power of what works *through* that technology – then paper, now electronic, once upon a time wood. Structuring powers attributed to the books of bookkeeping belong to unwritten human ways brought into being and kept in place (or not) by elementary material and moral arrangements. This is one lesson of the penny box. Box and book, *Büchse* and *Buch*, have in fact the same root: *Buche* (beech), the kind of wood commonly used in runic Europe for carving records to keep names and numbers and for carving out containers to keep things, eventually coins, as in the collection boxes in medieval churches which were typically of turned wood, as those of the early mining brotherhoods would have been before they were made of metal.[69] In a sense, box and book share this root because of accounting, which thus seems a function of using either.

This structure, the miners' chest, withstood three powerful countervailing forces from the sixteenth through the eighteenth centuries. First, the capitalisation of mining tended over time to turn artisanal communities into a proletariat.[70] Second, the Reformation dissolved the Church-chartered brotherhoods, and local governments expropriated their funds for the 'community chest' of poor relief. Yet miners' protest and solidarity reversed this, as we saw in Goslar in the 1530s. By and large, the miners' fraternities and their funds were reconstituted, without their religious function, as miners' societies. Third, state-building by rulers of mining territories could have dissolved miners' societies into generalised health and welfare administration, but ended up instead retaining the former within the latter and indeed mandating new societies.[71] Symbolically the state even joined the frat. That is why the penny box in Figure 12.1 bears a version of the Saxon coat of arms. Through three centuries of countervailing historical forces (capitalism, the Reformation, and state-building), the strong box held 'mining disease' together. This was a strength neither of metal, nor of miners – who were ever more subordinate – but of accountability rooted in the dependency of rulers and owners on a workforce (just) able and willing to do the very work that consumed it.

Notes

1 D. Rosner and G.E. Markowitz, *Deadly Dust: Silicosis and the Politics of Occupational Disease in Twentieth-Century America* (Princeton: Princeton University Press, 1991), p. 5. See generally P.-A. Rosental (ed.), *Silicosis: A World History* (Baltimore: Johns Hopkins University Press, 2017).
2 P.J. Weindling (ed.), *The Social History of Occupational Health* (London: Croom Helm, 1985); R. Cooter and B. Luckin (eds), *Accidents in History: Injuries, Fatalities and Social Relations* (Amsterdam: Rodopi, 1997); J.

Rainhorn and L. Bluma (eds), 'History of the workplace: Environment and health at stake', *European Review of History* 20:2 (2013) (special issue); T. Le Roux (ed.), *Risques industriels: Savoirs, régulations, politiques d'assistance, fin XVIIe – début XXe siècle* (Rennes: Presses Universitaires de Rennes, 2016).

3 For the nineteenth and twentieth centuries, these two histories are now being studied as one: L. Bluma, 'Die Objektivierung des bergmännischen Körpers: Praktiken der Sichtbarmachung im Kontext von Versicherungsrationalität und berufsspezifischen Krankheiten', in S. Nikolow (ed.), *Erkenne Dich selbst!: Strategien der Sichtbarmachung des Körpers im 20. Jahrhundert* (Cologne: Böhlau, 2015), pp. 269–85; J. Rainhorn (ed.), *Santé et travail à la mine: XIXe–XXIe siècle* (Villeneuve d'Ascq, 2016). For earlier periods, recent collective volumes contributing to both literatures include: J. Bair and W. Ingenhaeff (eds), *Bergvolk und Medizin* (Innsbruck: Berenkamp, 2005). Miners' societies and social insurance: C. Bartels (ed.), ... *höchst verpönte Selbst-Hülfe ... : zur Entstehung und Entwicklung der Sozialversicherung in Bergbau, Seefahrt und Eisenbahnwesen* (Bochum: Deutsches Bergbau Museum, 2012); U. Lauf, *Die Knappschaft: ein Streifzug durch tausend Jahre Sozialgeschichte* (Sankt Augustin: Asgard Verlag, 1994); M. Fessner, A. Bingener, and R. Slotta (eds), *Auf breiten Schultern: 750 Jahre Knappschaft; Katalog der Ausstellung des Deutschen Bergbau-Museums Bochum* (Bochum: Deutsches Bergbau Museum, 2010). Miners' diseases and health care: G. Rosen, *The History of Miners' Diseases: A Medical and Social Interpretation* (New York: Schuman, 1943); W. Kaiser and A. Völker (eds), *Montanmedizin und Bergbauwissenschaften* (Halle: Martin-Luther-University, 1987).

4 Brotherhoods appear to have relied on performative accounting rather than keeping registers of weekly contributions until they came under direct ducal administration or indeed much later; tellingly, the earliest extant registers are for Freiberg, that is, for the *Knappschaft* of the Saxon mining capital and administrative centre, of which the elector and dukes were made honorary members: Sächsisches Staatsarchiv, Bergarchiv Freiberg (hereafter: BAF), 40010 Bergamt Freiberg, No. 4400: Register der Bergknappschaft über Einnahme der Büchsenpfennige auf der Trinkstube, 1543–1561. *Büchsenpfennig* income is mentioned in general mining accounts as early as 1409: Fessner, Bingener, and Slotta (eds), *Auf breiten Schultern*, p. 113; written rules for weekly contribution date from as early as 1450 (Bruderschaft Altenberg); Bergordnung (hereafter: BO) Schneeberg 1471–72, §9, in H. Ermisch, *Das sächsische Bergrecht des Mittelalters* (Leipzig, 1887); BO Goslar 1476, §2, in T. Wagner (ed.), *Corpus juris metallici recentissimi et antiquioris: Sammlung der neuesten und*

älterer Berggesetze (Leipzig, 1791), col. 1030 (hereafter: Wagner); for many similar rules in the following centuries, see Wagner, index s.v. 'Knappschafts-Einrichtungen'; see C. Entzel, J. Deucerus, and A. von Schönberg, *Corpus juris & systema rerum metallicarum, oder Neu-verfasstes Berg-Buch* (Frankfurt, 1698) (hereafter: *Corpus*). On payday, see J. Vetter, *Die soziale und hygienische Lage der bergbauenden Bevölkerung des Erzgebirges in der ersten Hälfte des 16. Jahrhunderts* (Berlin: Limpert, 1940), p. 12.

5 With increasing administrative control in the sixteenth century, this function passed from brotherhood-elected heads to officials such as the *Berg-Meister* and *Zechen-Meister*: for example, Freiberger Knappschaftsordnung 1553, printed in A.F. Wappler, 'Über die Freiberger Berg-, Knapp- und Bruderschaft', *Mitteilungen des Freiberger Altertumsvereins* 37 (1901), 48–71, on 50–3, Art. 7.

6 See generally, H. Keller, 'Vom "heiligen Buch" zur "Buchführung": Lebensfunktionen der Schrift im Mittelalter', *Frühmittelalterliche Studien* 26 (1992), 1–31; J.A. Aho, *Confession and Bookkeeping: The Religious, Moral, and Rhetorical Roots of Modern Accounting* (New York: State University of New York Press, 2005); J. Soll, *The Reckoning: Financial Accountability and the Rise and Fall of Nations* (New York: Basic Books, 2014), ch. 2. Brotherhoods also had larger chests to hold weekly contributions and other income; Fessner, Bingener, and Slotta (eds), *Auf breiten Schultern*, pp. 208–9.

7 U. Lauf, 'Frühe Sozialeinrichtungen im Bergbau Goslars und ihre Spitäler', in Bair and Ingenhaeff (eds), *Bergvolk und Medizin*, pp. 194–200; see generally, I. Sahmland, 'Anfänge des "Betriebskrankenhauses" und erste Formen einer Krankenversicherung im 16. Jahrhundert', *Medizinhistorisches Journal* 22:1 (1987), 28–47.

8 C. Bartels, A. Bingener, and R. Slotta (eds), *Das Schwazer Bergbuch* (3 vols, Bochum, 2006); A. Bingener, 'Zur Entwicklung des Knappschaftswesens in Tirol', in Bartels (ed.), *Höchst verpönte Selbst-Hülfe*, pp. 26–45, 43–4.

9 BO Goslar 1538, in Wagner, cols 1046–7.

10 BO Goslar 1538, in Wagner, col. 1047: 'den schaden besehen'; 'uppe deme Rammelsberge vordoruen'.

11 Wagner, s.v. 'Knappschafts-Einrichtungen'; see Büchsenpfennig traditions and rules in Freiberger Knappschaftsordnung 1553, Art. 2 and Art. 6, Confirmation Knappschafts-Büchsenpfennige zu Marienberg 1553, and Alte Freibergischen Bergkgebreuche (Simon Bogner) 1567, Art. 39, Art. 131–2, printed in Wappler, 'Über die Freiberger Berg-, Knapp- und Bruderschaft', on pp. 50–5.

12 For episodes of refusal to contribute pennies and negligence in collecting them, see Lauf, *Knappschaft*.

13 See most recently J.A. Mendelsohn, 'Lepraschau als Urszene medizinischen Gutachtens' in A. Geisthövel and V. Hess (eds), *Medizinisches Gutachten: Geschichte einer neuzeitlichen Praxis* (Göttingen: Wallstein, 2017), pp. 43–69 and references therein.
14 C. Stein, *Negotiating the French Pox in Early Modern Germany* (Farnham: Ashgate, 2009); M.L. Hammond, 'Medical examination and poor relief in early modern Germany', *Social History of Medicine* 24:2 (2011), 244–59; miners' relief supplications have been sampled for the Harz region, c. 1570–1660: C. Küpper-Eichas, '"... und in solcher ihrer arbeit vielfältig zu schaden / und umb ihre Gesundheit kommen ...": Maßnahmen zur Gesundheits- und Sozialfürsorge im Harzer Bergrevier im 16. und frühen 17. Jahrhundert', in Bair and Ingenhaeff (eds), *Bergvolk und Medizin*, pp. 163–81, especially pp. 172–4.
15 For *Bergordnungen* especially rich in references to *besichtigen* and *besehen*, see Wagner: BO Schwarzburg 1533 (cols 1385, 1388–89, 1392, 1394, 1398); BO Hungary 1575 (col. 181) with Erläuterung alten BO Städte Schemnitz ... (cols 262–98, passim); BO Brandenburg 1619 (cols 435–6, 439, 449, 457, 459, 467–8).
16 Ermisch, *Das sächsische Bergrecht des Mittelalters*: Erste große BO Schneeberg 1492, §20, p. 109; Entwurf BO Schreckenberge 1499–1500, §63, pp. 132–3; Dritte Grosse BO Schneeberg 1500, §27, p. 152.
17 BO Goslar 1544 (Wagner, col. 1052).
18 Wagner, passim; Ermisch, *Das sächsische Bergrecht*, passim.
19 Some eighteenth-century records include this level of detail and require further study; this example is later: BAF, 40013 Bergamt Marienberg, No. 224: Bergphysikus des Bergamtes Marienberg, 1773–1800s, fols 214–24: 'Verzeichniß der Medicamente, welche namentlich benannte krank gewesenen Bergarbeiter im Quartal Reminiscere 1807 [?] und mit dem Erfolge allerseitiger Wiederherstellung, erhalten haben', clerk's copy of original by Physicus Dr. Christoph Conrad Steinmetz, dated Marienberg, 1 April 1806, on fol. 215r, entry No. 7: 'wegen eines rheumatisch Chronisch Schmerzens in der rechten Seite'; see also entry No. 2, fol. 214r: treatment 'wegen der Continuation seines gehabten Fiebers'.
20 As early as 1572, the Duke of Brunswick began appointing physicians on salary to treat miners; J.-T. Greuer, 'Die Oberharzer Knappschaftskassen vom 16. Jahrhundert bis zur Mitte des 19. Jahrhunderts ein Beitrag zur Sozialgeschichte der Oberharzer Bergleute' (Dissertation University at Göttingen, 1962), p. 120; Küpper-Eichas, 'und in solcher ihrer arbeit', pp. 175–7.
21 On *Bergsucht* as miners' own term: E. Rosner, 'Die Berufskrankheiten in der Predigtliteratur des 16. Jahrhunderts', *Sudhoffs Archiv für Geschichte der Medizin und der Naturwissenschaften* 41:3 (1957), 193–206, on 202;

on Paracelsus' experience of mining and his writing on mining disease: E. Rosner, 'Hohenheims Bergsuchtmonographie', *Medizinhistorisches Journal* 16:1–2 (1981), 20–52.

22 Supplication of 1659 quoted in Küpper-Eichas, 'und in solcher ihrer arbeit', p. 173; for lay diagnostic precision and imprecision in later letters of supplication in England, see S. King, *Sickness, Medical Welfare and the English Poor, 1750–1834* (Manchester: Manchester University Press, 2018), ch. 2.

23 F. Koelsch, 'Samuel Stockhausens Schrift über die Hüttenkatze, 1656', *Zentralblatt für Gewerbehygiene und Unfallverhütung* N.S. 1 (1924), 41–3, 76–8, 101–3.

24 Compare cross-occupational women's friendly societies defining illness 'in functional rather than medical terms': A.A. Rusnock and V.E. Dietz, 'Defining women's sickness and work: Female friendly societies in England, 1780–1830', *Journal of Women's History* 24:1 (2012), 60–85, on 61.

25 BAF, 40010 Bergamt Freiberg, Nr. 4402: Rechnung der Bergknappschaft, 1515–1604; recent comparative analysis and overview: A. Bingener, 'Das knappschaftliche Rechnungswesen vom 16. bis zum 18. Jahrhundert am Beispiel der Freiberger, Schneeberger und Johanngeorgenstädter Knappschaftsrechnungen', in Bartels (ed.), *Höchst verpönte Selbst-Hülfe*, pp. 64–87; Harz: Greuer, 'Die Oberharzer Knappschaftskassen'.

26 BO Goslar 1538, in Wagner as 'Bergordnung des Rathes zu Goslar', col. 1046; typically called 'Knappschaftsordnung'.

27 BAF, 40010 Bergamt Freiberg, No. 1203: Verzeichnis der bei der Bergknappschaft rückständigen Büchsenpfennige, February 1678.

28 Wagner: BO Kur Köln 1669, Part 7, Art. 36 (col. 870); quotations from BO Itter (Hessen-Darmstadt) 1718, Part I, Art. 11 (col. 697); for much later simulation detection in health insurance, see T.W. Guinnane and J. Streb, 'Moral hazard in a mutual health insurance system: German Knappschaften, 1867–1914', *Journal of Economic History* 71:1 (2011), 70–104; and the contribution of Helene Castenbrandt (Chapter 13) in this volume.

29 Niedersächsisches Landesarchiv, Bergarchiv Clausthal, Hann. 84 a Berg- und Forstamt Clausthal, Acc. 26, No. 1040: 'Rechnung ... Berg-, Pochwercks und Gnadenlöhner Patienten an Medicin verabfolget worden, de Quartal Luciae 1787', p. 1.

30 Stein, *Negotiating the French Pox*; O.P. Grell and A. Cunningham (eds), *Health Care and Poor Relief in Protestant Europe, 1500–1700* (London: Routledge, 1997).

31 BAF, 40001 Oberbergamt Freiberg, Nr. 707: Anstellung und Verpflichtung des Bergchirurgen für das Freiberger Revier, 1715–1837, fol. 20: miner's attestation, c. 1717.

32 Vetter, *Soziale und hygienische Lage*; S.C. Karant-Nunn, 'From adventurers to drones: the Saxon silver miners as an early proletariat', in T.M.

Safley and L.N. Rosenband (eds), *The Workplace Before the Factory: Artisans and Proletarians, 1500–1800* (Ithaca: Cornell University Press, 1993), pp. 73–99.
33 Vetter, *Soziale und hygienische Lage*, pp. 35–7.
34 Four elements: G. Agricola, *De re metallica*, trans. H. Hoover and L.H. Hoover (New York, 1950), Book IX, p. 379.
35 Or four weeks for a mine in a period of little or no yield; BO Joachimsthal 1518 Art. CV (Wagner, col. 4).
36 No such stipulation is found in Saxony's widely copied BO Annaberg 1509 (Ermisch, *Das sächsische Bergrecht*). The sickness benefit article of BO Joachimsthal 1518 was copied in the Harz in BO Bergwerke bey Gittel im Grunde 1524 Art. CV (Wagner, cols 1041–42); BO Joachimsthal 1548 Part II Art. 85 (*Corpus*, p. 61); Zinnbergwerksordnung Kingdom of Bohemia and Hungary 1548, Berg-Städte Art. XXI (*Corpus*, p. 120), Bergwerke Art. XLVIII (*Corpus*, p. 129); BO Nassau 1559 Art. LXV (Wagner, col. 786); BO Kur Trier 1564 Art. XVI §2 (Wagner, col. 961); BO Brandenburg 1619 Art. XXXV (Wagner, col. 452); and many more.
37 Wagner: BO Kur Trier 1564 Art XVI §1-§4 (col. 961); BO Tarnowitz (Silesia) 1599, Art. I (cols 1311–12), establishing 'Bruderbüchse' with weekly contributions by *Gewerken*, administrators, and 'workers'; General-Privilegium Cleve 1767 Art. VII (col. 1265–66); BO Magdeburg 1772 Ch. LXXVIII, §1 (col. 1227); BO Bayern 1784 Art. LIV (col. 362).
38 Quotation from U. Ellenbog, *Von den gifftigen besen Tempffen und Reüchen; der Metal, als Silber, Quecksilber, Bley und anders. So die Edlenhandt werck des Goltschmidens und ander arbaiter in des feürsich gebrauchen mussen. Wie sie sich da mit halten und die gift vertreibe solle* (Augsburg, 1524), sig. A1v; see E. Rosner, 'Ulrich Ellenbog und die Anfänge der Gewerbehygiene', *Sudhoffs Archiv für Geschichte der Medizin und der Naturwissenschaften* 38:2 (1954), 104–10.
39 U. Rülein von Calw, *Bergwerk- und Probierbüchlein: A Translation from the German*, trans. A. Grünhaldt Sisco and C.S. Smith (New York, 1949); G. Agricola, *Bermannus, sive de re metallica* (Basel, 1530).
40 H. Pforr, 'Der Freiberger Stadtphysikus Ulrich Rülein von Calw (1465–1523) als Wegbereiter der Bergbauwissenschaften und als Vorläufer von Georgius Agricola (1494–1555)', in W. Kaiser and A. Völker (eds), *Montanmedizin und Bergbauwissenschaften*, pp. 52–66.
41 T. von Hohenheim, *Von der Bergsucht und anderen Bergkrankheiten*, ed. by F. Koelsch (Berlin: Springer, 1925), p. 3.
42 Magnus Hundt, *Eyn Nutzliches Regiment sampt dem bericht der ertzney wider etzliche kra[n]ckheit d[er] brust, vn[d] sund[er]lich wid[er] de[n] huste[n], brust seuche, vn[d] beschweru[n]g des Adems* (Leipzig, 1529), p. 1v.

43 Ibid., pp. 15v–16v, 17r, 40v.
44 Rosner, 'Berufskrankheiten'.
45 Bonet managed to create two such *observationes* from passing references in Sennert and in a letter from Schenck to Thomas Bartholin: T. Bonet, *Sepulchretum sive anatomia practica ex cadaveribus morbo denatis* (2 vols, Geneva, 1679), vol. 2, Bk II, Section I, p. 404, Obs. XLIV–XLV.
46 Classical sources had no such category; Pliny the Elder and others compiled information on the dangers of mining and metalworking, and the medieval Hippocratic corpus included recipes against 'morbi metallici' or the ill effects of lead, mercury, and zinc, yet not even the erudite Agricola seems to have taken note of this; see V. Zimmermann, 'Ansätze zu einer Sozial- und Arbeitsmedizin am mittelalterlichen Arbeitsplatz', in B. Herrmann (ed.), *Mensch und Umwelt im Mittelalter* (Stuttgart: Deutsche Verlags-Anstalt, 1986), pp. 140–9.
47 Agricola, *De re metallica*, p. 214; I have inserted *tabes* from G. Agricola, *Georgii Agricolae De re metallica libri XII* (Basel, 1556), p. 172.
48 Rosner and Markowitz, *Deadly Dust*, p. 5.
49 Agricola, *De re metallica*, pp. 214–16.
50 Rosner, 'Berufskrankheiten', pp. 203–5; I. Sahmland, 'Gesundheitsschädigungen der Bergleute: Die Bedeutung der Bergpredigten des 16. bis frühen 18. Jahrhunderts als Quelle arbeitsmedizingeschichtlicher Fragestellungen', *Medizinhistorisches Journal* 23:3–4 (1988), 240–76.
51 BO Goslar 1538, in Wagner, col. 1047.
52 *Corpus* and Wagner, both passim (Schmelzer, Hütten).
53 F. Koelsch, 'Bemerkungen zum III. Buch' in Hohenheim, *Von der Bergsucht*, pp. 63–4; E. Rosner, 'Die Bedeutung des Annaberger Stadtarztes Martin Pansa für die Geschichte der Gewerbehygiene', *Sudhoffs Archiv für Geschichte der Medizin und der Naturwissenschaften* 37:3–4 (1953), 357–61.
54 For a series of examples, see F. Koelsch, 'Bemerkungen zum I. Buch' in Hohenheim, *Von der Bergsucht*, pp. 25–9.
55 See, for example, ibid., pp. 29–30.
56 See the contributions of Michael Stolberg (Chapter 1) and Philipp Rieder (Chapter 2) in this volume.
57 University Archive, Humboldt University Berlin, Grotjahn Papers 7: Nachlass Heinrich Grotjahn (1794–1872), No. 343: Patientenbuch Heinrich Grotjahns aus Schladen und Umgebung, 1833–1841, 946 pages, one page per patient with treatments listed and crossed out when paid.
58 M. Stolberg, 'Medizinische Loci communes: Formen und Funktionen einer ärztlichen Aufzeichnungspraxis im 16. und 17. Jahrhundert', *NTM: International Journal of History and Ethics of Natural Sciences, Technology*

and Medicine, 21:1 (2013), 37–60; V. Hess and J.A. Mendelsohn, 'Case and series: Medical knowledge and paper technology, 1600–1900', *History of Science*, 48:3–4 (2010), 287–314.

59 R. Schilling, *Johann Friedrich Glaser (1707–1789): Scharfrichtersohn und Stadtphysikus in Suhl* (Cologne: Böhlau, 2015), transcription from 1753 entries rendered into modern German on p. 43, my English translation.

60 BAF, 40006 Bergamt Altenberg, No. 290: Entlassung des Zwitterstock-Bergchirurgen Johann Heinrich Wendler durch den Zwitterstockfaktor, fols 3r–4v: 'Specificatio Derer innerl. Medic[amenten]: welche an E. Hoch und Wohlersehne Zwitter-Stocksgewerckschaft verunglückter Arbeitern geben worden müßen, in Quartal Crucis 1750', submitted by Gottfried Schäffer Berg Chirurgus, on fol. 3r.

61 Such invoicing reports appear to be no longer extant in series in the Bergarchiv Freiberg. Extant examples appear to be limited to copies filed in cases of disagreement or petition to the *Bergamt*. This particular such file (note 60 above) shows that invoicing reports were nonetheless kept for decades, as the file was begun in 1751 and includes copies of such documents from 1736.

62 BAF, 40001 Oberbergamt Freiberg, Nr. 707: Anstellung und Verpflichtung des Bergchirurgen für das Freiberger Revier, 1715–1837, fols 112r–113v: 'Es sind von an[no] 1757 bis 1758 von Gersdorffer Zeche Segen Gottes folgende daselbst anstehende Personen successive zu mir gekommen, mit Vergebung, wie sie in den Gruben verunglücket wären', submitted by Johann Gottfried Leuthold (?), 5 May 1759, entry No. 7 on fols 113r–v: 'Bei Besehung befunden'.

63 BAF, 40168 Grubenakten des Bergreviers Marienberg, No. 847: Schießwecken Fundgrube am Wildsberg bei Pobershau, 1727–1743, fol. 3r–v: surgeon's detailed report on injured miner Gotthard Seiffert, March 1734; fol. 4r: detailed report of Seiffert's long illness, with invoice, March 1735.

64 'Verzeichniß der Medicamente', 1806 (note 19 above), fol. 218r, entry No. 27.

65 In Altenberg he was Bergmeister and Zehntner; then in Freiberg, Bergmeister: *Königlich-Sächsischer Hof und Staats Kalender auf das Jahr 1805* (Leipzig, 1805), p. 109; *auf das Jahr 1809* (1809), p. 130.

66 'Verzeichniß der Medicamente', 1806 (note 19 above), fol. 223r, entry No. 60; see also No. 64.

67 BAF, 40169 Grubenakten des Bergreviers Schwarzenberg, No. 1053: Henneberger tiefer Erbstolln, fols 163–70: Begutachtung der Heilkosten des verunglückten Bergarbeiter Christian Friedrich Oeser aus Sosa durch den Amtsphysikus Forberger (1776), on fol. 163r; for an earlier example, see

No. 1340: Neue Brüderschaft Fundgrube: Almosen und Heilkosten für den verunglückten Bergarbeiter Christoph Friedrich Leuschner (1727).
68 Most recently emphasised in Soll, *The Reckoning*. See H.E. Lowood, 'The calculating forester: quantification, cameral science, and the emergence of scientific forestry management in Germany', in J.L. Heilbron (ed.), *The Quantifying Spirit in the 18th Century* (Berkeley: University of California Press, 1990), pp. 315–42; M. Power (ed.), *Accounting and Science: Natural Inquiry and Commercial Reason* (Cambridge: Cambridge University Press, 1996); A. Barrera-Osorio, *Experiencing Nature: The Spanish American Empire and the Early Scientific Revolution* (Austin: University of Texas Press, 2006); A. te Heesen, 'Accounting for the natural world: double-entry bookkeeping in the field', in L.L. Schiebinger and C. Swan (eds), *Colonial Botany: Science, Commerce, and Politics in the Early Modern World* (Philadelphia: University of Pennsylvania Press, 2007), pp. 237–51; A. Wakefield, *The Disordered Police State: German Cameralism as Science and Practice* (Chicago: University of Chicago Press, 2009).
69 Grimm, *Deutsches Wörterbuch*, s.v. *Büchse*, *Buch*; Lauf, 'Frühe Sozialeinrichtungen', p. 201.
70 See Karant-Nunn, 'From adventurers to drones'.
71 The *Knappschaften* of Joachimsthal and of Marienberg, for example, successfully retained administration of their own *Kasse* or *Büchsenpfennig* throughout the revolts and protests during and after the Peasants War of 1525: Vetter, *Soziale und hygienische Lage*, p. 27.

13

Administrating sickness: The workings of an all-female sickness fund, 1898–1931

Helene Castenbrandt

With the industrial revolution, mutual aid organisations grew in importance and several European countries saw a remarkable growth in the number of sickness funds, with membership increasing throughout the nineteenth century.[1] In general, the purpose of these funds was to ensure the economic stability of members and their families. They did this by providing monetary assistance in times of sickness and death. However, these organisations often found themselves in difficult economic circumstances and many sickness funds struggled in forming sustainable organisations. Some funds did not last for long, while others grew prosperous and continued for decades or even centuries. This unstable situation was especially the case in Sweden during the early twentieth century, when the Swedish sickness fund movement was expanding rapidly, with privately organised and often voluntary organisations. This chapter examines what characterised a successful voluntary sickness fund in early twentieth-century Sweden.

This chapter analyses the practices of one of the most successful voluntary sickness funds in the city of Gothenburg, the Seamstresses Sickness and Burial Fund (hereafter SSBK) during the period 1898–1931.[2] This sickness fund is a useful case study because it was one of only five all female sickness funds that existed in Gothenburg in 1901 and, of these five, SSBK lasted the longest.[3] At the time, Gothenburg had 128 sickness funds and 108 of them accepted only male members. So, from the outset, SSBK was at a disadvantage in an otherwise male-dominated movement, as it targeted low-paid working-class women. So how did this fund survive to become one of the few in Gothenburg that lasted into the reorganisation of Swedish sickness funds in the mid-1930s? Analysing SSBK's accounting practices reveals how a working-class organisation strove to improve the living conditions of its members during the first half of the twentieth century. The fund's longevity, at a time when the sickness fund movement in Sweden greatly expanded and many funds came and went, can help us understand the economic considerations and motives behind the building of a successful fund.

In assessing the fund's strategies, this chapter analyses archival material, including annual statistical reports as well as the minutes of the fund's member and board meetings. In order to understand the fund's economic considerations, SSBK will be examined as a *moral economy*. Since the works of E.P. Thompson and James C. Scott,[4] many scholars from different scientific fields have used and understood the term moral economy in slightly different ways. Here the term will be used as an analytic tool to identify the accounting practices in a specific social setting and attribute agency to those involved in creating these practices.[5] Interpreting an organisation as a moral economy helps us understand economic practices in civil society. A moral economy, with strong roots in the social world and organised around mutual aid, participates in economic practices that are governed not simply by capital accumulation.[6] The concept of moral economy can thus be used to understand the rationality behind efforts to build an organisation based on trust, as well as to act in accordance with not just statutory membership rights, but also values and responsibilities. I argue that a large part of SSBK's success lies in its actions as a moral economy and in the leadership of its highly devoted president of thirty-three years, Stina Fagerskog.

Previous research

The growth of sickness funds in Europe during the nineteenth century can be interpreted as a sign of rising living standards, as the working class could afford to think of the future and spend money on insurance.[7] It thereby also became a way for the respectable working class to be less dependent on poor relief and charity.[8] Not until the 1920s did the more prosperous middle class develop a greater interest in health insurance.[9]

For centuries, this voluntary sector of friendly societies, or dedicated sickness funds, together with the state, commercial stakeholders, as well as informal sectors (involving family, friends, and neighbours) provided welfare services. However, the distribution between these sectors changed over time and these shifts become especially evident when considering the expanding role of the state during the twentieth century.[10] Sickness funds in particular were generally mutual aid organisations funded by their members, but here too the variations were large. For example, in the Netherlands, as voluntary organisations expanded during the nineteenth century, commercial interests also grew in importance. While commercial insurance was practically non-existent around the year 1800, a century later it had come to comprise about a third of the market.[11] These mixed welfare economies exhibited various national traits depending on the nature and degree of government involvement.[12] For the voluntary sector, there was also a close relationship between philanthropy and mutual aid.[13] In Britain, especially female friendly societies were often closely tied to rich donors and were part of the philanthropic work of local elites.[14]

To become a successful and economically stable organisation, voluntary sickness funds needed rules and principles for dealing with *adverse selection* and *moral hazards*. Adverse selection concerns the selection of members. A problem facing voluntary sickness funds was that unhealthy workers might subscribe in greater numbers, whereas healthy workers could find it less interesting to join a fund or would leave a fund that had too many ailing members.[15] Funds therefore needed to carefully balance the influx of new members and make sure that members remained in the fund. These issues were dealt with in a number of ways. For example, recruitment in female funds was generally guided by the principle that young and unmarried women were good new recruits, as they would hopefully spend several years in the fund before needing benefits.[16]

The term moral hazard refers to the greater incentive of members to take sick leave compared to non-members. Funds needed to limit simple malingering or outright fraud, otherwise costs would increase and membership fees would need to be raised.[17] Rules usually limited the number of sick days members could take, imposed a few qualifying days at the start of each illness, and generally imposed a waiting period at the start of each new membership. There could also be restrictions regarding accidents and self-inflicted conditions, including venereal diseases.[18] Furthermore, the funds often imposed obligations on sick members. Female friendly societies in England generally defined what unpaid work a woman on benefits was allowed to do at home, stating whether or not she was allowed to cook or take care of her children. Some funds prohibited any type of housework, while other funds accepted that members did some domestic work as well as cared for their own children. In male societies, the obligations were usually altogether different, often stating that a member could not go outside at inappropriate times or be found drinking while on benefits.[19]

Scholars have noted the importance of the social aspect of voluntary sickness funds in dealing with adverse selection and moral hazards.[20] Voluntary funds with high levels of mutual responsibility seem to have had more inbuilt control over moral hazards and therefore needed fewer rules to counter fraud. In line with this, the economic historian John E. Murray has used aggregated data from Germany, Austria, France, Belgium, and Denmark for the period 1885–1908 to show that countries with compulsory sickness funds had higher sickness rates compared to countries with voluntary insurance schemes. He concludes that it was easier to claim benefits in the well-financed compulsory funds, while the more economically restrained voluntary funds were more reluctant to pay out compensation.[21]

A voluntary sickness fund's reputation was important and meant that funds could not simply rely on their economic viability. Instead, it was vitally important to uphold the moral conduct of fund members. Members needed to show good behaviour and there were often rules about moral conduct designed to preserve the society's good name. One issue that demonstrates the delicate balance that needed to be maintained was the custom of beer drinking and meetings at local pubs in British societies. In general, the working-class movement of friendly societies was seen as a good thing. However, beer drinking habits sometimes spurred concerns about the level of alcohol consumption during meetings and at other social gatherings.[22] This social side of friendly societies suggests that they comprised an important part of members' social lives and became far more than just insurance providers in the event of lost income in times of sickness. So even though this social aspect of friendly societies could raise concerns about members' moral conduct, it is also key to explaining the seemingly low level of fraud in sickness funds, given that dishonest behaviour could cost members both their reputation and their friends.[23] Maintaining one's good reputation was of crucial importance for the fund, collectively as well as for each individual member.

Although the rise of friendly societies began as a very male phenomenon, the number of female members grew over time. Women were, however, sometimes excluded on the grounds that they constituted a higher risk.[24] Nevertheless, many male-friendly societies in Great Britain began accepting female members by the end of the nineteenth century, although women were often so badly paid that they could not afford the membership fees in these funds.[25] Thus arose the need for all-female funds. Historian Daniel Weinbren has found that rich and influential men often held important positions in these female friendly societies. The board and treasury were in his findings run by men, often with close ties to the church. For example, in the Southill Female Friendly Society, which existed between 1844 and 1948, the vicar always held the position of treasurer. Also, in many funds the wife of the church clerk administered the collection of membership fees.[26] In contrast, historians Andrea Rusnock and Vivien Dietz, in a study of rules and regulations in English female friendly societies, find that men were largely absent from the administration of female funds. In fact, many rules stated that men were not even allowed to attend meetings. In these cases, it was women who made the rules, held the meetings, and decided about benefits.[27]

The expansion of the Swedish sickness fund movement

Before the introduction of compulsory national health insurance in 1955, Swedish sickness funds were mutual aid organisations with voluntary membership, or in some cases affiliated with larger workplaces. These privately organised funds sometimes had to compete for members, which often meant that they kept membership fees to a minimum.[28] Many white collar workers in Sweden received sick pay as part of their compensation, so it was mostly blue collar workers that drove the country's sickness fund movement. Even though the recruitment of members became more diversified over time, the split between blue and white collar workers persisted until the introduction of compulsory national health insurance.[29] As the number of sickness funds increased, the government began addressing their financial difficulties and sought to stabilise the market for sickness funds. For example, from 1892 the government supported funds that registered under Sweden's first sickness fund law. At this point, government control was still at a minimum, but registered funds were obligated to submit annual statistics, allowing the government to monitor the movement.[30]

The Swedish government adopted a middle way by providing private sickness funds with successively more government grants, thus transforming the hitherto mixed welfare economy into one that was increasingly dominated by the state and in which public insurance organisations did not compete on the open market. The new law regarding sickness funds from 1910 resulted in more government involvement, but the biggest intervention came with the 1931 law. In practice, the 1931 law went a long way toward creating the structure for a compulsory system, especially since funds could no longer choose their own members, but were instead required to admit all applicants that fit the health and age criteria within their assigned geographic area. When obligatory health insurance was introduced in 1955, the government more or less took over the structures that the 1931 law had created.[31]

Evidence for the rapid expansion of the Swedish sickness fund movement between 1900 and 1910 can be found in the expanding number of registered funds, going from 221 to 2,426, while membership between 1900 and 1950 increased from 260,000 to 3 million, which then accounted for 58 per cent of the population over 15 years old. During the expansion of sickness funds, the proportion of female members increased dramatically. Women constituted only 20 per cent of members in 1900, but by 1941 there were more female than male members.[32] Up until the 1930s, most Swedish sickness funds were small: in 1901, 80 per cent of the funds had no more than 200 members; and even by 1930, only 8 per cent of sickness funds had more than 1,000 members.[33] However, the legislative changes gradually created larger and more robust organizations, as shown for the city of Gothenburg in Figure 13.1.

Gothenburg followed the national trend with a continuous increase in members during the first half of the twentieth century, with members concentrated in fewer and fewer sickness funds following the legislative changes in 1910 and 1931.

Administrating sickness

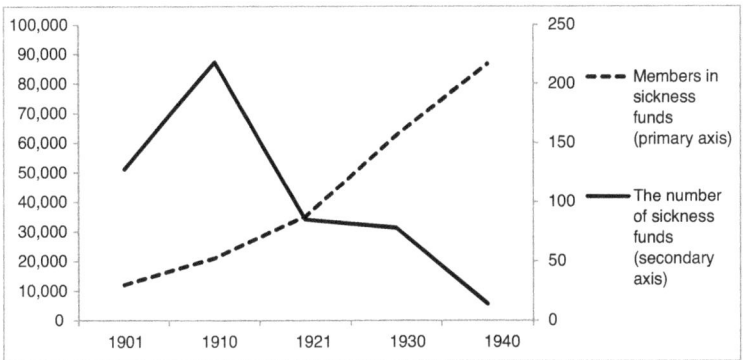

13.1 Members and sickness funds in Gothenburg, 1901–40.

The Seamstresses Sickness and Burial Fund (SSBK)

With the arduous working conditions for seamstresses in mind, the sickness and burial fund SSBK was funded in April 1898 as an organisation of mutual aid for female seamstresses in Gothenburg. The aim was to help seamstresses working from home or in factories in the city, although members were allowed to stay on even after a change in occupation. From 1923 they also accepted members from other occupational groups. From 1934 male members were accepted, in accordance with the 1931 law, and fifteen years later 10 per cent of the members were men. The fund operated until 1946 when it was absorbed into the central sickness fund covering the whole city of Gothenburg, which was in line with the general development at the time that saw all remaining sickness funds in Gothenburg transferred into the central fund between 1940 and 1950.

During its early years, the fund limited membership to no more than 200 members. However, this rule was soon abandoned and in 1913 the fund adopted several initiatives to greatly increase the number of members. Board members personally went out to workplaces and recruited new members, talking to workers as well as encouraging employers to persuade their workers to join the fund, and perhaps even to agree to pay for their workers' entrance fees. All members were asked to help recruit new members. Furthermore, SSBK often advertised for new members, as well as developed a form that made applying for membership easy, which was sent out to workplaces. As a result of these initiatives, many new members were recruited and other smaller funds were incorporated into SSBK. By 1919, the fund had almost 700 members and was the largest female sickness fund in Gothenburg, as well as one of the largest female funds in Sweden. Thereafter membership numbers stagnated, but by 1934 the number of members started to increase again after the admission process was again simplified using new application forms and with the board asking for a medical certificate only when considered necessary.[34]

The fund's economy

Attracting new and healthy members while retaining older ones was an important part of ensuring adequate revenue for the fund. At the start of the twentieth century, 77 per cent of the revenue was derived from membership fees, which later stabilised at around 60 to 65 per cent. The remaining income came mostly from government and municipal grants, and from interest on bank savings.[35] State and municipal subsidies to the fund increased up until 1920, but thereafter state contributions per member remained fairly stable. The fund also continuously received smaller donations, usually between 50 and 100 kronor, which they used to attract new members. The fund advertised in the local newspaper, sometimes alongside the announcement of the fund's monthly meeting, stating that donations had now made it possible to admit new members free of charge or even to conduct free health examinations. Larger donations also played a part in the fund's economic stability; for example, in 1901 the fund was bequeathed the sum of 5,000 kronor, which was used to begin building its reserves.[36] Since they had started out as a smaller fund, the benefits for sick pay, the costs for doctors' appointments, and the payments for funeral allowance fluctuated significantly from year to year. But even so, it was only occasionally that the fund had to rely on savings to cover losses (Figure 13.2).

Over the years, the fund accumulated substantial reserves. Its financial assets increased the most during the 1920s, despite the fact that the average yearly benefits disbursed to each member also rose during this period. Certainly, the subsidies from the state and municipality were important, but it was the fund's decision to start using a two-class system, allowing some members to be charged higher premiums, that

	1899	1911	1920	1930
Income				
Membership fees	283	2,915	6,667	12,693
Entrance fees, fines	10	88	299	359
Government and municipality grants	0	419	3,704	4,270
Various (interest, donations etc.)	884	856	1,447	2,311
Expenditure				
Sickness benefit (including maternal benefit)	256	1,665	5,340	8,767
Medical treatment	190	477	2,566	3,599
Funeral allowance		200	150	1,600
Board and auditors		263	1,965	2,205
Sick visitors			170	200
Various (rent, inventory, gifts etc.)	84	327	873	1,074
Total income	1,177	4,278	12,117	19,633
Total expenditure	530	2,932	11,064	17,444
Balance	647	1,346	1,053	2,189
Financial assets	1,516	12,001	29,357	60,741

13.2 Income, expenditure, and financial assets in SSBK 1899–1930.

contributed mostly to its accumulation of wealth. The fund had long resisted different membership classes, but in 1923 the two-class system was introduced. Class I paid a membership fee of 1 krona per month and Class II paid 1 krona and 75 öre. The majority of members chose to belong to Class II, giving them access to higher benefits.[37]

However, for many years most members in SSBK had not been able to afford higher fees, so as a guiding principle the fund had kept their fees low. In 1900, members paid only 50 öre per month and by 1914 only 85 öre.[38] For a long time, the fund was anxious to retain its low fees, and so, for example, when the fund registered under the 1910 law, it submitted statistics demonstrating that it was viable in spite of its very low fees.[39] In addition to membership fees, members paid a lump sum funeral fee, which in 1905 was set at 1 krona per year.[40] The fund also charged each member extra for funeral wreaths for members that had passed away.

The fund compensated funeral expenses, medication, hospital care, as well as sick and maternity leave. Each member had their own personal passbook, which they brought to the doctor and treasurer to be signed. Also, for visits to a physician, all members brought a form for the doctor to fill out, and by 1913 a special form had been developed to apply for maternal benefits. To claim benefits, a sick member needed to report directly to SSBK's chair and submit a medical certificate. Benefits were paid from the day after the illness was reported and collected at the treasurer's residence at specific times each week. All collected fees and benefit payments were recorded in the fund's account books, and the annual reports to the government had a unifying effect on this data collection. Information on what data to collect was circulated to all registered funds and SSBK kept its records in ways that made it easier to compile the annual statistical reports.

Long-term sickness cases

SSBK introduced several rules to counteract the potential economic burden of members afflicted with long-term illnesses. Such cases were a major concern of the fund because of the economic uncertainty and potential ruin that they entailed. The fund's responsibility for long-term cases was restricted to a maximum of ninety days during one year, which was a normal limit for Swedish sickness funds. However, in 1904 SSBK joined the central organisation for sickness funds in Gothenburg and members could, for an additional annual fee, gain the right to an extra seventy days of compensation. Once it became obligatory to belong to the central organisation in 1917, all members gained the right to a maximum of 160 days.[41]

Early detection of diseases was considered to be the most effective way to avoid long-term cases. In its early years, the fund had an agreement with one doctor who performed all the medical examinations on sick members. However, the fund suspected that members did not have enough confidence in him and that they therefore waited too long before they saw the doctor. Hence, from 1903 members were granted the right to freely choose which doctor they felt most comfortable with and then be compensated by the fund. There was a limit to the medical expenses that could be claimed each year, and to prevent physicians from overcharging for their services the central fund in Gothenburg in 1916 reached an agreement on fixed prices for members in sickness funds with many of the city's doctors.[42] The substantially lower number of sick days in 1903 compared to 1902 was seen by SSBK as a direct result of the decision to let members chose their doctor freely.[43]

The fund's expenditures for medical care also proved to be much less when members chose their own doctor rather than relying on physicians under yearly contract with SSBK. The issue was discussed regularly, but annual accounts showed it to be more economical. For example, in 1912 the fund spent in total 648 kronor on medical care, but for a yearly subscription with a doctor, at a rate of 4 kronor for each of the 338 members, the fund would instead have had to spend 1,352 kronor, more than double the amount. Also, in addition to early detection, it seemed that this arrangement encouraged members to go directly to a specialist, which was thought to speed up recovery. This also illustrates the inbuilt trust of the system. As members were given the right to choose their own doctor, the fund had no control over the physician's judgement about the need for sick leave.

To prevent long-term cases, in 1911 the fund decided that all prospective members should be examined by a specific doctor. Previously, new members had been allowed to submit a health certificate from any doctor. However, the fund's careful monitoring of members on sick leave had revealed that many members suffered from lung conditions and other chest-related ailments. So in 1912, they found a doctor specialising in chest illnesses whom they instructed to take the interests of the fund into account when issuing health certificates. Although this arrangement increasingly led to the exclusion of young women suffering from lung disease, it also likely helped improve the health of seamstresses as the doctor helped those that were found sick in getting into early treatment.[44]

An organisation led by its members

The fund was organised around its monthly meetings and for many years the fund had the privilege of using the congregation house of Oscar Fredrik parish for their meetings. The fund's good relations with the priest allowed it free use of the meeting room up until 1917, when larger premises were required to accommodate the expanding fund's meetings. At each general meeting, members heard reports on the fund's finances and on who had been sick since the last meeting; members took far-reaching decisions about difficult cases and about the fund's financial affairs. However, as the fund grew larger and its administration more professionalised, more and more issues were decided at its board meetings.

SSBK was structured around monthly social gatherings which also served as a kind of social control over its members. The custom of sponsoring a funeral wreath when members died shows that SSBK was not just an insurance scheme; it was also a social movement involving close relations and friendships. Also, besides handling the affairs of the fund, the monthly meetings became a way of informing members about the development of sickness funds in general. For example, the president, Stina Fagerskog, repeatedly lectured about the conferences and other meetings she attended on behalf of SSBK.

The fund was led entirely by its members and its first chair, Stina Fagerskog, served for thirty-three years. She devoted her life to the fund and administered it from her own home. Fagerskog was herself a seamstress. Born in the province of Värmland, she moved to the city of Gothenburg in 1881 and found work as a maid, but after a few years began working as a seamstress from her home.[45] As the fund's chair, she kept its archive at her home and maintained many of the fund's social connections.

Heavy obligations rested on the chair, but also on the treasurer and the rest of the board. The chair was preoccupied with the fund's general administration, with decisions regarding sick leave and benefit payments, and with promoting the fund and advising its members. After considerable deliberation, in 1916 the fund had a phone installed in Fagerskog's apartment making it easier for members to reach her if they needed to.[46] Board members received some compensation for their work, and as the fund expanded the level of compensation increased. Their remuneration grew from 75 kronor in 1900 to 600 kronor (of which around 300 went to the chair) in 1919. Apart from this, the chair also received other monetary compensation. From 1914, she received 180 kronor a year for hosting the fund's office. Also, since many members neglected to conduct their visits to sick members, the chair often had to step in. From 1918, Fagerskog therefore received 50 kronor, plus the fines from members who had neglected their visits, and by 1929 she received 200 kronor a year for this work. This meant that around 1920 the chair received about 600 kronor a year for her work. Compared to average wages for female workers in industry and craft-trades, this constituted about a third to a half of a year's wages.[47] Over time, the fund became a considerable source of income, which made it possible for her to devote much attention to its affairs.

The social dimension of the fund meant that many obligations also rested on members. Each member had to show up in person to receive benefits. Membership fees were paid at the monthly meetings, with the exception of July and August. The payments were collected at the end of the meeting and noted in each member's personal passbook. If a member did not show up at three consecutive meetings they would be disbarred from the fund. Members were also advised to bring exact change and if they missed a payment a small fine was assessed. For many years these meetings were held on Sundays, but in 1920 it was decided to meet on a weekday, and not until the implementation of the 1931 law could members choose to make their payment on any afternoon. All of these financial transactions between the fund and its members were noted in members' passbooks, and at the end of the year all books were collected for the annual audit. Members were fined if their books could not be collected.

Members also took turns visiting sick members. The visitors for the upcoming month were chosen at the monthly membership meetings and published in the local paper alongside the meeting announcement. Members were appointed for a month at a time and fined if they did not conduct their visits properly. As part of their obligations, visitors needed to compile a report that included who was reported sick, the type of illness they had, whether the member had reported herself well again, and whether someone had used up all their eligible sick days. These reports were read out at the membership meetings, where difficult cases were also openly discussed. As the fund grew in size and the executive board assumed greater responsibilities, these readings became obsolete, so to save time visitors' reports were, after 1912, summarised in a quarterly report and thereby became less personal. The visits were an important tool for the fund to ensure that members used their benefits according to the fund's rules and to monitor members' illnesses and other problems. Importantly, for these visits to run smoothly, members' names and addresses needed to be up to date. Given that their membership depended on fulfilling these obligations, it can be assumed that most members would have been diligent workers and that these social interactions would also have protected against moral hazard.

After reporting their illnesses to SSBK's chair, members on sick leave were subject to a strict regulatory regime. They were required to follow the doctor's instructions and do everything necessary to restore their health, as well as to remain in their homes.[48] Accordingly, the fund's visitors expected sick members to be home when they came calling. If that was not the case, the visitors were required to report the violation. The chair then usually consulted with the physician to determine whether sick leave should be withdrawn or not. However, there were exceptions to the rule about staying at home. If members were admitted to a hospital or other medical institution, they could receive their benefits as usual. Also, in some cases when the doctor had prescribed that the patient would benefit from recovery in the countryside, the fund agreed to continue payment. This exception gave raise to several discussions over the years. The issue was addressed for the first time in February 1902 when one member was staying in the countryside outside Gothenburg. A doctor had certified that her nervous condition and anaemia made it better for her not to be in the city. The fund agreed and granted her the money.[49] It was decided that benefits for the time spent in the countryside could be paid for fourteen days in advance. For a time thereafter, payments could be mailed, provided a new medical certificate was submitted to the fund each month.[50]

But not all requests were granted. For a disease such as pharyngitis, a stay in the countryside was not allowed, even with a doctor's certificate saying that it would be good for the patient.[51] Moreover, in 1916 a member asked for sick leave due to ear problems. However, the board decided against it by drawing a distinction between being sick and being fit for work, arguing that the member could work and at the same time be treated by a doctor.[52] Another issue involved maternity benefits. After a miscarriage, one member asked for her fourteen days of maternity leave. This sparked a discussion about whether or not miscarriages should be compensated with maternity benefit. Because the member and the board were unable to reach an agreement, a request was sent to the responsible public authority, *Socialstyrelsen*. Based on their answer, the fund decided that women could not claim any maternity benefits after miscarriages; however, they were eligible to receive sick leave for miscarriages that occurred after the fifth month.[53]

While it strictly monitored benefit claims, the fund also felt obligated to help its members above and beyond its statutory obligations. In such cases, the fund proved to be a very idealistic organisation. For instance, in times of surplus, it established an assistance-fund for members in need, allowing, for example, extra financial aid to old members at Christmas. One woman who received the assistance was old and sickly with no one to help her except for a brother and his daughter.[54] On several occasions, the fund also helped members in need with their membership fees. Members that had been sick for a longer period or had an unemployed husband could, after making a request, receive help in paying their fees.[55]

Women's rights

Women's rights became a central tenet of SSBK. The fund was politically involved in the larger sickness fund movement, focusing especially on women's rights, as well as in the general women's rights movement. In 1905, Stina Fagerskog attended her first national sickness fund congress on behalf of SSBK. Beforehand, SSBK advertised its participation in the local press in order to encourage other female funds to join in.[56] Fagerskog became a regular and active participant at congresses and national meetings and reported on her experiences at the fund's monthly meetings. She was involved as a representative on the board of the central organisation for sickness funds in Gothenburg and also served as one of their sick visitors. Fagerskog's ongoing engagement provided members of SSBK with a political platform and influence over the sickness fund movement. Moreover, SSBK maintained close ties with the women's rights movement, working with questions such as equal pension rights for women and men and women's suffrage.

One of the most important questions on SSBK's agenda involved benefits for maternal leave. From 1902, SSBK provided sick leave to women who, fourteen days after childbirth, still were unwell. Being an all-female fund, SSBK was concerned that members would leave the fund after they married and so this measure was designed to retain those members.[57] A few years later, in 1907, the fund went further and proposed actual benefits for maternity leave, both on a local and a national level, and became the first fund in Sweden to provide such benefits. SSBK's initiative to maternity benefits was recognised at the time; for example, on the tenth anniversary of the central organisation for sickness funds in Gothenburg in 1911, SSBK was asked to host a lecture on the issue. From 1908, married women in SSBK could claim fourteen days of maternity benefits after each childbirth. Although introduced as a way to make sure married women remained members, it was also a political statement about fairness and women's rights. But to receive maternity benefits women needed to be married, which was essential for the respectability of the fund. The important balancing act in this matter was especially noticeable in a discussion at one of the fund's meetings in 1911, when members agreed to grant maternity benefits to an unmarried woman. It was then clearly stated that the woman had been engaged, which, in line with the significance placed on the engagement in Swedish history, enabled her to be seen as a respectable woman.[58]

The fund's ideological grounding in women's rights can again be seen in another discussion in 1911, when a member suggested that married women should not be admitted to the fund. The member argued that married women should be provided for by their husbands. The suggestion was voted down after a heated discussion over the course of several membership and board meetings. Opponents of the proposal argued that, having initiated maternity benefits, to now refuse admission to married women would go against everything the fund stood for. It was stressed that the fund was supposed to serve all seamstresses, and should continue to do so.[59] This illustrates just how political funds like SSBK were: it was not just about providing sickness benefits, it was also about changing society and advancing the interests of working-class women.

Conclusion

When it was founded in 1898, SSBK was a small all-female and marginal sickness fund, but by the 1930s it had developed into one of the largest in the city of Gothenburg, with substantial financial reserves. The sickness fund movement greatly expanded in Sweden during the first half of the twentieth century and the number of female members rose substantially during that time. However, many funds struggled economically and did not last for long, so SSBK's success cannot be seen merely as a consequence of the sickness fund movement's expansion. Instead, its success should be attributed to other characteristics.

Much of the success had to do with the values and responsibilities upheld by SSBK's moral economy: its strong social ties, its emphasis on mutual aid, and its economic decision-making practices that went beyond mere capital accumulation. The anchor of this moral economy was the fund's first chair, Stina Fagerskog, who remained in office for thirty-three years. She was highly devoted to the fund and responsible not only for much of its day-to-day operations, but also for upholding the fund's social standing. She participated in national sickness fund congresses, served as the only female member on the board of the central sickness fund in Gothenburg, agitated for women's rights, and cultivated the fund's social alliances with important benefactors. SSBK was a sickness fund that covered funeral expenses, medical treatment, maternal benefits, and sick leave; but the fund also provided much more than just insurance against hard economic times.

Most importantly, the fund successfully attracted new members and retained old ones, thus continually expanding its memberships and spurring its economic growth. Donations often made it possible to offer free admission to the fund and free health checks, which were advertised in the local newspaper. Also, women found to be sick, and therefore excluded from the fund, were nevertheless given help in accessing treatment. Such efforts certainly enhanced the fund's social reputation. Furthermore, SSBK was an organisation that was led by its members and that relied on their involvement in operating the fund, such as visiting sick members and participating in meetings. Here, a sense of personal belonging and value can be seen as an important part of upholding members' engagement and ensuring their willingness to remain members. The fund's decision to become a strong voice for working-class women in the women's rights movement is likely to have played a part in this. The fund was a vigorous promoter within the male-dominated sickness fund movement, helping to initiate discussions on maternity benefits and actively participating in the general women's rights movement.

SSBK proved to be effective in reducing the costs of long-term cases, one of its greatest concerns. In 1903, hoping to improve early detection of illnesses, the fund decided that instead of it prescribing one doctor for all members, members could freely choose any doctor they felt comfortable with. The fund soon also found that this led to substantially lower annual treatment costs. The information the fund's visitors gathered about members' sickness claims revealed that many members suffered from chest-related ailments that often became chronic. Therefore, in 1911, the fund decided that instead of accepting health certificates from any doctor, they would have one specialist in lung and chest disorders perform all the examinations of prospective members. This allowed the fund to counter the negative effects of adverse selection and lower the number of members at risk of long-term illness.

Because the fund was built around mutual aid for mostly low-paid working-class seamstresses, it was eager to keep its fees and costs low, which made it rely heavily on membership participation. In this respect, the monthly meeting was an important collective forum for discussion. Participation was mandatory and if absent from three consecutive meetings, members risked exclusion. At the meetings, members discussed and were informed about wider developments in the sickness fund movement, about the work of SSBK in particular, and about the past month's sick members. An important part of the meetings involved paying the monthly fee. Since members long worked in the same business and belonged to the same social class, and some of them probably were colleagues, we can assume that they also enjoyed these meetings as opportunities to meet and socialise with theirs peers, which again would have added to their willingness to remain in the fund. Members were also obliged to visit sick members, with each month's visitors being announced at the meeting. The moral conduct of members was important and several rules governed their behaviour while on benefits. Members were required to remain at home so that they could receive the fund's visitors. Exceptions were made for hospital care and if the doctor had recommended a stay in the countryside. These visits were a way of verifying benefit claims, but also of gathering further information about the claims. These different social dimensions of the fund, involving members frequently meeting and fraternising with one another, can be viewed as an inbuilt control against moral hazard, but they also highlight how crucially important the social nature of the fund was to its success.

Notes

1 M.H.D. van Leeuwen, *Mutual Insurance 1550–2015: From Guild Welfare and Friendly Societies to Contemporary Micro–Insurers* (London: Palgrave Macmillan, 2016), pp. 121–2.

2 In Swedish: *Sömmerskornas sjuk- och begravningskassa*.
3 Kommerskollegium, *Arbetsstatistik. B, Registrerade sjukkassors verksamhet* (Stockholm: 1905–1912); Socialstyrelsen, *Registrerade sjukkassor* (Stockholm: 1915–1936); Pensionsstyrelsen, *Erkända sjukkassor år 1940, Sveriges officiella statistik: Försäkringsväsen* (Stockholm, 1943).
4 E.P. Thompson, 'The moral economy of the English crowd in the eighteenth century', *Past & Present* 50 (1971), 76–136; J.C. Scott, *The Moral Economy of the Peasant: Rebellion and Subsistence in Southeast Asia* (New Haven: Yale University Press, 1976).
5 D. Fassin, 'Moral economies revisited', *Annales. Histoire, Sciences Sociales* 64:6 (2009), 1237–66.
6 N. Götz, '"Moral economy": its conceptual history and analytical prospects', *Journal of Global Ethics* 11:2 (2015), 147–62; Fassin, 'Moral economies revisited'; S.C. Bolton and K. Laaser, 'Work, employment and society through the lens of moral economy', *Work, Employment and Society* 27:3 (2013), 508–25; J. Palomera and T. Vetta, 'Moral economy: Rethinking a radical concept', *Anthropological Theory* 16:4 (2016), 413–32.
7 Van Leeuwen, *Mutual Insurance*, p. 162.
8 E. Lord, 'The friendly society movement and the respectability of the rural working class', *Rural History* 8:2 (1997), 165–73, here 170; Van Leeuwen, *Mutual Insurance*, pp. 129–31; P. Shapely, 'The co-operative men's guild, citizenship and the limits of mutual aid', in A. Borsay and P. Shapely (eds), *Medicine, Charity and Mutual Aid, the Consumption of Health and Welfare in Britain, c. 1550–1950* (Aldershot: Ashgate Publishing, 2007), pp. 225–43, here p. 226.
9 M. Lengwiler, 'Competing appeals: the rise of mixed welfare economies in Europe, 1850–1945', in G. Clark (ed.), *The Appeal of Insurance* (Toronto: University of Toronto Press, 2010), pp. 173–200, here pp. 183, 188.
10 B. Harris and P. Bridgen, *Charity and Mutual Aid in Europe and North America since 1800* (New York: Routledge, 2007), pp. 1–10.
11 Van Leeuwen, *Mutual Insurance*, p. 122.
12 See Lengwiler, 'Competing appeals'.
13 See Harris and Bridgen, *Charity and Mutual Aid*.
14 D. Weinbren, 'The fraternity of female friendly societies', in M.F. Cross (ed.), *Gender and Fraternal Orders in Europe, 1300–2000* (Basingstoke: Palgrave Macmillan, 2010); M. Gorsky, B. Harris, and A. Hinde, 'Age, sickness and longevity in the late nineteenth and early twentieth centuries: evidence from the Hampshire Friendly Society', *Social Science History* 30:4 (2006), 571–600, here 574.
15 Van Leeuwen, *Mutual Insurance*, pp. 6–7.

16 A.A. Rusnock and V.E. Dietz, 'Defining women's sickness and work: Female friendly societies in England, 1780–1830', *Journal of Women's History* 24:1 (2012), 60–85, here 64–5, 76.
17 Van Leeuwen, *Mutual Insurance*, pp. 6–7.
18 Ibid., pp. 126–31.
19 Rusnock and Dietz, 'Defining women's sickness and work', 70–3.
20 L.F. Andersson and L. Eriksson, 'Sickness absence in compulsory and voluntary health insurance: the case of Sweden at the turn of the twentieth century', *Scandinavian Economic History Review* 65:1 (2017) 6–27, here 24; L. Nekby, 'Pure versus mutual health insurance: Evidence from Swedish historical data', *The Journal of Risk and Insurance* 71:1 (2004), 115–34.
21 J.E. Murray, 'Social insurance claims as morbidity estimates: Sickness or absence?' *Social History of Medicine* 16:2 (2003), 225–45.
22 Lord, 'The friendly society movement'.
23 Van Leeuwen, *Mutual Insurance*, p. 125.
24 L.-F. Andersson and L. Eriksson, 'Exclusion of women and organisational characteristics: Swedish mutual health insurance 1901–1910', *Business History* (2018), 1–27.
25 Weinbren, 'The fraternity of female friendly societies', p. 205.
26 Ibid.
27 Rusnock and Dietz, 'Defining women's sickness and work', 68.
28 P.G. Edebalk and J. Olofsson, 'Sickness benefits prior to the welfare state: the case of Sweden 1850–1950', *Scandinavian Journal of History* 24:3–4 (1999), 281–97, here 283–4.
29 P.G. Edebalk, 'Sjuklön och sjukpenning: 1955 års sjukförsäkringsreform och sjuklönefrågan', *Working-paper serien, Socialhögskolan, Lunds universitet* 4 (2005), 8–16; Edebalk and Olofsson, 'Sickness benefits prior to the welfare state', pp. 284, 287–9, 296.
30 H. Castenbrandt, 'Trends in morbidity: National statistics on sickness claims among the working population in Sweden, 1892–1954', *Economic History Review* 71:1 (2018), 213–235.
31 Ibid.
32 Ibid.
33 Kommerskollegium, *Arbetsstatistik. B. Registrerade sjukkassors verksamhet år 1901*; Socialstyrelsen, *Registrerade sjukkassor åren 1928–1930*.
34 H. Castenbrandt, B.A. Revuelta-Eugercios, and K. Torén, 'Differences in health: variation in health by age and gender among the working population in Gothenburg, Sweden, 1890–1950', *Social History of Medicine*, https://doi.org/10.1093/shm/hkz019.

35 Landsarkivet i Göteborg (hereafter GLA, Swedish National Archives), Sömmerskornas sjuk- och begravningskassa (hereafter SSBK), vol. 42, annual statistical reports.
36 GLA, SSBK, vol. 1, meeting minutes, 14 October 1900, annual report, 1901.
37 GLA, SSBK, vol. 4, meeting minutes, 18 September 1922, vol. 42, annual statistical report, 1923.
38 GLA, SSBK, vol. 42, annual statistical report.
39 GLA, SSBK, vol. 2, board minutes, 20 May 1913.
40 GLA, SSBK, vol. 1, meeting minutes, 14 February 1904, 10 April 1904, 9 October 1904, 8 January 1905.
41 GLA, SSBK, vol. 1, meeting minutes, 9 October 1904; annual report 1904, vol. 2, 12 January 1913; vol. 3, meeting minutes, 12 November 1916; vol. 4, board minutes, 13 January 1918.
42 GLA, SSBK, vol. 3, board minutes, 7 September 1916; meeting minutes, 10 September 1916.
43 GLA, SSBK, vol. 1, meeting minutes, 14 December 1902; annual reports, 1903 and 1904.
44 GLA, SSBK, vol. 2, meeting minutes, 9 April 1911, 11 February 1912, 12 January 1913.
45 Population censuses (1880, 1900, 1910), available online: https://sok.riksarkivet.se/folkrakningar [accessed in May 2017]; Church books: Norra Råda, Göteborgs Haga, Göteborgs Kristine och Göteborgs domkyrkoförsamling, available online: www.arkivdigital.se [accessed in November 2017].
46 GLA, SSBK, vol. 3, meeting minutes, 10 May 1914, 12 August 1916, 8 October 1916.
47 *Lönestatistisk årsbok för Sverige*, 1929 (Stockholm, 1931), pp. 46–51.
48 Castenbrandt, Revuelta-Eugercios, and Torén, 'Differences in health.'
49 GLA, SSBK, vol. 1, meeting minutes, 9 February 1902.
50 GLA, SSBK, vol. 1, meeting minutes, 13 September 1903.
51 GLA, SSBK, vol. 1, meeting minutes, 14 June 1903, 10 September 1905.
52 GLA, SSBK, vol. 3, board minutes, 5 April 1916.
53 GLA, SSBK, vol. 3, board minutes, 5 April 1916, 7 September 1916.
54 GLA, SSBK, vol. 5, board minutes, 4 December 1933, 22 March 1934.
55 GLA, SSBK, vol. 5, board minutes, 20 March 1933, 15 June 1933, 15 March 1934.
56 GLA, SSBK, vol. 1, meeting minutes, 14 May 1905.

57 GLA, SSBK, vol. 1, meeting minutes, 14 September 1902.
58 GLA, SSBK, vol. 2, board minutes, 6 December 1911. Other scholars have likewise pointed out that rules governing maternal benefits were designed to ensure funds' respectability, see Weinbren, 'The fraternity of female friendly societies', p. 211; Rusnock and Dietz, 'Defining women's sickness and work', 75.
59 GLA, SSBK, vol. 2, meeting minutes, 9 April 1911.

14

The health of nations: International health accounting in historical perspective, 1925–2011

Christopher Sirrs

The need for countries to reliably measure and compare health spending is somewhat obvious today. By accounting for health, governments can identify how money flows through their health systems: who funds health care and who provides it; how much money is being spent; and on what. In this way, governments can adjust their priorities, evaluate the impact of interventions, improve services, and address various structural problems.[1] In practically all countries, improving the distribution of resources and containing costs is a top priority, while in others, especially in the global South, improving access to health care, fairness in financing, and tackling health inequalities are also important considerations. By relating health spending to key outcome indicators, such as healthy life expectancy (HALE), national health accounting allows the assessment of health systems performance, a task which in recent decades has fallen to international organisations including the World Health Organisation (WHO) and World Bank.[2] By accounting for national health spending systematically, governments can tap into an invaluable store of international policy experience.

Perhaps understandably, the complexity of health systems and methodological problems surrounding national health accounting have undermined attempts to compare health expenditures globally over the last century. While the Organisation for Economic Co-operation and Development (OECD) has maintained a database of health spending for its member states since 1985, it was only in 1999 that WHO established a comparable worldwide database.[3] Even today, significant problems attend the comparison of national health expenditures, with frequent data gaps and adjustment needed to ensure compatibility. For many countries, including those yet to produce dedicated National Health Accounts (NHAs), the best WHO can do is provide 'best estimates'.[4] These problems aside, WHO's database has become a definitive resource on national health expenditures, making global inefficiencies and disparities in health financing visible. For example, 82 per cent of health expenditure worldwide in 2011 was in well-developed OECD countries.[5]

This chapter traces the history of 'international' health accounting: organised attempts to measure and compare health spending across national boundaries, including the rules and conventions that ensure the coherence of this information. Although a comprehensive system of health accounts has been established only recently, it has had various precursors over the twentieth century.[6] I trace its antecedents through the work of various international organisations, including the League of Nations Health Organisation (LNHO), the United Nations, the International Labour Organisation (ILO), the OECD, and the World Bank. My analysis is bookended by two landmark publications: the first LNHO *International Health Yearbook* in 1925, which contained crude government health budgets, and the latest system of health accounts (SHA) in 2011, which provides the underlying framework for WHO's Global Health Expenditure Database.[7] In presenting a history of international health accounting, I describe the evolving role of health financing in global health and highlight the development of accounting technologies, such as standardised tables and accounting manuals, which have facilitated measurement and comparison. The chapter begins with an overview of the existing historiography on international health accounting before turning to a chronological survey of the major concepts and technologies that have shaped its development. It concludes with a discussion of major themes, including the political agendas of the main actors, and the problematisation of financing in global health.

International health accounting in global health governance

Considering how important international comparisons of health spending are in contemporary health policy, remarkably little has been written on health accounting from an international perspective.[8] The origins of international health accounting have been alluded to in numerous articles on *national* health accounting: how particular countries have measured health spending, usually from the perspectives of policy analysis and strategic health system governance.[9] The accounting framework that surrounds these activities internationally, however, has been examined only superficially. The global politics which drive international health accounting have been neglected in favour of a focus on the practical and methodological dimensions of national health accounts. Important historical publications which have advanced international knowledge on health financing have featured, but only as milestones on the road to present-day knowledge. The key institutions and individuals who helped shape the international framework barely figure. The health financing literature tends to take a superficial view of measures such as health expenditure, interpreting them as self-evident and instrumental rather than as politically and socially mediated representations.

Thus, this chapter connects with a wider critical literature on indicators as instruments of global governance; for example, the use of gross domestic product (GDP) to compare and rank countries based on notions of economic development.[10] Indicators promulgated by international bodies are rarely simple metrics, but vehicles for global power, contention, and debate.[11] Political scientists have shown how indicators can exert disciplinary power over actors, formulate organisational identities, articulate notions of transparency and scientific authority, and simplify decision making by reducing decisions to a basic set of procedures or mathematical formulae.[12] Indicators may even create the phenomena they seek to measure.[13] This chapter also speaks to a wider history of statistics and accounting. This book shows how international health accounting forms part of a long lineage of accounting practices connected to health. Tables, for example, have been central to health accounting for many centuries: recording births, deaths, illnesses, payments, and hospital resources. In the twenty-first century, tables (or spreadsheets) continue to be the health accounting technology *par excellence*, vital to recording health expenditure.[14]

In epistemological terms, notions of objectivity and virtue have long been reflected in accounting cultures, as other chapters of this book demonstrate. International health accounting, however, is an intriguing counterpoint, because the discipline is patently incomplete. Methodological issues and a lack of systematic data have not prevented the use of comparative health expenditure data in global governance.[15] Conceptually, too, international health accounting echoes earlier accounting practices: in the early twentieth century, measurement of national income helped shape the notion of an 'economy'.[16] Later in the century, measurement of national health spending helped support the idea of the 'health system'. My assertion is that international health accounting has not merely *analysed* health systems, but *constituted* them, visualising their shape and defining their boundaries in national and functional terms.

An uncertain quantity: measuring health spending before the Second World War (1925–45)

Established at the beginning of the twentieth century, the first international health organisations were not concerned with health spending. The financing of health services was an uncertain quantity, largely of domestic interest to health practitioners or government officials, rather than an informed international readership. Not only was the role of such statistics in international health unclear, but they could not be clearly related to health outcomes. Instead, these organisations, such as the Office International D'Hygiène Publique, were preoccupied with accounting for disease: compiling mortality and morbidity statistics, overseeing international sanitary regulations, and providing quarantine assistance to governments.[17]

It was not until the 1920s, following the establishment of the LNHO, that the scope of international health statistics broadened to address wider issues of health services' organisation and administration. Under its medical director, Ludwik Rajchman, the LNHO initiated an unprecedented drive to compile data on such subjects as health personnel, hospitals, disease control programmes, and health budgets. These were presented in a pioneering series of statistical annuals, the *International Health Yearbooks*.[18] The *Yearbooks* were designed to allow interested readers (principally health practitioners and government officials) to take a broad overview of public health developments around the world. Guided by a vision of 'progress', they were intended to inspire international action on public health. Each volume consisted of a series of country reports prepared by domestic experts. These included a statistical portion (vital and epidemiological statistics as well as health services and personnel), a descriptive portion (narrative accounts of recent events and trends, such as legislation), and a budgeting portion (health spending by central and regional authorities).[19]

Unfortunately, while each report followed the same general outline, they were otherwise unrelated. The reports were not comparable, since international standards on the causes of death were rudimentary, and those on health services and financing were non-existent. Data collection for the *Yearbooks* was difficult, costly, and time-consuming. The requisite infrastructure was absent in many countries, and language barriers further complicated efforts.[20] From 1927, the League established model tables to improve the comparability of numerical data. However, gaps and inconsistencies persisted. And while nearly forty countries contributed to the final volume in 1930, the *Yearbooks* remained distinctly Eurocentric.[21]

Health budgets occupied an unusual position in the *Yearbooks*. Considered neither 'statistical' nor 'descriptive', they constituted an anomalous third category.[22] This difficulty stemmed from the complexity of presenting and analysing figures on health spending. As a guidance document for authors explained, 'the public health budget is usually a complex affair, and it is almost always difficult to secure from the report a picture of the actual public health expenditure in a given country'.[23] First, health budgets were presented in native currencies. This meant that figures could not be compared without being converted. Second, due to differences in accounting conventions and the structure of health services between countries, it was difficult to disaggregate health spending in a common way. What countries counted as a 'health expenditure' varied enormously: some countries presented their budgets with considerable precision, others provided only elementary breakdowns (see Figure 14.1). This disparity reflected not only differences in national enthusiasm towards the *Yearbooks*, but also the problem of disambiguating 'health' spending from other government expenditures: in many countries, health spending was reflected in the budgets of several government departments. Without a common definition of 'health', it was impossible to compare health spending reliably. Above all, however, the budgets were difficult because they were a novel feature of international statistics. The practical use of the budgets was unclear. Yet, as Iris Borowy argues, their ultimate value was that they could be seen and scrutinised.[24] The budgets signalled that finance was a consideration in

— 285 —

B. Public Health Development in Germany during 1926,

BY PROFESSOR BERNARD MÖLLERS (BERLIN).

I. BUDGETS FOR 1927.

1. *The Public Health Budget of the Reich.*

In the draft budget of the Reich Ministry of the Interior for the financial year 1927, the estimates are as follows:

(a) GENERAL APPROPRIATIONS FOR PUBLIC EDUCATION AND SCHOOLS.

Marks

For the promotion of gymnastics and sport (subsidies to the chief associations of the Reich concerned with gymnastics, sports and walking excursions; subsidies granted to representative sports institutions) 1,000,000
(same amount as in the preceding year)

Encouragement of efforts which aim at the moral improvement of the population and, in particular, of young persons, in so far as these efforts are of general importance (encouragement of welfare institutions and associations, particularly of those working for the young) 300,000
(same amount as in the preceding year)

(b) PUBLIC HEALTH.

Encouragement of work of general importance, directed towards the improvement of health conditions among the people, especially among the young, and, particularly, welfare work in connection with the health of infants, children and cripples, as well as popular teaching of hygiene 500,000
(same amount as in the preceding year)

Credits for the temperance campaign and the campaign against affections connected with alcoholism (tuberculosis, venereal diseases, care of persons suffering from mental disease and lunatics) 1,800,000
(same amount as in the preceding year)

The ordinary budget of the Reich Ministry of the Interior in respect of salaries and personal and material expenses amounts to 1,440,981
(1,303,083 M. in the preceding year)

14.1 Health budgets in the *International Health Yearbooks*. Left: Germany, 1927 (extract); right: Italy, 1928

INTERNATIONAL HEALTH YEAR-BOOK 1928

The new *Police Act (Consolidated)* of November 6th, 1927, enacted two important provisions affecting this trade ; one making it compulsory for physicians and surgeons to notify cases of chronic alcoholism or drug-poisoning to the police, and the other prescribing the permanent closing of houses of prostitution where poisonous or narcotic drugs are supplied or kept, or the use thereof encouraged.

6. SUPERVISION OF TREATMENT CENTRES, PRE-NATAL CLINICS, HEROIC REMEDIES, AND ADVERTISEMENTS FOR THE SALE OF MEDICINES.

By the Law of June 23rd, 1927, No. 1070, many new rules for supervision in these matters were enacted with a view to safeguarding health and, in certain cases, decency and public morals.

VI. BUDGET.

The following tables summarise the principal items of expenditure in respect of health services incurred by the Ministry of the Interior and other Ministries, and by the provinces and communes, under the laws in force.

(A) EXPENDITURE INCURRED FOR THE PUBLIC HEALTH SERVICES BY THE MINISTRY OF THE INTERIOR DURING THE FINANCIAL YEAR JULY 1ST, 1926, TO JUNE 30TH, 1927.

Nature of expenditure	Lire
1. General expenses, personnel, inspections and upkeep of laboratories ..	9,857,777
2. General and international prophylaxis	5,175,000
3. Special prophylaxis (pellagra, venereal disease, tuberculosis, malaria, trachoma, leprosy, cancer, wet-nursing) ..	16,285,670
4. Prophylaxis of epizootic diseases	1,657,894
5. Sanitation and improvement works ..	7,769,123
Total	40,745,464

(B) HEALTH EXPENDITURE SANCTIONED IN THE BUDGETS OF THE FOLLOWING MINISTRIES.

	Lire
Ministry of Public Works [1]	100,000,000
Ministry of War [2]	63,338,369
Ministry of Marine [2]	8,160,001
Ministry of Air [2]	3,967,410
Ministry of National Economy [3]	45,554,252
Ministry of Communications [2]	5,995,235
Total	227,015,267

(C) EXPENDITURE IN RESPECT OF LOCAL POLICE AND SANITATION SERVICES, PROVIDED FOR IN THE PROVINCIAL AND COMMUNAL BUDGET ESTIMATES UNDER THE LAW ORGANISING THE PROTECTION OF PUBLIC HEALTH OF DECEMBER 22ND, 1888.

	Lire
Provincial Administrations [4]	23,749,800
Communal Administrations [5]	693,013,784

Rome, July 1928.

[1] Drainage of swamps and marshlands.
[2] Medical service.
[3] Grants for reducing the causes of pellagra and for minor improvement works and agricultural improvements in the Agro Romano.
[4] Provision of vaccine lymph, medical examinations in epidemics and epizootics, contributions to salaries of provincial veterinary officers, health and prophylaxis laboratories, contributions to provincial anti-tuberculosis associations, cancer campaign, etc., (figures for 1926).
[5] Service of urban scavenging, health service for the poor, medical treatment and assistance, vaccination burial, supervision, health supervision, etc. (figures for 1925).

public health and that figures on spending were needed alongside traditional metrics such as mortality. In this way, the budgets created the precedent for more systematic attempts at health accounting later in the century.

If finance had an uncertain status in international health, then it assumed a pressing importance during the Great Depression. As governments cut public health spending, officials grappled with complex problems of health service organisation and administration. In 1933, a joint ILO/LNHO expert committee argued that 'compulsory sickness insurance must be regarded as the most appropriate and rational method of organising the protection of the working classes'.[25] Suddenly, money – and how it could be marshalled – became a major health policy issue.

In the USA, a Committee on the Costs of Medical Care (CCMC) was formed in 1927 to consider ways of improving access to health care.[26] Highlighting major inequities in the distribution of medical costs across American society, its 1932 report presented essentially the world's first national health accounts. It estimated total expenditure on medical care, both public and private ($3.7 billion), and the share of health spending as a percentage of national income (4 per cent).[27] The report formed part of a progressive-era push for national health insurance, with the CCMC recommending cost-sharing, including federal aid and compulsory health insurance.[28]

While the format of the accounts was not considered especially innovative, it set a precedent for the visual representation of health spending. Presented via a bi-dimensional matrix, or table, the report modelled the flow of funds through the American health system: where the money came from (what is now referred to as 'sources'), such as patients, industry, and government, and what it was being spent on ('uses'), such as physicians, hospitals, and public health.[29] Bi-dimensional matrices continue to underpin NHAs today. For the first time, the health sector's contribution to national income had been quantified. However, the concept of national income remained ambiguous.[30] It was not until 1934 that the economist Simon Kuznets defined gross national product (GNP), thus establishing a common basis for countries to compare social expenditures.[31] Later, the vast logistical demands of the Second World War promoted a concerted effort to measure national income and relate it to the constituent transactions making up the economy. It was from this further strand of work that international health accounting stemmed.[32]

Starting with the League of Nations, work on a system of national accounts (SNA) was passed to the UN, which published its first national accounting manual in 1953.[33] The SNA was principally designed to measure economic inputs and outputs: the flow of money through the economy, from production to consumption. The 1953 manual outlined a system of six separate accounts and twelve supporting tables that represented the economy. Health or medicine featured in four of these tables, including the industrial origin of GDP and the composition of private consumption expenditure. Unfortunately, while the SNA provided rudimentary figures on health spending, it was highly generalised, constructing broad aggregates which were unsuitable for detailed analysis of health spending. For example, school medical services were counted under education rather than health.[34] More seriously, health was considered from the viewpoint of consumption – as a 'good'. Consequently, the economic effects of improvements in population health were not considered; effectively, the SNA measured the value of *inputs* in health, such as physicians and hospitals, rather than the value of *outputs*, i.e., 'health' itself.[35]

Financing health systems (1945–70)

The end of the Second World War marked a major turning point in the development of international health accounting. The reorganisation of health systems and the growth of welfare states stimulated a wide-ranging search for new and better models of financing health care. As the international organisation with primary responsibility for workers' rights and social insurance, the ILO – established in 1919 – was at the centre of this movement. At high-level meetings, the ILO facilitated international exchanges of social security expertise, but also had considerable autonomy to shape the policy agenda. Officials such as Laura Bodmer, an economist working in its Social Security Division, promoted a model of health care that was comprehensive in scope and universal in coverage, funded by general taxation.[36] It was in this dynamic postwar context that health spending was further problematised: in order to expand health coverage to entire populations, what was the most effective financing model?

The need for detailed cross-national comparisons became more acute as concerns about health care costs grew. In 1956, Hernán Romero Cordero, a WHO consultant, expressed alarm at increasing costs worldwide, especially hospital costs. For him it was apparent that that 'Better health conditions do not make health cheaper'.[37] The International Social Security Association was also anxious about the growing cost of pharmaceuticals.[38] Responding to these concerns in 1959, Bodmer penned a ground-breaking report comparing medical care costs under the social security systems of thirteen countries, including West Germany, New Zealand, and England and Wales. These were compared with costs under a system with predominantly private funding, the USA (see Figure 14.2).[39] Bodmer found that, contrary to expectation, costs under social security systems were relatively stable, and only in two instances, France and Italy, had they greatly increased, mainly due to inflation and the expansion of benefits. In fact, under the taxpayer-funded system in England and Wales, the cost per capita of providing services decreased between 1945 and 1955. Bodmer's sights were fixed firmly on the USA, which vehemently defended its voluntary insurance model. Bodmer argued that while social security permitted wider access to health care, 'it [did] not appear [...] to have been more expensive ... than care privately obtained, or provided at the expense of public funds, in the United States'.[40] Thus, the ILO's health accounting did not occur in a political vacuum. Rather, the ILO chose its comparator and arranged its data in a manner that supported its political position: that comprehensive social security was the best way to protect populations from socio-economic risks.

In terms of accounting technologies, Bodmer relied on estimates of national income and social security medical expenditure. To ensure comparability, health spending was expressed in three ways: as a proportion of national income per capita, an annual reference wage, and the national income per economically active person. This circumvented the problems of currency conversion that undermined the LNHO *Yearbooks*, allowing broad trends in health spending to be determined. While the calculated figures were ultimately relative, this permitted the construction of comparative tables representing the *sources* and *uses* of health expenditure. In this sense, Bodmer's study can be considered the first true exercise in international health accounting.

14.2 Comparative tables of health expenditure in *The Cost of Medical Care*

Within WHO, established in 1948, interest in health financing was initially marginal. The WHO's constitution adopted a holistic definition of health as 'a state of complete physical, mental and social well-being'; but considering the political sensitivity attached to social security in the 1950s, WHO avoided directly tackling the economic determinants of health.[41] Instead, it supported vertical interventions against specific diseases, such as malaria. Revealingly, health spending did not appear in WHO's annual statistics until the 1990s. Rather, they focused on vital and epidemiological statistics and, from the 1950s, health services personnel and institutions.[42] This neglect reflected not only WHO's vertical focus, but also the problematic status of health financing in international health. Health financing was not just politically controversial, it was considered tangential to WHO's primary mission: 'the attainment by all peoples of the highest possible level of health'.[43] Accordingly, it was left to other organisations.

This is not to say WHO's interest in health financing was non-existent. Rather, it emerged in response to more logistical concerns, such as health planning in the global South. The WHO's work on health planning and financing was mutually reinforcing, in the sense that the long-term planning of health programmes by countries required an understanding of how financial, human, and other resources were distributed. In the 1960s, Brian Abel-Smith, Reader of Social Administration at the London School of Economics, brought a crucial economic perspective to these areas. In *Paying for Health Services*, Abel-Smith built on the UN system of national accounts, constructing an 'international language of health-service finance' to classify and compare health spending.[44] His framework was applied to six countries with different models of organising and financing health care: Ceylon (Sri Lanka), Chile, Czechoslovakia, Israel, Sweden, and the USA.

The report's major innovation was that while the ILO's report was mainly based on existing data and expenditures under social security programmes, *Paying for Health Services* relied on new data collected by questionnaire, and notionally covered entire health systems. To do this, Abel-Smith provided a working definition of 'health services', subdivided into medical care services, public health services, and research and training. Respondents had to supply data meeting these classifications.[45] From this raw data, Abel-Smith could derive total spending on health services as a proportion of national income (gross national expenditure), and thus, for the first time, draw direct comparisons between the *actual* health spending of countries. In 1967, Abel-Smith's pilot study was extended to thirty different countries, including Kenya and Tanganyika (Tanzania).[46] In addition, the study used a more detailed questionnaire to parse health spending through six inter-related tables. In effect, these tables were the first internationally comparable system of health accounts: bi-dimensional matrices disaggregated the sources of health expenditure into a series of predefined uses.

Perhaps the most important outcome of Abel-Smith's research was the observation that a country's 'need' for health services, expressed in terms of mortality, bore little relation to health spending. The countries with the highest mortality, and supposedly greatest 'need' for health care, tended to spend the least on health services, while those with the lowest mortality, and thus the least 'need', tended to spend the most. The implication was that an array of factors influenced spending, including culture.[47] This had profound consequences for health planning, determining the proportion of national resources countries were willing to devote to health. It also shone light on the expense of systems such as the USA, reinforcing the claim that publicly funded systems were more efficient and effective.

Reforming health systems (1970–2000)

By the 1970s, concern about the rising costs of health care reached new heights. Inflation, prompted by the rising cost of oil, generated a crisis in post-Second World War welfare states, attracting renewed political attention to the need to contain health systems. Within public health, tightened belts encouraged a search for new metrics to represent health status and evaluate interventions. These included the Quality-Adjusted Life Year (QALY), described by the Harvard academics Richard Zeckhauser and Donald Shepard in 1976.[48] These metrics defined illness and disability as an economic 'disutility', susceptible to improvement through effective medical care. Money (cost) assumed a profound importance in determining the most cost-effective interventions. Hence, financial resources became a recognised 'input' to an overall calculation of health: the marriage of expenditure and epidemiology.

Within international organisations such as the OECD, the policy agenda turned to questions of efficiency and health system reform. A 'think-tank' of predominantly developed nations, the OECD exercised its influence chiefly through its facilitation of a 'global policy network', allowing member countries to exchange experiences in various fields.[49] The OECD's interest in health was largely dictated by its concern with economic and social policy, which by the 1970s revolved around controlling rising social expenditures. This interest was expressed in the report *Public Expenditure on Health*, part of a wider study of government expenditure and resource allocation.[50] Subsequently, the OECD began to focus more directly on health, promoting system reform as well as more efficient and effective health financing.[51] This remit relied on member states being able to exchange accurate data on health spending, but by this point very few countries had produced dedicated NHAs.

From 1985, the OECD began to compile a database with figures on health spending for some countries dating back to 1960.[52] Initially disseminated on paper, from 1991 the health database was distributed electronically via floppy disk and CD-ROM, providing the impetus for many countries to standardise their health accounting frameworks.[53] The OECD's methodology differed significantly from the UN and WHO. First, it initially relied on 'massaging' existing data that was routinely produced by governments, instead of analysing new data submitted by questionnaire. Second, the focus was on elaborating the SNA rather than establishing a new basis for health accounting.[54] In the 1980s, the French economist Alain Foulon proposed a methodology to define health more precisely in the SNA, relying on the generation of additional tables and the development of 'satellite health accounts'.[55] Foulon's methodology informed the OECD's work, but it ultimately required new data which the Organisation was unwilling to process.[56] Finally, OECD accounting was fundamentally exploratory, designed to avoid 'conceptual procrastination' among policymakers and to stimulate the production of more accurate statistics.

The OECD was guided by a philosophy of 'learning-by-doing' whereby it cooperated with members to reduce statistical discrepancies. Thus, the OECD essentially aimed at adequacy rather than completeness, believing that the data would improve over time.[57] While the data were imperfect, they nonetheless revealed widespread variation among member countries in terms of health spending, prices, and utilisation, with the US emerging as a 'persistent outlier'.[58] By the 1990s, economists increasingly recognised the futility of adapting the SNA for use in measuring health spending. Even in developed countries, routine production of NHAs was disappointing, and in developing countries the lack of statistical capacity was an additional factor, with most data on health spending available only in the 'grey literature' of international donors. This prompted calls for a dedicated system of health accounts.[59]

The OECD's expertise in health accounting placed it in an opportune position to begin the construction of an accounting manual, beginning in 1996.[60] Published in 2000, the System of Health Accounts (SHA) established a new international basis for measuring and comparing health spending. Central to its methodology was a 'tri-axial' system for recording spending, promulgated via an International Classification of Health Accounts (ICHAs). Previously, NHAs had tended to break down health spending in two dimensions: sources and uses.[61] The new ICHA introduced an additional dimension, 'health care function', that significantly improved comparison. Instead of deriving health spending from national accounts, the SHA established ten new tables that measured more narrowly financial flows through the health system. From these tables, important aggregates could be calculated, such as total expenditure on health, which could be mapped onto major economic aggregates in the SNA.

Monitoring health systems (1990–2016)

Despite the creation of a new comparative framework, international health accounting continued to reflect the interests of the global North. Issues central to developing countries, such as the role of external resources (donor loans and funds), were not considered, even though they were integral to monitoring the impact of interventions and measuring health system performance.[62] It was largely for this reason that the World Bank's role in international health accounting grew. By the 1990s, it had become the dominant external funder of health in developing countries, displacing the WHO as the principal driver of global health policy.

Founded in 1944, the World Bank was initially designed to assist the reconstruction of war-torn Europe. Its interest in population health started in 1970, when it approved a loan to Jamaica to assist with family planning. Under the presidency of Robert McNamara, the former US Defence Secretary, the World Bank's interest in health blossomed. While it initially refrained from providing direct loans to the health sector, by the 1980s it began to do so under the rationale that it could lend vital health programming expertise.[63] However, this lending soon became conditional on various changes in national governance, such as cuts in public spending, privatisation, and civil service reform. Health lending became an instrument of the World Bank and International Monetary Fund's structural adjustment agenda, with the Bank directing its lending towards specific cost-effective interventions that reflected these priorities.[64]

As part of this transformation, in 1992 the World Bank initiated a programme to measure the 'global burden of disease'. Its rationale was not only to formulate a composite index of mortality and morbidity that could gauge the extent and severity of ill-health around the world, but to establish a practical outcome measure that could evaluate the cost-effectiveness of interventions.[65] This new metric, first described in the World Bank's 1993 report *Investing in Health*, was the disability-adjusted life year (DALY), formulated by the health economists Christopher Murray and Alan Lopez.[66] For the first time, information on health financing and outcomes could be related systematically within populations and this information fed back into health policy to assess health system performance.

Investing in Health was the first systematic effort to collect health expenditure data for low income countries.[67] It argued that governments should open up health financing to greater competition and that scarce government funds should be directed to the most cost-effective interventions, such as preventing infectious disease.[68] By this point, health economists recognised that health outcomes in countries were not perfectly correlated with health spending: for countries at a similar level of development, they could differ dramatically, with some countries getting considerably more 'bang for their buck' than others. The implication for international development was that health sectors needed reform to better match disease priorities. For this to happen, however, donors and recipients needed better information on health spending and outcomes. In this way, international health accounting became an instrument of global health governance: accounting assured accountability. With the DALY, the link between expenditure and epidemiology was made explicit, enabling policymakers to direct national resources to interventions, such as immunisation, that were the most cost-effective in terms of reducing aggregate years of life lost to disease.[69] While previously, the link between national health expenditure and population health had been tenuous, under the World Bank it assumed a critical dimension. Health expenditure could serve as an indicator of health and development and, combined with the DALY, define global health priorities.

From the late 1990s, World Bank reports included health spending data.[70] To construct this database, the World Bank relied on existing data sources (including the OECD Health Database), national accounts, and government surveys. In 2003, the World Bank collaborated with the WHO and USAID to produce a national accounting guide for developing countries (the Producers Guide), addressing the systemic problems that undermined national health accounting in these countries.[71]

In the twenty-first century, technological developments such as the Internet have accelerated the processes by which health finance statistics are compiled and disseminated. Furthermore, international health accounting has become truly international, with the caveat that many countries have still to produce NHAs. As the institutional landscape of global health has become more complex, a variety of bodies, from aid organisations to 'philanthrocapitalists', now have a stake in the accounting process.

By 1999, sufficient data was available for the WHO to construct its own database. This later surfaced online as the Global Health Expenditure Database (GHED), part of the Global Health Observatory (see Figure 14.3). Covering all WHO member states, the GHED is updated annually, drawing upon information collected from national statistical agencies, questionnaires, and other official sources. The GHED is one of the main inputs to the WHO's annual statistical publications. In turn, it provides input to the work of other organisations, such as the UN, demonstrating the increasing globalisation and interconnectivity of health accounting in the present century.[72]

This interconnectivity can be seen in the latest accounting standards. From 2007 a group of accounting experts from the WHO, OECD, and Eurostat cooperated to create the latest revision of the SHA: SHA 2011. This facilitated a more comprehensive picture of health systems by detailing a wider range of providers and health care functions. It also developed greater understanding of the sources of health spending by providing new classifications for health financing agents and the revenues of health financing schemes. Most notably, the SHA 2011 developed new 'analytical interfaces' that allowed analysts to visualise health systems from the perspectives of provision, consumption, and financing.[73]

The politics and technology of international health accounting

Evidently, the development of international health accounting has been a complex and multi-pronged affair. A range of international organisations, with a variety of motives, have had a stake in its evolution. At the most basic level, the particular calculative practices and accounting 'vehicles' used to measure and compare health spending have been informed by practical realities. The availability of data, most obviously, has dictated the methodologies that organisations have used to analyse health spending. International health accounting has also been shaped by various functional and policy 'needs': the need for countries to learn from each other, to disaggregate health spending into analytically useful categories, to develop indicators to evaluate health spending, and to monitor health systems performance. At the heart of international health accounting has also been a desire to develop a common language of health systems finance.

Countries	2000	2001	2002	2003	2004	2005	2006	2007	2008	2009	2010	2011	2012	2013	2014	2015
United States of America	13	13	14	14	15	15	15	15	15	16	16	16	16	16	17	17
France	10	10	10	10	10	10	10	10	10	11	11	11	11	11	11	11
Germany	10	10	10	10	10	10	10	10	10	11	11	11	11	11	11	11
United Kingdom	6	6	7	7	7	7	7	7	8	9	9	8	8	10	10	10
Republic of Korea	4	5	4	5	5	5	5	6	6	6	7	7	7	7	7	7

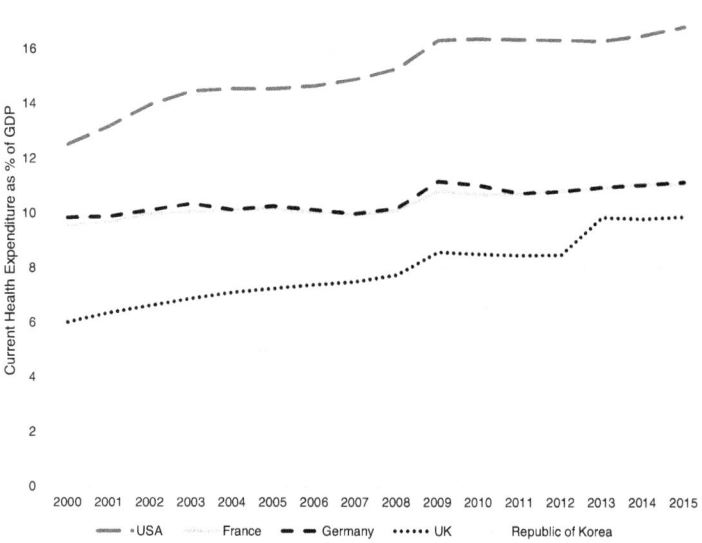

14.3 Example of comparative health expenditure data from the WHO Global Health Expenditure Database: Current health expenditure as a percentage of gross domestic product, selected OECD countries, 2000–15

Behind these superficial explanations, however, lie more nuanced political realities. International health accounting has been shaped by the aims and worldviews of the institutions doing the accounting. In the LNHO, it was accounting for 'progress'. Under Rajchman, the LNHO sought to stake out its authority as the world's leading health organisation and pushed the envelope of what international health statistics entailed. For the CCMC and ILO, health accounting took place against the drive to promote compulsory sickness insurance. For WHO after 1948, it was concern about rising costs and the need to support health planning in developing countries. For the OECD, it was about system reform; for the World Bank, it was fundamentally about making better lending decisions. There is a sense in which international health accounting has been self-reinforcing: as ever more detailed measures and comparisons have been produced, the demand for more sophisticated accounting systems has grown, which in turn has stimulated more detailed measures and comparisons. Through this circular accounting, the existing policy 'needs' of international actors have been legitimised, while new 'needs' (such as performance monitoring) have been facilitated.

An institutional focus might suggest that international health accounting has been performed for separate, institutionally-specific reasons. But this fails to tell the whole story. As this chapter has suggested, international organisations increasingly work together to develop statistics on health spending. To develop an accurate picture, international organisations rely on data produced by other organisations. The professional movement of expert international health accountants also implies that we cannot think about health accounting in institutional silos: one of the key architects of the SHA, Jean-Pierre Poullier, subsequently moved to WHO. The water is further muddied when we consider the role of these international 'accountants' alongside national statistical agencies and experts, who have their own reasons for constructing health accounts, such as financial prudence, health planning, and general administration. In constructing NHAs, some international bodies have worked more closely alongside governments (for example, WHO), others more remotely (for example, the OECD). In this respect, international health accounting is best seen as a negotiation between national and international policy levels.

A variety of accounting technologies have underpinned the systematisation of health accounting. Standardised tables have attempted to present data in a uniform format. Common units, such as total expenditure on health as a percentage of GDP, have been developed to express health spending in a consistent 'currency'. Questionnaires have been used to collect figures on health spending according to a predetermined system and idea of what constitutes the health system. Finally, accounting manuals have laid down rules and conventions that guide data collection by national authorities. By establishing norms and standards, organisations such as the OECD and WHO have encouraged countries to report data in a consistent way. Historical experience, however, reveals that this power has been applied inconsistently. The current focus by experts on the need to 'institutionalise' health accounting within countries reflects how many countries have resisted, neglected, or had difficulty applying concepts and systems promoted from above.[74]

Perhaps the greatest influence international organisations have wielded is conceptual. In standardising national health accounting, international organisations have in turn constructed their object of analysis: the health system. The proto-NHAs developed by the CCMC in the 1920s visualised the health system in just two dimensions: sources and uses. Seventy years later, the SHA defined the health system in functional terms according to health care function, source of finance, and provider.

What is further apparent is just how central finance has become to global health, and how health spending has come to stand in for the health (or ill-health) of systems, and by extension the health (or ill-health) of the populations they serve. When lending decisions need to be made, when resources need to be allocated, when performance needs to be assessed, it is to spending – not just traditional measures such as mortality and morbidity – that experts now turn. It is not that such information used to be irrelevant; indeed, as the LNHO *Yearbooks* reveal, it was always central. However, developments over the twentieth century problematised health spending and positioned it as a key policy issue. For example, the Great Depression raised questions about how health services should be effectively organised and financed, leading to calls for compulsory sickness insurance. Following the Second World War, cost pressures transformed what was previously a fiscal imperative to record health budgets into a more deep-seated desire to guide resource allocation decisions. If, for the LNHO, the numbers meant little beyond their immediate domestic and fiscal context, for organisations in the latter twentieth century, such as the OECD and World Bank, they served a deeper purpose, used to monitor systems performance and influence lending decisions. The key point is that these monetary figures could never directly construct or constitute 'health' on their own; they have always been an imperfect mirror for what is, by any account, a highly complex and fuzzy phenomenon. However, by the late twentieth century, comparative health expenditure data had become an invaluable input into global decisions about health. Financial aggregates, such as total expenditure on health, joined metrics derived from epidemiology – such as life expectancy – as key indicators to assess the health of nations.

This prompts a final question: how has changing technology influenced international health accounting? While the computer played an increasingly important role in international health from the 1960s, the medium for international health accounting remained fundamentally paper-based until the mid 1980s, when the OECD began to compile their electronic database. Paper technology has increasingly given way to digital technology, and data on national health spending today is much more widely accessible through the Internet, able to reach expert communities beyond the traditional constituencies of international organisations, national governments, and academics. Thus, national health spending has arguably become more politically transparent, though experts such as economists still play a central role in negotiating the mass of information now available. At the same time, the underlying rationale of international health accounting – to record, process, and analyse – has remained similar. With the exception perhaps of the LNHO, international health accounting has rarely been performed simply to *record* health expenditure. Instead, it has been performed to *transform* this data into something useful for policymakers. Older technologies such as bi-dimensional tables continue to play a fundamental role in international health accounting.

What is abundantly clear is that the intellectual development of international health accounting has been slow and difficult. It is only recently that a coherent international framework for measuring and comparing health spending has been established; and even today, problems with statistical capacity in many countries inhibit the routine production of NHAs. International health accounting thus continues to be a discipline under formation, despite the combined efforts of a multitude of organisations over the last century. While information on health spending has undoubtedly improved, this is by no means a straightforward story of success.

Notes

1 A. Maeda, M. Harrit, S. Mabuchi, B. Siadat, and S. Nagpal, *Creating Evidence for Better Health Financing Decisions* (Washington DC: The World Bank, 2012), p. xviii; J.-P. Poullier, P. Hernández, and K. Kawabata, 'National health accounts: Concepts, data sources, and methodology', in C.J. Murray and David B. Evans (eds), *Health Systems Performance Assessment: Debates, Methods and Empiricism* (Geneva: WHO, 2003).
2 WHO, *The World Health Report 2000: Health Systems: Improving Performance* (Geneva: WHO, 2000); World Bank, *World Development Report 1993: Investing in Health* (Oxford: Oxford University Press, 1993).
3 C. Gillion, G. Schieber, and J.-P. Poullier, *Measuring Health Care 1960–1983*, Social Policy Studies, No. 2 (Paris: OECD, 1985); WHO, 'General statistical procedures used to construct WHO health expenditure database', 2012, http://apps.who.int/entity/nha/expenditure_database/estimation.pdf?ua=1 [accessed 2 June 2016].
4 WHO, 'General statistical procedures', p. 11.
5 WHO, *Global Health Expenditure Atlas* (Geneva: WHO, 2014), pp. 3–4.
6 OECD, *A System of Health Accounts* (Paris: OECD, 2000).
7 OECD, Eurostat and WHO, *A System of Health Accounts 2011 Edition* (Paris: OECD Publishing, 2011).
8 An important exception is M. Schneider, 'National health accounts: A tool for international comparison of health spending', in T.R. Marmor, R. Freeman, and K.H.G. Okma (eds), *Comparative Studies and the Politics of Modern Medical Care* (New Haven: Yale University Press, 2009), pp. 319–45.
9 C. J. Murray, R. Govindaraj, and P. Musgrove, 'National health expenditures: A global analysis', *Bulletin of the World Health Organization* 72:4 (1994), 623–37; P. Berman, 'What can the U.S. learn from national health accounting elsewhere?' *Health Care Financing Review* 21:2 (1999), 47–63; B. Fetter, 'Origins and elaboration of the National Health Accounts, 1926–2006', *Health Care Financing Review* 28:1 (2006), 53–67.
10 L. Fioramonti, *Gross Domestic Problem: The Politics Behind the World's Most Powerful Number* (London: Zed Books, 2013).

11 K.E. Davis, A. Fisher, B. Kingsbury, and S.E. Merry (eds), *Governance by Indicators: Global Power through Quantification and Ranking* (Oxford: Oxford University Press, 2012); L. Fioramonti, *How Numbers Rule The World: The Use and Abuse of Statistics in Global Politics* (London: Zed Books, 2014); A. Cooley and J. Snyder (eds), *Ranking the World: Grading States as a Tool of Global Governance* (Cambridge: Cambridge University Press, 2015).
12 K.E. Davis, B. Kingsbury, and S. Engle Merry, 'Indicators as a technology of global governance', *Law & Society Review* 46:1 (2012), 71–104.
13 S. Engle Merry, 'Measuring the world: Indicators, human rights, and global governance', *Current Anthropology* 52:S3 (2011), S83–95.
14 A. Rusnock, *Vital Accounts: Quantifying Health and Population in Eighteenth-Century England and France* (Cambridge: Cambridge University Press, 2002). See also Rusnock's Chapter 8 on smallpox vaccination in this volume.
15 T.M. Porter, *Trust in Numbers: The Pursuit of Objectivity in Science and Public Life* (Princeton: Princeton University Press, 1995); I. Hacking, *The Taming of Chance* (Cambridge: Cambridge University Press, 1990); M. Poovey, *A History of the Modern Fact: Problems of Knowledge in the Sciences of Wealth and Society* (Chicago: University of Chicago Press, 1998).
16 J.A. Tooze, *Statistics and the German State, 1900–1945: The Making of Modern Economic Knowledge* (Cambridge: Cambridge University Press, 2001), p. 9.
17 P. Weindling (ed.), *International Health Organisations and Movements, 1918–1939* (Cambridge: Cambridge University Press, 1995); I. Borowy, *Coming to Terms with World Health: The League of Nations Health Organisation 1921–1946* (Frankfurt: Peter Lang, 2009).
18 Borowy, *Coming to Terms with World Health*; I. Borowy, 'World health in a book—the International Health Yearbooks', in I. Borowy and W.D. Gruner (eds), *Facing Illness in Troubled Times: Health in Europe in the Interwar Years 1918–1939* (Frankfurt: Peter Lang, 2005).
19 League of Nations archive, Geneva, R5902/8A/12452/10022, 'Suggestions to authors of the Reports for the International Health Year Book', 1929.
20 Borowy, 'World health in a book'.
21 Ibid.
22 League of Nations archive, Geneva, R5902/8A/12452/10022, 'Suggestions to authors of the Reports for the International Health Year Book', 1929.
23 Ibid.
24 Borowy, 'World health in a book'.

25 ILO archive, Geneva, SI 21/7/2/3, 'The best methods of safeguarding the public health during the depression', 1933, p. 18. For other models of insurance, see the contributions of Castenbrandt (Chapter 13) and Mendelsohn (Chapter 12) in this volume.
26 Fetter, 'Origins and elaboration of the National Health Accounts', 53–67.
27 Ibid.; Committee on the Costs of Medical Care, *Medical Care for the American People. The Final Report of the Committee on the Costs of Medical Care, Adopted October 31, 1932* (Chicago: University of Chicago Press, 1932).
28 J.S. Ross, 'The Committee on the Costs of Medical Care and the history of health insurance in the United States', *Einstein Quarterly* 19:3 (2002), 129–34.
29 Fetter, 'Origins and elaboration of the National Health Accounts', 55.
30 Ibid.
31 Fioramonti, *Gross Domestic Problem*.
32 Ibid.; Berman, 'What can the U.S. learn from national health accounting elsewhere', pp. 47–63.
33 United Nations, *Measurement of National Income and the Construction of Social Accounts. Report of the Sub-Committee on National Income Statistics of the League of Nations Committee of Statistical Experts*, Studies and Reports on Statistical Methods No. 7 (Geneva: United Nations, 1947); United Nations, *A System of National Accounts and Supporting Tables*, Studies in Methods No. 2 (New York: United Nations, 1953).
34 Gillion et al., *Measuring Health Care*; A. Foulon, 'Proposals for a homogenous treatment of health expenditures in the national accounts', *Review of Income & Wealth* 28:1 (1982), 45–70.
35 W.D. Nordhaus, 'The health of nations: The contribution of improved health to living standards' (February 2002), www.nber.org/papers/w8818 [accessed 17 June 2020].
36 M. Gorsky and C. Sirrs, 'The rise and fall of "universal health coverage" as a goal of international health politics, 1925–52', *American Journal of Public Health* 108:3 (2018), 334–42; S. Kott, 'Une "communauté épistémique" du social? Experts de l'OIT et internationalisation des politiques socialises dans l'entre-deux-guerres', *Genèses* 71:2 (2008), 26–46.
37 WHO archive, Geneva, WHO/OMC/26, H. Romero, 'An approach to the problem of costs and financing of medical care services' (8 August 1956), p. 4.
38 ILO, *The Cost of Medical Care* (Geneva: ILO, 1959).
39 Ibid.
40 Ibid., p. 156.

41 WHO, 'Constitution of the World Health Organisation', in *Basic Documents. Forty-Eighth Edition. Including Amendments Adopted up to 31 December 2014* (Geneva: WHO, 2014), pp. 1–19; J.A. Gillespie, 'Social medicine, social security and international health, 1940–60', in Esteban Rodríguez Ocaña (ed.), *The Politics of the Healthy Life: An International Perspective* (Sheffield, UK: European Association for the History of Medicine and Health Publications, 2002), pp. 219–39.
42 M. Gorsky and C. Sirrs, 'World health by place: The politics of international health system metrics, 1924–c.2000', *Journal of Global History* 12:3 (2017), 361–85.
43 WHO, 'Constitution of the World Health Organisation', pp. 1–19.
44 B. Abel-Smith, *Paying for Health Services: A Study of the Costs and Sources of Finance in Six Countries* (Geneva: WHO, 1963), p. 9.
45 Ibid.
46 B. Abel-Smith, *An International Study of Health Expenditure and its Relevance for Health Planning* (Geneva: WHO, 1967).
47 Ibid., pp. 95–6.
48 R. Zeckhauser and D. Shepard, 'Where now for saving lives?', *Law and Contemporary Problems* 40:4 (1976), 5–45.
49 P. Carroll and A. Kellow, *The OECD: A Study of Organisational Adaptation* (Cheltenham, UK: Edward Elgar Publishing, 2011); A. Kaasch, *Shaping Global Health Policy: Global Social Policy Actors and Ideas about Health Care Systems* (Basingstoke: Palgrave Macmillan, 2015).
50 OECD, *Public Expenditure on Health*, Studies in Resource Allocation, No. 4 (Paris: OECD, 1977); Kaasch, *Shaping Global Health Policy*.
51 See, e.g. OECD, *Health Care Systems in Transition: The Search for Efficiency*, Social Policy Studies No. 7 (Paris: OECD, 1990); OECD, *The Reform of Health Care Systems: A Review of Seventeen OECD Countries* (Paris: OECD, 1994).
52 Gillion et al., *Measuring Health Care*.
53 M.-C. Canaud, OECD, personal communication.
54 J.-P. Poullier, 'OECD experiences with the initiation and coordination of health indicator systems, with special emphasis on interinstitutional coordination and comparability', in D. Schwefel (ed.), *Indicators and Trends in Health and Health Care*, Health Systems Research (Berlin: Springer Verlag, 1987), pp. 23–36.
55 Foulon, 'Proposals for a homogeneous treatment of health expenditures', pp. 45–70.
56 Poullier, 'OECD experiences', pp. 23–36.
57 Ibid.

58 Gillion et al., *Measuring Health Care*; OECD, *OECD Health Systems*, Health Policy Studies No. 3, 2 vols (Paris: OECD, 1993), vol. I, p. 14.
59 R.P. Rannan-Eliya and P. Berman, 'National health accounts in developing countries: Improving the foundation, data for decision-making project', 1993, https://www.hsph.harvard.edu/ihsg/publications/ pdf/No-2.pdf [accessed 17 June 2020].
60 OECD, *A System of Health Accounts*.
61 Ibid., pp. 11–12.
62 Poullier, Hernández, and Kawabata, 'National health accounts'.
63 K. Buse, 'Spotlight on international organizations: The World Bank', *Health Policy and Planning* 9:1 (1994), 95–9; A.S. Preker and R.G.A. Feachem, 'The role of the World Bank in facilitating health sector reform', in Z. Feachem, M. Hensher, and L. Rose (eds), *Implementing Health Sector Reform in Central Asia: Papers from an EDI Health Policy Seminar Held in Ashgabat, Turkmenistan, June 1996*, EDI Learning Resources Series (Washington, DC: World Bank, 1999), pp. 143–6; K. Lee, *The World Health Organization (WHO)* (Oxford: Taylor and Francis, 2008).
64 World Bank, *Financing Health in Developing Countries: An Agenda for Reform* (Washington, DC: World Bank 1987); Buse, 'Spotlight on international organizations', 95–9.
65 J.N. Smith, *Epic Measures: One Doctor. Seven Billion Patients* (New York: HarperWave, 2015).
66 C.J. Murray, 'Quantifying the burden of disease: The technical basis for disability-adjusted life years', *Bulletin of the World Health Organization* 72:3 (1994), 429–45; C.J. Murray, J. Kreuser, and W. Whang, 'Cost-effectiveness analysis and policy choices: Investing in health systems', *Bulletin of the World Health Organization* 72:4 (1994), 663; World Bank, *World Development Report 1993: Investing in Health*; C.J. Murray and A.K. Acharya, 'Understanding DALYs', *Journal of Health Economics* 16:6 (1997), 703–30.
67 G.J. Schieber and A. Maeda, 'A curmudgeon's guide to financing health care in developing countries', in G.J. Schieber (ed.), *Innovations in Health Care Financing. Proceedings of a World Bank Conference, March 10–11, 1997*, World Bank Discussion Paper No. 365 (Washington: World Bank, 1997), p. 5.
68 World Bank, *World Development Report 1993: Investing in Health*, p. iii.
69 Nitsan Chorev, *The World Health Organization between North and South* (Ithaca: Cornell University Press, 2012).
70 Public expenditure on health featured in the World Development Indicators from the 1980s.
71 World Bank, WHO and The United States Agency for International Development, *Guide to Producing National Health Accounts with Special*

Applications for Low-Income and Middle-Income Countries (Geneva: WHO, 2003).
72 WHO, 'General statistical procedures'.
73 OECD, Eurostat and WHO, *A System of Health Accounts 2011 Edition*, p. 21.
74 J.A. Price, L. Guinness, W. Irava, I. Khan, A. Asante, and V. Wiseman, 'How to do (or not to do) ... Translation of National Health Accounts data to evidence for policy making in a low resourced setting', *Health Policy and Planning* 31:4 (2016), 472–81.

Index

Abel-Smith, Brian 370
account book 3, 5, 21, 22, 36, 41, 43, 45, 46, 57–9, 63, 74, 76, 158, 218, 260, 262, 271–2, 313, 346
accountability 15, 143, 167, 172–3, 183, 190, 209, 247, 292, 297, 308, 324, 328, 374
(being) accountable 10, 16, 42, 50, 123, 167, 272–4
accountant 7, 10, 14, 22, 84, 95, 115, 119, 129, 133, 148, 177–9, 182–4, 254–5, 268–73, 288, 377
  see also bookkeeper
accumulation (of)
  capital 20, 338, 345, 352
  data 192
  knowledge 91
Addington, John 217–18, 220, 222
Agricola, Georgius 318, 320–1
Allen, Frederick M. 86
allocation 22, 23, 149, 152, 154, 159–60, 312, 314, 371, 379
annual
  account 3, 4, 285, 347
  budget 112, 116, 145, 177–9

  report 42, 145, 149, 190, 194, 196, 212, 325, 338, 346
  statistics 342, 369
antidepressant 230–2, 234–6, 238–47
  see also drug; pharmaceutical; remedy/ies
army 109, 224, 284–7, 289–90, 292–6
assessment 48, 191, 239, 241–2, 246, 249, 359
Assistance Médicale Gratuite (AMG) 146
Assistance Obligatoire (AO) 146
asylum 18, 19, 111, 168, 189–205
  Bethlem, Royal Asylum London 190, 202–3
  Hanwell 193, 196, 202–3
  (in) Ohio 195–7
  Worcester 193, 196–7
  see also care; hospital, mental asylum
audit 148, 313–14, 326, 349
Awl, William M. 195–6, 199

balance/to balance
  information/outcome 231, 235–7, 247, 339–40

Index

life/soul 20
money/finance 13, 113, 119, 128, 149, 167, 170, 178–9, 182–3, 198, 204, 269, 289, 305
physiological 4, 5, 15, 95, 112, 256, 263
benefit, to benefit
benefit (profit) 8, 21, 23, 40, 148, 174, 176, 183, 195–6, 214, 239, 248, 292
sickness/social benefit 212, 313, 339–41, 344–6, 348–54, 368
therapeutic benefit 91, 95, 231, 238, 244, 246, 317, 350
Bilguer, Johann Ulrich 296–7
Blumenberg, Hans 15
bookkeeper 10, 167, 177–8, 180, 230, 249, 268, 271
see also accountant
bookkeeping 8, 10–12, 15, 17, 19, 21, 23, 24, 36, 42, 46, 47, 50, 63, 111, 168, 170, 175, 178–9, 181–2, 231, 235, 239, 246, 248, 256, 271, 273, 287, 289, 307, 313, 327
see also double-entry (bookkeeping); hospital, accounting
Bothmer, Friedrich Johann von 286, 290
brotherhood (fraternity/ies) 22, 308–9, 313, 315–16, 319, 321, 328
Bruynoghe, Richard 169
budget
(to) budget 18, 112
consumption 116, 118, 125
(national) health 12, 17, 23, 360, 362–6, 378

government/state 112
Offices of NIH 256, 260
see also annual, budget; hospital, budget
Burdett, Henry 9, 129, 143, 149
business management *see* management

care
asylum 190, 195–8, 204
care to cure 114, 133, 144, 151, 157–60, 167
charitable 311
health/healthcare (macro) 8, 9, 14, 23, 41, 124, 160, 167–8, 174, 181, 183, 209, 306, 312, 315, 320, 359, 366–8, 370–2, 375, 378
health care institutions/hospital care 9, 19, 90, 115, 123, 133, 144, 146, 152, 155, 157–8, 167, 182, 184, 211, 287, 345, 354
medical care (individual, patient care) 17, 62, 124, 128, 132, 143–4, 146, 151, 167–8, 174–5, 178, 182–3, 209, 211–13, 286, 288, 308–10, 314, 325, 346–7, 366, 368, 370–1
military health care (macro) 283–6, 297
self-care 93, 314
case
(of a patient) 83–7, 89–91, 95, 99, 101, 147–8, 151, 155–6, 159, 193, 199–201, 210, 213, 218, 220–1, 243, 245, 312, 314, 320, 323–4, 326, 346–7, 349–50, 353

history 71, 89, 191, 193, 219–20, 224, 294, 296, 298, 319, 326
record/file 84, 86, 120–3, 130, 194, 324
  see also patient, file
report 323, 326
Case Report Form (CRF) 233–7
casebook 193
casenotes 71, 193, 324
charity 10, 11, 37, 151, 155, 157, 160, 210, 212, 215, 224, 314–15, 338
chart 18, 83, 85
Ciba/Ciba-Geigy 231–2, 236–44, 246–7, 249
classification 22
  of patients 288
  of data 18, 82, 200, 370
  of disease 12, 322
clerk 119, 120, 128, 132, 158, 221, 288, 341
clinical
  accounting 8, 231, 236, 238, 241, 246–7
  data (facts) 236, 240 (244), 246 (248), 264, 272
  demonstration (as source of income) 169–70
  examination 98
  knowledge 249, 295
  marketing see marketing
  medicine 6, 18
  notebook see notebook
  practice 151, 295
  research 19, 176, 230–3, 240–1, 243, 245–6, 249, 266
  science 264
  service 176
  trial 14, 15, 17, 21, 230, 232–4, 237–8, 241, 244, 246–9
  see also practice

Clinical Center, NIH 23, 254–63, 266–74
(to) collect/collection of
  data 4, 7, 13, 17, 20, 83, 88, 89, 95, 98, 101, 154, 220, 237, 289–90, 292, 294, 298, 346, 363, 370, 374–5, 378
  lymph 213, 216
  money/fees 20, 22, 63, 66, 74, 149, 154, 168, 170–1, 174–7, 183, 209, 328, 341, 346, 349
  objects 13, 20
Committee on the Costs of Medical Care (CCMC) 366, 377–8
compensation 22, 75, 284, 289, 292, 306, 340–1, 346, 348
confession 42, 43, 189, 191, 193–4
Conolly, John 196, 202
control
  (to) control 5, 8, 58, 89, 101, 148, 167, 169, 171, 174, 178, 182–3, 189, 200, 222, 234, 285–7, 289–90, 292, 298, 340, 347, 362, 371
  government 342
  'normal control' 23, 254–5, 263, 266–8, 273–4
  self-control 84, 95, 98
  social 347
  technology 247
  see also moral, control
Craushaar, Johann Georg 286–7, 300
cure
  care to cure see care
  cure (remedy) 58, 92, 123, 151, 189–90, 195–6
  to cure 4, 43, 44, 57, 93, 143, 147, 190, 192, 198–202, 204, 211
  cure rate 4, 21, 125, 198–202
    see also daily rate; daily catering rate; prix de journée

daily catering rate 124, 127
  see also cure, cure rate; day rate; daily rate; fee, hospital; *prix de journeé*
daily rate 125–6, 128–30, 149, 154–6, 287–8
  see also cure, cure rate; day rate; daily catering rate; fee, hospital; *prix de journeé*
data 11, 13, 14, 16–18, 21, 42, 57, 62–6, 75, 82, 85, 88–92, 95, 98, 101, 125, 127, 131, 145, 178, 189–92, 194, 196–7, 200–1, 230, 232, 237–9, 242, 244, 246, 265, 290–8, 360–3, 368, 370–2, 374–9
  see also clinical, data (facts); collect/ collection of, data; patient, data
database 359–60, 371, 374–5, 379
decision 6, 21, 157, 160, 167, 175, 183, 203, 212, 238, 240, 247, 254, 268, 344, 346–8, 353, 361, 377–9
decision-making (making of decisions) 7, 14, 24, 182, 240, 247, 295, 313, 352, 361
depression
  economic 99, 152, 366, 378
  (mental disease) 233–5, 237, 241–6
Despine, Joseph 58–64, 66, 69–71, 74–6
diabetes 5, 19, 21, 82–8, 90–3,
diabetic arithmetic 97
diet
  Allen/starvation 86
  extra/special 120, 124, 128, 288
  patient's 4, 5, 94–8, 111–12, 116, 120–2, 124, 127, 131, 263, 288, 293, 316

dietary
  classes/scheme 124–5, 127–8, 131
  prescription 83
  regime 85, 89, 93, 112, 115–16, 120
  schedule 116–18, 120–2, 127, 129–30
  treatment 85
donation 3, 4, 10, 20, 21, 101, 146, 152, 154, 158, 210, 214, 223, 344–5, 353
  see also economy, gift/philanthropic
donor 3, 4, 10, 20, 143, 145, 159, 172, 212, 339, 372, 374
  see also funder
double-entry (bookkeeping) 5, 8, 20, 42, 179, 313, 327
drug 5, 17, 85, 92, 168–9, 230–9, 245–9
  see also antidepressant; pharmaceutical; remedy/ies

economisation (of medicine) 3, 6, 13, 23, 111
economy
  body 111, 122, 283–4, 292, 297–8
  divine 10, 20
  gift/philanthropic 10, 20, 183
  moral 10, 143, 338, 352
efficiency
  economic/financial 3, 24, 133, 160, 297
  of government actions 23, 371
  therapeutic 85, 96, 297
Eller, Johann Theodor 109, 111, 116, 130
epidemiology 6, 294, 371, 374, 379
Esse, Carl Heinrich 115–16, 120, 122, 127, 131–2

evaluation 17, 83, 85, 89, 99, 101, 231, 237, 241, 245–6, 310–11, 326
examination 86, 88, 90–3, 95–6, 98, 100–1, 168, 191, 232, 234, 310, 312, 326, 344, 346, 354
expert 89, 132, 182–3, 201, 203, 263, 268, 306, 311, 322, 362, 375, 377–9
expertise 22, 58, 75, 148, 197, 307, 367, 372–3

Fagerskog, Stina 338, 348, 351, 353
Falkovsky, Nicholas 178–9
Farr, William 202–3
fee
  doctor's 35, 41, 48, 49, 56, 69, 98, 148, 309–10, 314, 316–17
  hospital/patient 112–14, 123–4, 126–7, 131, 146, 152, 155, 168–71, 174, 176–7, 182–3
  insurance/sickness fund 21, 168, 175–7, 339, 341, 343–6, 349, 351, 354
  see also cure, cure rate; daily (catering) rate; day rate; *prix de journeé*
field hospital *see* hospital
file *see* case, record/file; patient, file
Finzel, Hiob 20, 36–41, 43–50
Foucault, Michel 7, 8, 16, 272
fraternity/ies 308–9, 314, 328
  see also brotherhood
fraud 287–8, 290, 292, 339
  see also moral, hazard (also includes defraud, fraudulent)
friendly society/ies 9, 19, 123, 150, 308, 338–41

fund(s)
  charitable 146, 210, 328
  government 172, 374
  hospital 159, 172, 204, 288, 292
  (health care) insurance 21, 130
  NIH 260
  pension 292
  public 172, 189, 210, 368
  research 152, 169
  RJS 214, 216, 224
  sick(ness)/health 154, 174, 307–12, 314–17, 321–2, 324, 326, 328, 337–54
  see also hospital, funding; subscription
funder 148, 154, 160, 373
  see also donor
fundraising 172–3, 210

Geigy/Ciba-Geigy *see* Ciba/Ciba-Geigy
God 10, 11, 16, 21, 43, 44–7, 50, 51, 66, 74, 195, 231, 315
good medical practice 4, 24, 123
gout 5, 318, 323
government
  authorities 84
  central/national 190, 379
  local/municipal 11, 124, 197, 328
  officials 362
  regulation 23
  see also fund(s), government
governmentality 8
Gross Domestic Product (GDP)/Gross National Product (GNP) 361, 366–7, 376, 378

Hamilton Rating Scale for Depression (HRSD) 235–8
Harder, Bruce (NIH) 257, 262–4, 269, 271

Index

health care
  in general/system 8, 9, 23, 41, 160, 167–8, 174, 181, 183, 209, 283, 306, 359, 366–8, 370–2, 375, 378
  institutions 19, 115, 133
  of patients 155
  see also insurance; dietary, classes/scheme
health economics 5, 12, 132–3
hospice 117, 143, 146, 149, 155–7, 168
hospital
  accounting/accounts/bookkeeping 6, 8–12, 111–12, 119, 125–6, 131–3, 143–5, 149, 160, 178–9, 180–1, 212, 287, 289–90
  administration 10, 112, 120, 123, 132, 167–8, 175, 177, 182, 286–8
  board 20, 168, 181–2
  budget 12, 119, 151
  charitable 9, 144–6, 152
  economics 22, 111–12, 132
  economy 17, 111–12, 114, 115–16, 118–19, 123, 125, 130, 132–3, 285, 289
  field 283–90, 292–8
  finances 9, 11, 22, 132, 144, 152, 160, 166, 171, 178, 285, 290, 368
  food/kitchen 111–12, 114, 116–15, 127–32, 151, 153, 158, 166, 318
  funding 9
  inspector 109, 111, 115–16, 119, 122, 125, 130, 132
  local hospital commission (F) 146, 148–50, 153, 156–7
  management/governance 21, 22, 112, 115, 119, 126, 131–2, 167, 175, 183
  see also management (of), hospital
  maternity hospital 158
  mental 200
  see also asylum
  miners hospital 309
  military 109, 112, 166, 284, 288
  municipal hospital 109, 127, 145, 155, 289
  officials 116, 132, 285
  (for-)profit hospital 3
  public 168
  report 132, 143, 194, 295, 297
  staff 117, 119–20, 125, 127, 129, 151–2, 158
  voluntary (in GB) 9, 10, 123, 129, 143–9, 154, 172, 209, 211–12
  see also care, health care institutions; fee, hospital; report; service
hospitals
  Charité Hospital, Berlin (G) 1, 19, 109–31, 156, 294
  Düsseldorf Community Hospital (G) 129
  Le Havre (F) 144, 146, 150, 156–7, 159
  (in) Leeds (General Infirmary LGI) 144, 147–8, 150, 153, 155, 158–9
  Leuven University Hospital (B) 19, 22, 166–84
  (in) Lille (F) 144–6, 148, 150, 152–3, 156, 159
  London Foundling Hospital 212
  London Smallpox and Inoculation Hospitals 220
  Rouen (F) 144, 159

Sheffield 144, 153–4, 158–9
St. Pieters (B) 166, 168, 181
St. Raphael (B) 166–8, 170–1
household
  economics 131
  economy 111, 114, 118–19, 131

indigent patients 73, 124, 126, 146, 148, 150–1, 156–7, 168–70, 174, 176, 189, 195
infirmary/ies *see* hospitals
injury/ies 146, 150, 285, 289, 295–8, 311, 313, 315, 326
inoculation 58, 60, 63, 210, 213–14, 216, 218–20, 223, 231
  see also vaccination; vaccine
inspection (medical) 203, 222, 310–11, 313, 326
Institute of Cancer (of Leuven University Hospitals) 170–3, 178–9, 180
insurance
  health/sickness 9, 18, 21, 22, 123–6, 130, 151, 153, 159, 173–4, 176, 338, 340–2, 348, 353, 366, 368, 377–8
  life 17, 21, 84, 86–90, 101, 203
  medicine 18
  private (companies) 8, 18, 19, 63, 316, 339
  social (social security) 157, 159, 307–8, 367
  see also friendly societies; fund(s); fund(s), insurance/sickness fund; national health, insurance
international health
  accounting 360–2, 367–8, 373–5, 377, 379–80
  organisations 362
  statistics 362, 377

yearbook 360, 362–5
  see also national health
International Labour Organisation (ILO) 360, 366–8, 370, 377
invalids, invalidity 22, 111, 113–14, 116, 123, 143, 285, 295, 297–8

Jenner, Edward 209–10, 213, 215, 219–21, 223
Joslin, Elliot Proctor 19, 21, 82–101
Joslin Diabetes Center (JDC) 84
journal (practice, accounting) 36, 38, 41–3, 45, 47, 49, 290, 294, 298

League of Nations Health Organisation (LNHO) 360, 362–3, 366–8, 377–9
ledger 5, 17, 18, 20, 21, 42, 43, 57–67, 70, 71, 73–5, 82, 83, 131, 256, 262, 264, 267, 323
Levoprotiline® 233–4, 236, 238, 246–7, 249
(to) list 4, 5, 7, 13, 21, 60, 62–4, 69, 94, 113, 118, 120–1, 124, 126–7, 129, 145, 158, 210, 212, 214, 216, 218–22, 231–2, 234–6, 246, 265, 283, 285–7, 289–92, 314, 323
Ludiomil® 236, 240–3, 245–6, 249

management (of) 6, 42, 115, 175, 196, 306
  behavioural 197
  business 14, 131
  cases 83, 101
  Ciba/Ciba-Geigy 235, 238–9

health 18, 83, 85, 96, 101
hospital 10, 115, 119, 125–6, 145, 148, 158, 193
   see also hospital, administration; hospital, management
information/data 14, 96, 240
resources 14, 112, 116, 123, 310
scientific 175
system 85
techniques 120, 167
manpower 283–4, 288–9, 292, 297–8
marketing 75, 230–3, 236, 238–42, 245–9
market
   drug 5, 23, 231–2, 236, 238–41, 243–7
   medical/health 5, 12, 19, 23, 56, 57, 71, 74–6, 268, 339, 342
   see also moral, market
Maisin, Joseph 170, 172, 178, 182
metabolism 4, 18, 84, 89, 101, 256
Mennonite (church) 22, 23, 254–7, 259–62, 264–6, 268–75
merchant 42–5, 58, 231, 313
military
   hospital
      see also hospital
   medicine/health 283–4, 294, 297
   patients 155
miners 19, 22, 159, 307–22, 324–8
miners' society/ies 307, 309–14, 316–18, 324, 326, 328
   see also brotherhood; fraternity/ies
mining 22, 37, 307–26, 328
miners/mining disease 305, 307, 312, 314–17, 319, 321–2, 328
   see also silicosis

moral
   aspects/implications (related to/of accounting) 3, 4, 13, 20–1, 42–4, 50, 83, 258, 260, 262, 273, 275, 292, 308, 310–11, 327
   compte moral 145
   conduct 340, 354
   control 21, 24, 340
   dimension (of accounting) 4, 18–20, 24, 101
   economy see economy, moral
   hazard 339–40, 349, 354
      see also fraud
   market (for healthy human subjects) 256, 262, 272–3
   'moral treatment' (in asylum) 197, 203
   value 290, 310
morbidity (statistics) 293–8, 362, 373, 378
mortality (statistics) 6, 86, 118, 202, 212, 221, 223, 293–8, 362, 366, 370, 373, 378

national health 11, 359–60, 361–2, 366, 374, 379
   accounting 359, 361, 374, 378
   budgets 12, 17, 23
   Insurance Act 9, 152
   Insurance (D) 9
   Insurance (S) 341
   see also international health
National Health Accounts (NHA) 360–1, 366, 371–2, 374, 377–8, 380
National Institutes of Health (NIH) 23, 254–62, 264, 266, 268–70, 272–4
Naunyn, Bernhard 84, 88
notebook 17, 18, 21, 22, 41, 62, 71, 95

obligation
  professional 37, 176
  charitable/social 43, 148, 160, 197, 339–40, 348–50
observation 12, 73, 82, 85, 87, 90, 148, 170, 191–2, 199, 218, 230–5, 237, 265, 292–7, 319–20, 322, 325, 370
occupational
  disease/illness 22, 306, 320–2
  health 18, 305, 307, 318, 322
Odier, Louis 56, 58, 59, 62, 63, 66–76
Office International D'Hygiène Publique 362
Organisation for Economic Co-operation and Development (OECD) 359–60, 371–2, 374–9

paper machine 167, 179
paper technology 6, 12, 17–19, 24, 73, 119, 122, 173, 242, 283, 298, 379
paper tool 5, 50, 210, 220, 224, 269
paperwork 12, 111–12, 125, 129, 184, 232–3
Paracelsus, Theophrastus von Hohenheim 312, 318, 320–2
patient
  account 13, 21, 201, 204
  data 14, 82, 83, 130, 190, 193
  file 83, 84
  record 83, 101, 212
  see also case
pharmaceutical 64, 151, 231–2, 239–40, 245, 368
  companies 18, 230, 247
  formulas 70
  industry 143
  revolution 230, 249

  sales 238
  see also antidepressant; drug; remedy/ies; therapeutic
philanthropic
  gift 173, 223
  public 155
  see also economy, gift
philanthropist 159
philanthropy 9, 11, 211, 339
Pichollet, Catherin 57, 58, 62–6, 69–71, 74–6
political arithmetic 6, 18
  see also statistics, vital
poor box 1–3, 13, 22
practice
  medical (therapeutic) 4, 12, 14, 19, 22, 24, 35–6, 50, 85, 96, 101, 131, 133, 209–10, 217–18, 220–1, 236, 240–5, 274, 284, 292, 295–7, 306, 311, 318, 322–3
  physician's/private 17–19, 21, 22, 36, 46, 49, 50, 56–8, 62, 63, 66, 68, 71, 73–5, 82, 83, 86, 90–2, 148, 190, 242
  see also practitioner
  see also clinical, practice; good medical practice
practitioner 18, 35, 41, 57–9, 63, 64, 70, 73–6, 82, 90, 101, 130, 152, 209, 212, 220, 241, 243–4, 271, 284, 297–8, 309, 317, 323–4, 362
prevention 5, 94, 288, 292
Pringle, John 292–4, 297
prix de journeé 144–5, 150, 155–7, 159–60, 169
  see also cure, cure rate; day rate; daily (catering) rate; fee, hospital
procurement 119, 259–62, 274

professionalisation 8, 14, 167, 268
professionalise 111, 131, 158, 175, 182, 347
public health 6, 86, 130, 201, 204, 209, 247, 249, 284, 362–3, 366, 370–1
  budget 363
  institutions 17, 18, 284
  physician/officer 190, 192
  see also welfare

quantification 6, 18, 231, 268, 298

radiotherapy 169–70, 172, 180–1
Rainsford, William 82, 92, 95–7, 99
Rationarium praxeos medicae 17, 36, 38, 39, 41, 43–7, 50
  see also account book
record
  financial 113, 145, 269, 328, 346
  medical 22, 38, 63, 83, 86, 92, 99, 101, 189–94, 200, 210, 212, 214, 292, 294, 298, 312, 323
recordkeeping 5, 60, 82–4, 96, 189, 193, 212, 272, 290, 323
register 7, 210–12, 217–20, 222, 224, 314, 323–4, 327
regulation 219, 305
  drug 230, 249
  government/state 8, 12, 23, 257, 273, 294, 362
  institutional 115, 153, 288, 326, 341
  research 274
remedy/ies 18, 21, 48, 64, 70, 71, 73, 85, 124, 203, 318, 323
  see also antidepressant; pharmaceutical

report 18, 63, 85, 127, 167, 173, 179, 183, 211, 221, 269, 271, 284
  financial 145, 180, 183, 210, 269, 271–2, 347
  health 362–3, 366, 368, 370–1, 373–4
  medical 58, 95, 191, 195, 198, 345, 349
  public 10
  regular (daily, weekly, monthly, quarterly) 119–20, 179, 210, 215, 269, 290, 324, 326, 349
  statistical 338, 346
  see also annual, report; case, report; Case Report Form; hospital, report
resource(s) 7, 10, 14, 22, 23, 91, 114, 123, 125, 131, 133, 152, 154–5, 160, 166, 176, 237, 239, 257–8, 260, 284, 298, 312–13, 325, 359–61, 370–1, 373–4, 378–9
risk 182, 235, 306, 310, 316, 341, 354, 368
  benefit ratio 231, 238, 246
  calculation 6, 14
  factor 91, 273
Royal Audit Chamber (Prussian) 125
Royal Jennerian Society for the Extermination of Small Pox (RJS) 209–11, 213–24

Schueren, Gerard van der 170, 175–9, 181–4
Seamstresses Sickness and Burial Fund (SSBK) 337–8, 343–9, 351–4
service
  administrative/bookkeeping 171, 177–9

396 Index

clinical/hospice/hospital 146, 175–6, 178–9, 181–3, 212
health 173, 359, 362–3, 366, 368–70, 378
maternity 145
medical/health 23, 41, 44, 47, 48, 56, 57, 59, 60, 62–4, 68, 70, 75–7, 124–5, 130, 144, 148, 151, 158, 160, 166, 168, 170–1, 177, 181–3, 216, 324, 346, 367, 370
military 285, 294, 298
voluntary 22, 254, 257, 259, 262–8, 270, 273, 275
see also welfare service
'sick visits' 21, 345, 348
silicosis 305–6
see also miners/mining disease
smallpox 60, 114, 147, 209–10, 212–13, 220–1, 223
Smith, Samuel Hanbury 196, 198
Smucker, Esther (addressed as Esther) 254–8, 260, 262–9, 271–3, 275
Social Service Agency (Leuven) 168
Sombart, Werner 6
statistics 6, 7, 13, 87, 89, 190–2, 194, 200–3, 284, 296–7, 345, 361–3, 372, 374, 377
asylum 190, 200–2
epidemiological 362, 369
health 17, 200, 362, 377
hospital 118
medical 18, 86, 231, 284, 297, 298
population 23
vital 6, 17, 99, 298, 362, 369
see also annual, statistics; morbidity; mortality
subscription 20, 69, 113, 146, 154, 159, 172–3, 209–14, 223, 347

surgeon 48, 57, 62, 70, 71, 75, 111–13, 116, 118, 120, 122, 209, 212–16, 218, 224, 285–6, 288, 294–7, 322, 326
System of National Accounts (SNA) 367, 370–2

table (also tableau) 4, 5, 7, 13, 16–18, 66, 85, 97, 98, 116–21, 126–8, 130–1, 190–1, 194, 196, 198–9, 216, 218–20, 222, 224, 290, 231, 241–2, 283, 289–92, 360–1, 363, 366–70, 372, 378–9
table (menus in hospitals, first, second, third) 120–1, 127–8
technology
control 247
financial/accounting 3, 14, 16, 132, 327, 361
medical 23, 132, 158
see also paper technology
therapeutic 22
adjustment 96, 99
agent 231
approach 5, 85, 89, 91, 93, 94, 294
class/systematisation 94, 239
development 86, 90
effect 238, 246
indication 238
intervention 88, 294, 297
outcome/success 39, 86, 95, 296
practice/measure 36, 89, 101
rationality/ies 83, 84
research 262
revolution 248
routine 89
standard 84
see also antidepressant; drug; pharmaceutical; remedy/ies

Index

therapy 5, 83, 84, 86, 91, 93, 95, 99, 101, 130, 151, 231, 245
  see also radiotherapy
transformation 4, 8, 14, 21, 116, 130, 144, 159, 167, 233, 240-1, 373

vaccination 209-11, 213-16, 218-24
  see also inoculation
vaccine 19, 209-11, 213-16, 218-24
  see also inoculation
Vismann, Cornelia 16

Waeyenbergh, Honoré van 166, 170, 172, 175, 181-2

Warye, Mary (addressed as Mary) 254-8, 260, 262-4, 266-9, 271-3, 275
Weber, Max 6, 46
welfare 10, 11, 120, 130, 209, 339
  administration 328
  authority/ies 123, 192
  economy/ies 339, 342
  state 9, 167, 367, 371
  service 339
Woodville, William 220
World Bank 359-60, 373-4, 377-9
World Health Organisation (WHO) 17, 359-60, 368-9, 371, 373-8

EU authorised representative for GPSR:
Easy Access System Europe, Mustamäe tee 50,
10621 Tallinn, Estonia
gpsr.requests@easproject.com

www.ingramcontent.com/pod-product-compliance
Ingram Content Group UK Ltd.
Pitfield, Milton Keynes, MK11 3LW, UK
UKHW021830210426
5322IPUK00004B/115